301120 24475730

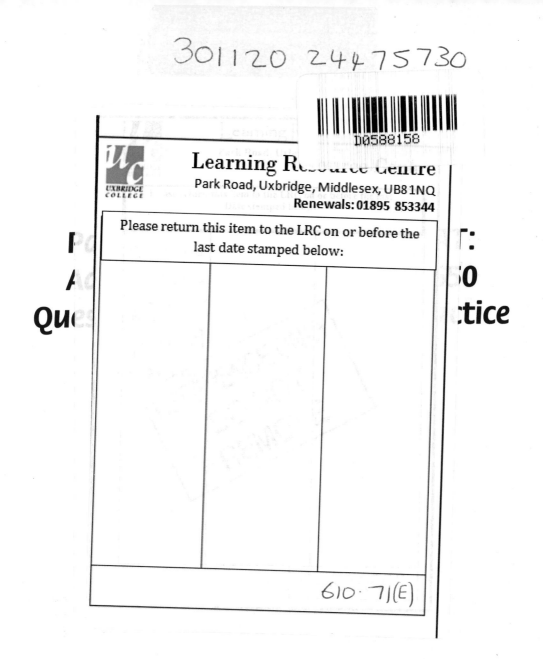

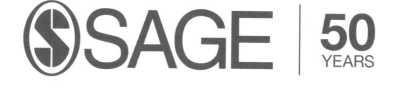

SAGE was founded in 1965 by Sara Miller McCune to support the dissemination of usable knowledge by publishing innovative and high-quality research and teaching content. Today, we publish more than 750 journals, including those of more than 300 learned societies, more than 800 new books per year, and a growing range of library products including archives, data, case studies, reports, conference highlights, and video. SAGE remains majority-owned by our founder, and after Sara's lifetime will become owned by a charitable trust that secures our continued independence.

Los Angeles | London | Washington DC | New Delhi | Singapore

Passing the UKCAT and BMAT: Advice, Guidance and over 650 Questions for Revision and Practice

Rosalie Hutton, Glenn Hutton and Felicity Taylor

Ninth edition

Los Angeles | London | New Delhi
Singapore | Washington DC

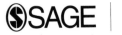

Learning Matters
An imprint of SAGE Publications Ltd
1 Oliver's Yard
55 City Road
London EC1Y 1SP

SAGE Publications Inc.
2455 Teller Road
Thousand Oaks, California 91320

SAGE Publications India Pvt Ltd
B 1/I 1 Mohan Cooperative Industrial Area
Mathura Road
New Delhi 110 044

SAGE Publications Asia-Pacific Pte Ltd
3 Church Street
#10-04 Samsung Hub
Singapore 049483

Editor: Amy Thornton
Production Controller: Chris Marke
Marketing Manager: Catherine Slinn
Cover Design: Wendy Scott
Typeset by: C&M Digitals (P) Ltd, Chennai, India
Printed in Great Britain by: Henry Ling Limited
at the Dorset Press, Dorchester, DT1 1HD

© 2015 Rosalie Hutton, Glenn Hutton and
Felicity Taylor

First published in 2006
Reprinted in 2006 (twice)
Second edition published in 2007
Reprinted in 2007 (three times)
Third edition published in 2008
Reprinted in 2008 (twice)
Fourth edition published in 2009
Reprinted in 2009
Fifth edition published in 2010
Reprinted in 2010
Sixth edition published in 2011
Reprinted in 2011
Seventh edition published in 2012
Eighth edition published in 2013
Ninth edition published in 2015

Library of Congress Control Number: 2014958164
British Library Cataloguing in Publication Data

A catalogue record for this book is available from the
British Library

ISBN 978-1-4739-0261-9 (pbk)
ISBN 978-1-4739-0260-2

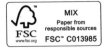

At SAGE we take sustainability seriously. Most of our products are printed in the UK using FSC papers and boards.
When we print overseas we ensure sustainable papers are used as measured by the Egmont grading system.
We undertake an annual audit to monitor our sustainability.

Contents

Part IV: Preparing for the BioMedical Admissions Test (BMAT)

Acknowledgements

The publisher and authors would like to thank the following for permission to reproduce extracts:

The British Psychological Society – Extract from Patrick Packwood, 'Enabling dyslexics to cope in employment' (2006) *Selection & Development Review* 22(1).

Oxford University Press – Extract from Fraser Sampson, *Blackstone's Police Manual, Volume 4: General Police Duties* (2005).

Every effort has been made to contact copyright holders for their permission to reproduce extracts contained in this book. Apologies are offered for any errors or omissions, which will be rectified in future editions.

FT: To my parents and Damian

RH and GH: To the memory of Martin Orme, Jessie Mary Orme and Hazel Orme

Part I
Introduction

As competition for university places continues to increase, admissions tutors are requiring more detailed assessment of students applying to university, in order to best discover their suitability for studying at undergraduate level. Nowhere has this extra burden of assessment been felt more keenly than in applying to read medicine, dentistry and veterinary science/ medicine: due to the huge numbers of high-quality applicants competing for each available place, with often nothing to choose between candidates in terms of exam results, the schools have turned towards alternative methods of assessing candidates' aptitudes. The first test to come into existence was the BioMedical Admissions Test (BMAT), which combines aptitude tests with an assessment of scientific knowledge and reasoning skills. At the five medical and veterinary schools that currently use the BMAT, it has proved very successful in providing a more in-depth description of candidates' strengths and weaknesses, allowing admissions tutors to use this information as part of their selection process.

The second test that has been developed is the UK Clinical Aptitude Test (UKCAT). The UKCAT aims to test verbal reasoning, quantitative reasoning, abstract reasoning, decision analysis and situational judgement rather than scientific knowledge. Unlike its cousin the BMAT, the UKCAT has been taken up by the majority of UK medical schools and some dentistry schools, so it is likely that, if you are intending to apply to university to read medicine or dentistry, you will have to sit the UKCAT. Although now well established, the UKCAT continues to create a large amount of anxiety. Some candidates will have to sit both the BMAT and UKCAT and may feel unsure how they will manage to prepare for both tests while still keeping up with their normal studies.

This book has been designed to assist you to prepare for both the BMAT and UKCAT exams by helping you to familiarise yourself with the types of questions used, and how to solve them. The developers of both the BMAT and UKCAT advise that their tests cannot be revised for, but it is certain that they can definitely be prepared for: a familiarity with what you will meet in the test and a knowledge of what is required of you, combined with confidence in answering the questions, will enable you to fulfil your full potential and will remove a lot of the unnecessary anxiety and stress these tests generate.

Part I of this book introduces you to the tests.

In Part II of this book you will find detailed instructions on how to prepare for the UKCAT exam, including analysis of the types of questions you will encounter, practice tests and worked examples so that you can understand where mistakes are made and how to avoid them yourself.

Part III of this book provides over 300 practice questions for the UKCAT, across the five subtests, verbal reasoning, quantitative reasoning, abstract reasoning, situational judgement test and decision analysis. The answers and detailed rationale for each question are included to help you develop your understanding. Working through the questions in these chapters will help you to practise your UKCAT skills and exam technique, develop a better understanding of the areas being tested and enable you to reach your potential.

Finally, Part IV tackles the BMAT, providing examples and exam-style tests so that you can familiarise yourself with the standard required and build your confidence prior to the test. In this part there is also a detailed discussion regarding the essay section, with tips on how to research, plan and write the perfect essay.

While this book cannot promise you a guaranteed pass on the UKCAT and BMAT, if you follow the advice it offers and practise the questions it contains, we can promise that you will be much better prepared for the tests – which will permit you to achieve your best possible result.

All *about the* tests

The general and administrative information about the tests can be found on the UKCAT website (www.ukcat.ac.uk). This includes details of those universities requiring applicants to sit the UKCAT and/or BMAT, the dates when these tests are administered and registration for the tests.

All *about the* UKCAT

Introduced in 2006, the UKCAT is an aptitude test designed to assess whether or not you have the appropriate professional attitude, mental abilities and problem-solving skills that will be necessary for a successful career in medicine or dentistry. It's used by a selection of medical schools as part of the application procedure (i.e. they look at your personal statement, your predicted grades and your teacher reference too) and they may use it to help to decide whether to call you for interview or offer you a place.

As you can see from all the universities that require it, you're probably going to have to sit the UKCAT. The need for the UKCAT has arisen mainly out of the continuing increase in immensely well-qualified candidates applying for medicine, leaving admissions tutors with little to distinguish one candidate from another. The UKCAT does not include any questions that require science or A-level knowledge: think of it like an IQ or mental ability test. However, like anything in life, practice makes perfect, and you'll probably want to practise the types of questions likely to come up. You can look at the ones on the website (www.ukcat.ac.uk) and also use all the ones in this book.

In terms of the test administration, all the details can be found on the website. You can sit the test any time you want in the given period. There is a fee for the test which differs depending on when you take it. Bursaries will be available for those in financial need (make sure you apply via the website before you register to sit the test). There is also a version of the test, the UKCATSEN, which provides additional time for candidates with disabilities or medical conditions.

You will sit the test at a registered centre using a computer, and in total it will take just over 120 minutes. Each UKCAT subtest is separately timed, meaning you cannot overrun on one area and make it up in another. Results are available immediately, in theory enabling you to take your result into consideration before you have to submit your UCAS application form. However, there is no clear guidance available as to what constitutes a 'good' score, so I would consider it wise to see your result as part of your assessment and continue with your application to medical or dental school whatever the result.

There is no negative marking, and the computer will automatically scale your correct responses to give you a score between 300 and 900 in each of the first four subtests. In the past, the national average has been in the range of 2,400–2,500. UKCAT passes your score to the universities who require it and they use it as part of your admission assessment, along with your GCSE and A-level grades and your personal statement.

Unfortunately, there is no universal magic score on the UKCAT that guarantees an interview or a university place, although many universities use the same cut-off, below which you would not be considered further. For example, St Andrew's School of Medicine states on their website that candidates with a score less than a predetermined cut-off between 2,400 and 2,500 (not including the scores from the Situational Judgement Test) will not be considered for interview, although a score above this does not guarantee interview or entry. They then use your UKCAT score for ranking candidates post-interview, making up 15 per cent of your admissions score. Other universities give similar advice, but most just state that the UKCAT test is required without providing any further advice on score. In these circumstances it would seem sensible to continue with your application as planned.

All about the BMAT

The BMAT is a little older than its cousin, the UKCAT. It has been around for a number of years and is required for students applying to the medicine, veterinary medicine and related courses such as biomedical sciences listed on page 357.

The BMAT consists of three sections, and is a paper exam sat at your school or local test centre. You'll sit this in November, so it shouldn't clash with the UKCAT. The first paper tests problem-solving and analysing arguments; the second tests your science and maths knowledge; and the third tests your ability to create structured, coherent arguments in an essay format. All the information you need regarding the test, including practice papers, sample answers and arrangements for sitting the test, is available on the BMAT website (www. admissionstestingservice.org) which should be your first point of call for all your test queries. A point to note is that the entrance fee rises for late entries.

There's a lot you can do to prepare for the BMAT, which is why you will find a detailed section later in this book telling you just how to approach the questions and with lots of examples for you to practise. Before the UKCAT came along, students used to get very stressed over the idea of the BMAT, but now you have the UKCAT to worry about too.

Oxford, Cambridge, UCL and Imperial all have a reputation among students as being 'hard' to get into, and by allowing themselves to have a different test from all the other medical schools they probably haven't helped their cause any. But the BMAT is a sensible test once you get the hang of it, so don't let it put you off applying to those universities.

Courses not requiring tests

Some of you may have noticed that there are a few medical schools offering standard entry courses which require neither the BMAT nor the UKCAT (for reasons unknown to us mere mortals). Some among you may now be hatching a plan for an application which requires no tests by applying to these medical schools. We wouldn't advise you to go down that route, mainly because these schools are likely to have lots of people applying to them as an 'insurance' place in case they fail the UKCAT, so they may already be extra-competitive to get into. Additionally, there isn't much point in applying to a medical school you don't particularly want to go to merely to avoid a test which, with a bit of work, you can ace anyway.

Instead of thinking about the tests as a negative part of your application, look at them as having the potential to help you. The very fact you own this book indicates that you are committed to lots of hard work and preparation for the BMAT/UKCAT. If this is the case, then your test result will actually give you an advantage over everyone else, rather than it hampering your application. Just be sure to follow the advice and practise the questions in the second, third and fourth parts of this book.

Time management for the BMAT and UKCAT

By reading this book you will begin to understand the style and scope of the UKCAT and BMAT examination questions, and will hopefully realise that most of the questions do not present an intellectual challenge greater than that of your A-level courses. This is not to say that the exams are a walkover: the difficulty of these tests comes from the fact that the time allowed for their completion is extremely short, and that each of the subtests is individually timed and scored, preventing you from making up for lost time in areas of the test which you find easier. Until you have taken some mock examinations you won't really appreciate how difficult it is to answer all of the questions in the time available, and you certainly won't have much time (if any) for checking your answers. So throughout your preparation for the UKCAT and BMAT you need to focus on working accurately under time pressure and improving your performance in your weakest parts of the papers. Every year, even the most diligent students emerge from the examination room feeling that the exam was more difficult than they had expected and anxious that they didn't manage to complete or check all of their answers to the best of their ability. This is the challenge of the UKCAT and BMAT exams, and it is helpful to think of this situation as a mark of a successful examination method rather than a failure of the candidate. After all, there isn't much point taking an extra examination if there is no scope for stretching the very best students.

Below are a number of suggestions to help you to prepare yourself for the time pressure you will encounter in the UKCAT and BMAT examinations: as always, adequate preparation and practice will help to increase your confidence and alleviate much of the anxiety and stress of the exams.

Attempt practice papers with 10 per cent less time allowance

It is much less stressful doing a practice paper sitting in your bedroom with the cat in your lap and a plate of chocolate digestives within easy reach than it is doing the real thing in a cold school assembly hall with 40 other stressed-out candidates. To take account of this panic factor, always give yourself 10 per cent less time when you are doing the practice papers than you will be allowed for the real thing. Hopefully, by the time you get to the real exam you will be so efficient that you can use this 'free time' for checking or reattempting tricky questions.

Attempt the practice papers 'blind'

Often it is tempting to have a look through the practice papers before you actually have a go at them: if you do this, then your brain becomes familiar with the problems and may even start to solve them subconsciously before you actually come to sit the paper, hence the time pressure feels less acute. In short, it is easy to answer a question once you have seen it before (and may even have half-glanced at the answer while looking at another solution).

Have an order

The biggest cause of panic for most students is when turning over the paper and feeling they can't answer the first question, or the second, or the fifth, tenth, etc. This triggers a spiral of panic which can be extremely costly time-wise. Having a set order to how you tackle the paper really assists in helping you to achieve a sense of control. Whether you attempt the questions in the order they come, take the biology questions first in the BMAT or tackle the hardest/longest ones first/last in the UKCAT subsections, always keep this same order when practising sample papers and then you won't feel so phased in the exam room when you come across a tough first question.

Become a confident guesser

The fact that there is no negative marking on the BMAT and UKCAT means that even if you haven't a clue as to the answer, then you have approximately a 20 per cent chance of getting it right. That means, in a trade-off between spending the dying seconds of the exam trying to work out a complex bit of algebra, or answering an easy question and guessing a hard one, then it's worth a guess every time. This feels very strange for students used to carefully working out each answer, but the exams are constructed so as to allow for intelligent guesswork. This is something that you can practise with sample papers: never look up the answer to a question you can't do until you've made a guess at it – you will find in time that you develop a sixth sense for canny guesses.

Use the clock

In the actual UKCAT test you have a handy timer which starts counting down at the start of every section. With each section individually timed, you know exactly how much you have left. Don't be put off by the ticking clock; try to ignore it while answering each question, but do glance at it from time to time so you know when you have one or two minutes left. You won't have the time to go back to check your answers, but if things are getting tight you can at least have the time to make guesses on the last few questions rather than be timed out.

Read the instructions

Make sure that when you answer questions you do not lose marks by failing to read the question properly. In the BMAT marks are often lost by students failing to mark 'all that apply'. In the UKCAT the instructions for that question can be found in the bottom left of the screen, e.g. 'select the best response'.

Resources

You'll find practice questions for the UKCAT in Parts II and III of this book, and practice questions for the BMAT in Part IV. Included below is a selection of links that previous students have found useful. Remember, however, that these tests are only part of your application, and you shouldn't neglect your studies or your extracurricular activities for test revision, as these attributes are just as important to your application.

UKCAT

www.ukcat.ac.uk – specimen questions are available on the website, and you are strongly advised to do the online familiarity tutorial which provides a mock-up of how the computer test will look and operate. You can also see reports of past years' results.

www.onexamination.com/ukcat/ – offers limited practice questions to entice you to buy its question bank. It offers a one-month access package for around £26. Some students who want more practice find it useful.

BMAT

www.admissionstestingservice.org – this website has been updated and is much easier to use than previously. It has a specimen and past paper for each of the test sections, complete with answers and explanations. It also has examples of the answer papers, which it is good to familiarise yourself with, as well as an interesting piece of research from 2005 which shows your chance of getting a first at Cambridge based on your BMAT score.

www.ucl.ac.uk/lapt/bmat/ – an excellent free resource from UCL with a fair number of BMAT-style questions. It also gives you the answers as you go along. Just be aware that the 'confidence' rating to your answers isn't part of the actual test.

Good luck with the tests and your future career.

Part II
Preparing for the UK Clinical Aptitude Test (UKCAT)

This part of the book will help you to:

- understand the purpose and the format of the UK Clinical Aptitude Test (UKCAT);

- understand the format and design of multiple-choice questions;

- understand the different elements of the UKCAT and how to tackle them;

- prepare for the test using appropriate aptitude, reasoning and judgement questions.

Introduction

As with the BioMedical Admissions Test (BMAT), or other entry examination requirements, the UKCAT is designed to help universities to make more informed choices among the many highly-qualified applicants who apply for medical and dental degree programmes. The test has been designed to assess those skills, traits and behaviours that identify individuals who will be successful in clinical careers.

The UKCAT is an on-screen examination and comprises several subtests: Verbal Reasoning, Quantitative Reasoning, Abstract Reasoning, Decision Analysis and Situational Judgement. Each of these subtests will be in a multiple-choice format and timed separately. The overall examination is to be delivered in two hours. There are two versions of the UKCAT: the standard UKCAT and UKCATSEN (Special Educational Needs). The UKCATSEN is a longer version of the UKCAT intended for candidates who require special arrangements due to a documented medical condition or disability.

According to Pearson VUE, the test designers, 'The test will not contain any curriculum nor any science content; nor can it be revised for. It will focus on exploring the cognitive powers of candidates and other attributes considered to be valuable to health care professionals.'

The types of test being presented by Pearson VUE have been in existence for many decades and are used widely in the selection, assessment and development of staff. None of these commercially available tests claims to have a curriculum content and none can specifically be revised for. However, it has been demonstrated that practising such tests does increase both levels of competence and performance. It also helps to reduce anxiety levels in that applicants are not faced with the unknown.

For those of you who are 'fortunate' enough to be sitting both the UKCAT and BMAT, there is some overlap in the areas being assessed. The BMAT has three sections: Aptitude and Skills,

Scientific Knowledge and Applications, and a Writing Task. The Aptitude and Skills section includes three separate tests: problem-solving, understanding argument, and data analysis and influence. The problem-solving element contains some numerical-type, multiple-choice questions that are of a similar format to those in the UKCAT Quantitative Reasoning subtest. There are also some numerical-type questions within the Scientific Knowledge and Applications section of the BMAT. In relation to understanding argument, this may also have some parallels with the UKCAT Verbal Reasoning subtest.

Format and design of multiple-choice questions

This section provides a brief overview of multiple-choice question tests and then examines their format and design and, in particular, the design being suggested for use in the UKCAT.

Which of the following is true of multiple-choice tests and questions?

A   The tests are very simplistic.

B   The questions are easy to answer.

C   The tests are a poor substitute for real examinations.

D   A good guessing strategy will always get you a decent mark.

E   None of the above.

The answer, of course, is E – none of the above.

Multiple-choice tests have a very good track record in the field of assessment and, particularly, in selection. Multiple-choice questioning is a technique that simply tests the candidates' knowledge and understanding of a particular subject on the date of the test. They make candidates read and think, but not write, about the question set, contrary to the case with essay-type questions.

It is true that there have been a number of long-held criticisms – and myths – about multiple-choice tests. For one, it has been a criticism that they are too simple-minded and trivial. What this observation really means is that it is perfectly obvious to the candidate what he or she has to do. There are no marks for working out what the examiner wants – it's obvious. But this is not the same as saying that the answer is obvious – far from it.

In addition, multiple-choice questions are often referred to by students as being 'multiple-guess' questions, on the basis that the right answer lies in one of the options given and therefore you have a good mathematical chance of happening upon the right answer. Although systematic and even completely random guessing does occur in multiple-choice tests, their effects can be minimised and their use identified by properly constructed, presented and timed tests. The people who design and analyse multiple-choice tests are often just as interested in what wrong answers you give as the right ones. This is because, apart from other things, patterns can be discerned and compared with others taking the same test, and tendencies towards certain answers (e.g. always choosing option B) will stand out.

In short, guessing is easy to spot and unlikely to succeed. Given that the purpose of the UKCAT is to inform the overall decision-making process in selecting you over your fellow applicants (rather than your simply achieving a good score), relying on guesswork is a poor strategy.

Multiple-choice tests are used extensively both in Europe and the USA, from staged tests in schools to university selection and assessment, to some of the most complex and high-stake professional trade qualifications. The strength of these tests is that they can provide fair and objective testing on a huge scale at small cost, in the sense that their administration is standardised and their developers can demonstrate that the results are not going to vary according to the marker – a criticism of essay-type tests. The format and design of the multiple-choice questions used for the UKCAT will undoubtedly follow the general educational model.

The following description of the format and design of multiple-choice questions has been informed by two publications. First, *Assessment and Testing: A Survey of Research* (University of Cambridge Local Examinations Syndicate, 1995). The University of Cambridge Local Examinations Syndicate has been in existence for over 150 years and prepares examinations for more than 100 countries. Second, *Constructing Written Test Questions for the Basic Clinical Sciences* (second edition, Susan M. Case and David B. Swanson, National Board of Medical Examiners, 1998). The National Board of Medical Examiners, which is based in the USA, uses multiple-choice questions to test in excess of 100,000 medical students each year, including foreign doctors, at numerous sites throughout the world.

In all, multiple-choice testing – properly conducted – is well established, well respected and well used across the professional assessment world.

Multiple-choice questions: 'one best answer' format

There are a number of different formats that can be used for multiple-choice tests but the most common format is that taken from the 'one best answer' family. Generally, this is the format used in the UKCAT subtests and is discussed in detail below in relation to each of the four subtests. However, before looking at the specific subtests it is useful first to understand the general structure of the 'one best answer' format.

The 'one best answer' format is also known as 'A-type questions' and it is the most widely used format in multiple-choice tests. This format makes explicit the number of choices to be selected, and it usually consists of a *stem* and a *lead-in question*, followed by a series of *choices*, normally between three and five. To demonstrate this we will use a simple example taken from a typical numerical aptitude test.

Stem

The stem is usually a set of circumstances that can be presented in a number of different ways. The circumstances may be presented in a few simple sentences (as a document, a letter or some form of pictorial display) or may be presented in a longer passage (such as a newspaper article or an extract from a book or periodical). The stem provides all the information for the question that will follow.

A simple numerical aptitude stem could be:

A college had 20,000 students in 1999. Of these students, 8,000 studied a science subject.

Lead-in question

The lead-in question identifies the exact answer the examiner requires from the circumstances provided in the stem. For example, the lead-in question for the stem example given above would be:

What is the approximate ratio of students studying science to the total number of students at the college?

Choices

The choices provided will always consist of **one** correct answer. The remainder are incorrect answers, often referred to as 'distracters'.

For example, typical choices for the stem and lead-in question example given above could be:

A   2:3

B   2:5

C   3:2

D   3:5

Answer and rationale

Answer B is correct: 2:5.

Ratios: rule
A ratio allows one quantity to be compared with another quantity. Any two numbers can be compared by writing them alongside each other, with the numbers separated by a ratio sign (:).

To work out the ratio of students studying science to the total number of students at the college:

Step 1: write the figures separated by the ratio sign with the number being compared first, so here 8,000:20,000.

Step 2: cancel these figures down if possible. Here they can be cancelled to 8:20 by dividing by 1000 and then further cancelled by dividing both numbers by 4 to obtain 2:5.

Step 3: the ratio of students studying science compared with the total number of students at the college is 2:5.

Format of the Verbal Reasoning subtest

This subtest assesses your ability to think logically about written information and to arrive at a reasoned conclusion.

Stem

This stem will consist of reading passages usually taken from books, magazines, periodicals, pamphlets or newspapers.

Lead-in question

For each of the stems, there will be four separate lead-in statements. These statements will relate to the reading passage, and you will be required to determine whether the statement is true or false, or whether you cannot determine if the statement is true or false.

Choices

There will be three choices for each question: True, False or Can't Tell. Again, only **one** of these choices will be the correct answer and the remaining two choices will be incorrect.

Format of the Quantitative Reasoning subtest

This subtest assesses your ability to solve numerical problems. The format of the Quantitative Reasoning subtest is very similar to that described in the example above.

Stem

The stem will consist of tables, charts and/or graphs.

Lead-in question

For each of the stems (i.e. the tables, charts and/or graphs), there will be four separate lead-in questions.

Choices

There will be five choices for each question: A, B, C, D and E. Remember, there is only **one** correct answer and the remaining four choices will be incorrect.

Format of the Abstract Reasoning subtest

This subtest assesses your ability to infer relationships from information by convergent and divergent thinking.

Stem

The stem will consist of a pair of shapes known as 'Set A' and 'Set B'.

Lead-in question

For each pair of Set A and Set B shapes, there will be five 'test shapes' which represent five lead-in questions.

Choices

For each of the five test shapes there will be three choices: Set A, Set B or Neither Set. Only **one** of the three choices is correct.

Format of the Decision Analysis subtest

This subtest assesses your ability to decipher and make sense of coded information and to make judgements which cannot be based on logical deduction alone.

Stem

In the stem you will be presented with one scenario and a significant amount of information together with terms that become progressively more complex and ambiguous.

Lead-in question

There will be 26 separate lead-in questions based on the one scenario.

Choices

There will be either four or five choices for each question: A, B, C, D and/or E. Whereas in the Quantitative Reasoning subtest only **one** answer is correct, in the Decision Analysis subtest there may be **more than one** answer that is correct. This should be clearly indicated in the lead-in question.

Format of the Situational Judgement Test

This test measures your capacity to understand real-world situations and to identify critical factors and appropriate behaviour in dealing with them. The test assesses integrity, perspective taking and team involvement.

Stem

In the stem you will be presented with one reasonably short scenario. In total there are 20 of these scenarios included in the test.

Lead-in question

For each of the stems there will generally be between two and six questions with a total of 67 questions in all across the 20 scenarios.

Choices

This assessment consists of two sets of questions. In the first set you will be asked to rate the **appropriateness** of a series of options in response to the scenario. In the second set you will be asked to rate the **importance** of a series of options in response to the scenario.

How to approach multiple-choice questions

Whatever the purpose or the design of the test, it is worth bearing in mind some general rules to follow when answering multiple-choice questions. Clearly, your score should be higher if you attempt to answer all the questions in the test and avoid wild guessing. However, if you are running out of time you may attempt some 'educated' guesses but, where five options are available, this may prove difficult. If there are questions you are unsure of, you can place a mark against them for reviewing later.

Although it is often repeated at every level of testing and assessment in every walk of life, it is nevertheless worth reiterating – always read the questions carefully. It may help to read them more than once to avoid misreading a critical word(s). With the verbal reasoning and problem-solving tests in the UKCAT, careful reading of the words presented is crucial.

Where all the options, or some of the options, begin with the same word(s), or appear very similar, be sure to mark the correct option.

In relation to the Verbal Reasoning subtest, do not use your own knowledge or experience of the subject matter to influence your answers – even if your knowledge contradicts that of the author. The concept of this subtest is not to test individual prior knowledge – it is to present everyone competing against you with the same opportunity to demonstrate his or her skills and aptitudes. As such your answers should relate directly to:

- your understanding of the passage you have read; and
- the way in which the author has presented it to you, the reader.

Examine each passage to extract the main ideas and avoid making hasty conclusions.

The following five chapters contain details of the five UKCAT subtests and provide practice tests for each. By working through these chapters you will not only familiarise yourself with the format of these tests but will also speed up your reactions and give yourself the confidence to handle successfully the differing styles of questions involved.

Chapter 1
The Verbal Reasoning subtest

This chapter will help you to:

- understand the purpose and the format of verbal reasoning tests;
- prepare for the Verbal Reasoning subtest using general verbal reasoning questions;
- test your knowledge and understanding of verbal reasoning-type questions;
- identify those verbal reasoning skills where development is required.

Introduction

Pearson VUE describes the purpose of this subtest as follows: 'The Verbal Reasoning subtest assesses a candidate's ability to read and think carefully about information presented in passages.'

In the commercial world, the Verbal Reasoning subtest described by Pearson VUE is a classic critical reasoning test. The notion that we all have 'thinking skills' or 'core skills' that should be transferable to all subject areas has attracted a great deal of academic interest. One of these 'core skills' is called 'critical thinking' and the vast number of books on the subject testifies to the interest in – and complexity of – the subject. Critical thinking is fundamentally concerned with the way arguments are structured and produced by whatever media: discussion, debate, a paper, a report, an article or an essay. The following are the generally accepted criteria for critical thinking.

- The ability to differentiate between facts and opinions.
- The ability to examine assumptions.
- Being open-minded as you search for explanations, causes and solutions.
- Being aware of valid or invalid argument forms.
- Staying focused on the whole picture, while examining the specifics.
- Verifying sources.
- Deducing and judging deductions.
- Inducing and judging inductions.
- Making value judgements.
- Defining terms and judging definitions.
- Deciding on actions.
- Being objective.
- A willingness and ability always to look at alternatives.

The above is not meant to be an exhaustive list of all the criteria of critical thinking, but it provides an overview of some of the basic principles that underpin the Verbal Reasoning subtest.

When making selection decisions – whether they are for training, further education or for job appointments – the area of critical thinking/reasoning is deemed to be very important. This is largely because these skills are important in performing the roles themselves, particularly those in management. Graduate/managerial-level aptitude tests of verbal reasoning, which are basically assessing the understanding of words, grammar, spelling, word relationships, etc., may provide an objective assessment of a candidate's verbal ability.

However, these types of test are seen by some to lack face validity (that is, they do not appear to be job related) when used for graduate/managerial roles. People of this level often object to being given 'IQ tests' and prefer an assessment that appears to replicate, to some extent, the content of the job (i.e. critically evaluating reports). It is also believed by some that classic verbal reasoning tests do not provide an indication of an individual's ability to think critically. Therefore, psychometrists have developed what are generally called critical reasoning tests, which are similar in format to the UKCAT.

This chapter provides you with an opportunity to test your understanding and knowledge of the range of questions you are likely to be presented with in this UKCAT subtest. By taking this opportunity, you should be able to identify areas where you may need some development.

Verbal Reasoning subtest

Before attempting the practice questions you should find it beneficial to work through the following example questions. These passages and questions are formatted along the lines used in the UKCAT, using the response options of True, False or Can't Tell. The answers and the rationales for the correct answers follow each question.

The first passage is a relatively short paragraph followed by just one question. Subsequent passages will increase in size and the number of questions will increase to a maximum of four. The final passage, with its four questions, will serve as a 'trial run' prior to attempting the Verbal Reasoning practice subtest. This staged approach should develop your understanding of how this type of reasoning test is structured, and should also develop your confidence and ability when answering the questions.

Passages, response formats and example questions

The passages are normally extracts taken from various books, magazines, periodicals, pamphlets and newspapers. These passages are not a test of knowledge and may not include any medical or scientific-type matters. Each of the passages is intended to convey information or to persuade the reader of a point of view. You must assume that what is stated in each passage is factual and avoid drawing on your own knowledge or experience of any of the topics, which may contradict that of the author. Drawing on this assumption, read the passage carefully and decide whether the statement is True or False, or whether you Can't Tell without more information.

The definitions to be applied to each statement are as follows.

- *True*: this means that the statement is actually made in the passage, that it is implied or follows logically from the information in the passage.

- *False*: this means that the statement directly contradicts a statement made in, implied by or following logically from the passage.

- *Can't Tell*: this means that there is insufficient information in the passage to arrive at a firm conclusion as to whether the statement is true or false.

Example questions

Example passage I: European Convention on Human Rights: Article 10 (Freedom of Expression)

Article 10(2) clearly allows for an individual's freedom of expression to be curtailed under a number of circumstances, including the prevention of disorder or crime and the protection of morals. Balancing these competing needs is one area where the European Court of Human Rights has allowed a reasonable 'margin of appreciation'. Nevertheless, any restrictions on an individual's freedom of expression will be narrowly construed and closely scrutinised. Demonstrators may be able to rely on Article 10 as a defence to a charge under the Public Order Act 1986 and hunt saboteurs bound over to keep the peace by magistrates have been able to show their rights have thereby been unjustifiably restricted.

Source: Blackstone's Police Manual, Volume 4: General Police Duties, Oxford University Press, 2009. By permission of Oxford University Press.

Example passage I: question 1
Hunt saboteurs who have invoked Article 10 of the Convention have been released from being bound over to keep the peace.

A True

B False

C Can't Tell

Answer: True

In the final sentence, it is stated that hunt saboteurs who have been bound over to keep the peace have shown that their rights have been unjustifiably restricted by this order. The reference at the start of this sentence to the possible use of Article 10 as a defence by demonstrators implies that these hunt saboteurs were able to show the illegality of the binding over order by invoking Article 10. Having successfully shown its illegality, it follows logically that they would have been released from the order. It is therefore true to say that hunt saboteurs who have invoked Article 10 of the Convention have been released from being bound over to keep the peace.

Example passage II: National Minimum Wage

National Minimum Wage (NMW) was 7 years old on 1 April 2006 and since its introduction up until 2006 it continued to increase each year. When first introduced, the minimum wage stood at £3.60 per hour while by 2006, for workers aged 22 and above, this has now risen to £5.05 per hour (£5.35 from 1 October 2006). The rate for workers aged 18–21 and those on a Government-approved training scheme has also increased from £3.00 per hour in 1999 to £4.25 by April 2006. And in addition a rate of £3.00 per hour was introduced on 1 October 2004 (£3.30 from 1 October 2006) for workers under 18 who are above compulsory school leaving age.

Source: HM Revenue and Customs Employer Bulletin, April 2006, Issue 23.

Example passage II: question 1
Workers aged 21 did not have as big an increase in the minimum wage between 1999 and 2006 as those who are aged 22.

A True

B False

C Can't Tell

Answer: True

In 1999 the minimum wage was £3.60 per hour and by 2006, for workers aged 22, it has risen to £5.05 per hour, an increase of £1.45. For workers aged 18–21 it had risen from £3.00 per hour in 1999 to £4.25 per hour in 2006, an increase of £1.25. Therefore the increase in the minimum wage for those aged 22 is £0.20 more than for those aged 21.

Example passage II: question 2
Since 1 October 1999 the rate for workers aged 16–18 has been £3.00 per hour.

A True

B False

C Can't Tell

Answer: Can't Tell

The passage states that 'a rate of £3.00 per hour was introduced on 1 October 2004 ... for workers under 18 who are above compulsory school leaving age'. However, the passage does not tell you what compulsory school leaving age is. Although you may personally know what this is, it is not stated in the passage and therefore you cannot determine the answer without further information. In addition, the passage states the rate introduced in 2004 – without further information, we cannot determine what the rate was for this group before that date.

Example passage III: withdrawal symptoms

The health Bill that came into force in summer 2007, provided that all enclosed public spaces and workplaces in England would be smoke-free. The Bill covered virtually all workplaces, including offices, manufacturing plants, schools, shops, restaurants and voluntary workplaces. Vehicles – as enclosed workplaces – were also caught by the ban. The only exemptions were workplaces where people also lived, such as prisons, oil-rigs, residential care homes and designated hotel bedrooms. But as in Scotland, the no-smoking law for England did not say whether organisations should extend the ban to outdoor premises, erect smoking shelters, continue to allow customary smoking breaks, or outlaw smoking altogether. One of the keys to successfully implementing changes to smoking policies is consultation, which gives staff time to assimilate the reasons, benefits and timescales involved. Three months' consultation, followed by three months' notice of policy change would not be unusual, according to lawyers.

Source: 'Withdrawal symptoms' (Penny Cottee, *People Management*, 4 May 2006). © People Management.

Example passage III: question 1

Staff working at hotels who 'lived in' would not be subject to the same no-smoking requirements as the other guests in the hotel.

A True

B False

C Can't Tell

Answer: True

One of the exemptions was workplaces where people also lived, and this included designated hotel bedrooms. It is logical to assume that staff bedrooms are separate within a hotel and therefore would not be subject to any 'smoke-free' requirement. In any event, if staff were making use of hotel rooms these could be designated as 'smoking' if necessary.

Example passage III: question 2

The new health Bill requires that organisations provide three months' consultation before implementing the no-smoking policy.

A True

B False

C Can't Tell

Answer: False

The passage does not state that it is a specific requirement of the Bill to provide three months' consultation. It is only according to lawyers and, one assumes, best practice that three months' consultation, followed by three months' notice of policy change, would not be unusual.

Example passage III: question 3

It will be the responsibility of organisations themselves to introduce and enforce the new no-smoking law in the workplace.

A   True

B   False

C   Can't Tell

Answer: Can't Tell

From the tenet of the passage it is logical to assume that the introduction of a smoke-free workplace will be the responsibility of individual organisations. However, it is not as clear-cut in relation to the enforcement issue. The Bill may contain both a vicarious liability on the part of the organisation as well as a liability in relation to the individual 'breaking the law' (i.e. smoking in the workplace).

Example passage IV: enabling dyslexics to cope in employment

Sequencing difficulties affect the ability to plan and organise work, and express ideas on paper and verbally. Inaccuracies may occur in word processing or writing, typically involving letters, or words appearing in the wrong order, and words being left out or repeated. Written letters are often the mirror or reverse image of those they should have used, i.e. d for b, p for q, p for b, n for u, m for w. Rotation of numbers and letters through 180 degrees may occur, e.g. 6 to 9, b to q, p to d, n to u and a to e. Curved characters may be reproduced as similar ones with straight strokes, e.g. u as v, 2 as z, s as 5 and 8 as B. Common tools to help with spelling and grammar problems, such as dictionaries, thesauri and spell checkers, can be difficult for dyslexics to use.

Source: 'Enabling dyslexics to cope in employment' (Patrick Packwood, *Selection & Development Review* 22(1), 2006). © The British Psychological Society, 2006.

Example passage IV: question 1

Dictionaries, thesauri and spell checkers do not help dyslexics with sequencing problems.

A   True

B   False

C   Can't Tell

Answer: False

The passage actually states that 'dictionaries, thesauri and spell checkers can be difficult for dyslexics to use'. It does not say that they do not help dyslexics with sequencing problems – therefore the answer is False.

Example passage IV: question 2

Common problems in relation to letters can be where dyslexics include the letter 'n', which, if written, could actually be a 'u' or even a 'v' dependent on their particular difficulties with sequencing.

A True

B False

C Can't Tell

Answer: Can't Tell

In the passage it states that written letters are often the mirror or reverse image of those they should have used, and provides the example of 'n' for 'u'. The passage also discusses curved characters being reproduced as similar ones with straight strokes, and provides the example of 'u' being written as 'v'. Whether or not an 'n' could be reproduced as a 'v' is not discussed, but it may be that a dyslexic with image and curved character problems could write 'v' from an initial 'n'. More information would be required before a definitive True or False answer could be given.

Example passage IV: question 3

Considering written letters are often the mirror or reverse image of those they should have used, some people with dyslexia may write 'b' for 'd', or 'w' for 'm'.

A True

B False

C Can't Tell

Answer: True

The letters 'b' for 'd' and 'w' for 'm' are still mirror or reverse images and, although these have not been used by the author in his examples, he does use 'd' for 'b' and 'm' for 'w' which can logically be transposed.

Example passage IV: question 4

Dyslexics with sequencing problems may find it difficult to provide a coherent structure when writing an essay or presenting a research paper.

A True

B False

C Can't Tell

Answer: True

The passage specifically states that 'Sequencing difficulties affect the ability to plan and organise work and express ideas on paper and verbally.' It can be assumed, therefore, that dyslexics with sequencing problems would find difficulty in structuring an essay or presenting a research paper.

Verbal Reasoning practice subtest

The Verbal Reasoning subtest is an on-screen test that consists of 44 items associated with 11 reading passages. For each reading passage there are four questions in the form of statements. Three answer options are provided for each statement: True, False, Can't Tell.

Only one of these options is correct. A period of 22 minutes is allowed for the subtest, with one minute for instruction and the remaining 21 minutes for items.

If the reader wants to simulate 'test conditions', he or she is advised to use rough paper to mark down his or her choice for each of the questions (i.e. True, False or Can't Tell).

The correct answer and rationale to each of the questions are given in the section following the practice subtest.

Passage I: political and social influences on health

The social model of health says that 50 per cent of our health is determined by wider determinants, such as where we live, what our income is relative to other people and what level of education we have. Political and social factors which influence health are not isolated, but interplay in a complex way. For example, research shows that female contraception usage in developed Indian states (e.g. Tamil Nadu) is significantly higher than in less developed states (e.g. Bihar). Both socioeconomic status and husband's education are strongly associated with family planning in both states. Religion and caste are associated with family planning in Bihar but not in Tamil Nadu. What explains these differences? It seems that women's education is the key factor: women in states like Tamil Nadu enjoy higher education status and autonomy. On the other hand, women in northern states such as Bihar are strongly subject to traditional conservatism, are predominantly less educated and less likely to work outside their homes. Tamil Nadu has one of the most efficient governance structures in India and the least corrupt state bureaucracy. Bihar, on the other hand, is viewed by many as being misruled.

Source: Health, Behaviour and Society: Clinical Medicine in Context © Jennifer Cleland and Philip Cotton. Learning Matters, 2011.

Passage I: question 1

There is a very complex interaction of factors that contribute to health.

A   True

B   False

C   Can't Tell

Passage I: question 2

In Tamil Nadu female contraception usage is greater than male contraception usage.

A True

B False

C Can't Tell

Passage I: question 3

Unlike women in Tamil Nadu, those who live in Bihar are not allowed to work outside their homes.

A True

B False

C Can't Tell

Passage I: question 4

States that are misruled and have inefficient governance structures and corrupt bureaucracies are likely to be poorly associated with family planning.

A True

B False

C Can't Tell

Passage II: the funding debate

Funding of higher education has long been an issue in many countries. This is a contentious matter as only a minority of the population directly participate; in Britain this is approximately 40 per cent. England has seen a significant change in higher education funding in recent years with the introduction of variable tuition fees for students. Previously the state subsidised higher education for many students, depending on their family's financial income. Prior to 2006, tuition fees were set at the same amount for all institutions. Now individual universities can choose how much students can pay for tuition (to attend). Increasingly fierce competition for students had led to some institutions lowering their fees to attract more of them. Welsh students are effectively exempt from top-up fees if they stay in Wales, because they receive a non-means tested grant from the Welsh Government. In Scotland, students have to make no personal contribution to fees except when studying for a second degree or postgraduate award. Alongside tuition fees from students, each institution receives a grant from the respective country's Higher Education Funding Council based on the number of students registered. Those offering professional courses also receive grants from the relevant professional funding bodies (for example, teacher training degrees are funded by the Teacher Development Agency).

Source: Global Issues and Comparative Education © Wendy Bignold and Liz Gayton. Learning Matters, 2009.

Passage II: question 5

Students who are seeking a career as a teacher, in any subject, receive government funding if undertaking a teacher training degree programme.

A   True

B   False

C   Can't Tell

Passage II: question 6

Higher education students from lower socioeconomic backgrounds pay lower tuition fees than the better off.

A   True

B   False

C   Can't Tell

Passage II: question 7

Generally, students in England pay higher tuition fees than their counterparts in Wales or Scotland.

A   True

B   False

C   Can't Tell

Passage II: question 8

Students undertaking a first degree in Scotland pay no tuition fees as long as they stay in Scotland for the duration of their degree programme.

A   True

B   False

C   Can't Tell

Passage III: can adult learners be confrontational too?

One of the questions our 100 teachers were asked was about the relationship between learners' age and negative behaviour. It is often assumed that it is only the younger, 16–19 (and now perhaps 14–19), age group which presents a challenge to classroom management in post-compulsory education/training. However, one third of the teachers who responded to this question replied that they had experienced or observed difficult or negative behaviour from adult learners (that is, those over 21) as well as from the younger (14–19) age group. Perhaps we should not be surprised by this. The policies and practices which impact on adult learners are much the same as those which affect learners in their teens. And with adult learners, there may be added pressures of time, of family or financial responsibilities, and of anxieties about returning to education or training. Moreover, for the teacher, the idea of issuing rules to an adult learner, or challenging their behaviour or pulling them up on their language or attitude may somehow be more complicated than if the learner was a 16 year old. Whether this is right or wrong is not at issue here. What is important in our current context is that they may feel as though challenging behaviour from an adult is more difficult to deal with than challenging behaviour from a young learner, particularly if the adult in question is older than you are.

Source: Managing Behaviour in the Lifelong Learning Sector © Susan Wallace. Learning Matters, 2002.

Passage III: question 9
Two-thirds of teachers surveyed have not experienced or observed difficult or negative behaviour from learners aged over 21.

A True

B False

C Can't Tell

Passage III: question 10
The behaviour of adult learners can be as challenging as that of learners in their teens.

A True

B False

C Can't Tell

Passage III: question 11
Due to the added pressures experienced by adults, teaching adult learners is far more difficult than teaching learners in their teens.

A True

B False

C Can't Tell

Passage III: question 12
Policies and practices in relation to dealing with the negative behaviour of young learners are different from those for dealing with adult learners' negative behaviour.

A   True

B   False

C   Can't Tell

Passage IV: ethics and mental health law

In historical terms mental health law (and other social legislation, such as the Poor Law) were consistent with teleological ethics. The end justifies the means, and although mental health issues were perceived socially as moral conditions, it was ethically acceptable to segregate the mentally ill from general society for the protection of both. As treatment and understanding of mental health conditions developed, so did the ethics of psychiatric intervention, and whereas teleology remained the dominant school of thought, there was more consideration of the individual as a person, rather than a problem. The development of social welfare, and more humanistic approaches to those who were considered vulnerable, were reinforced by the establishment of the civil rights and user movements. Today's mental health and mental capacity legislation has both teleological and deontological elements. Although a paternalistic theme persists that emphasises protection of the individual and a degree of control which is teleological in nature, the strengthening of service user rights and increased levels of involvement make the distinction that in some situations the means cannot be justified by the end, and an individual's rights are sacrosanct, a view that belongs to the school of deontological ethics.

Source: Values and Ethics in Mental Health Practice © Daisy Bogg. Learning Matters, 2010.

Passage IV: question 13

Due to the establishment of the civil rights and user movements, the personal freedom of the mentally ill now takes precedence over the previous overarching moral system.

A   True

B   False

C   Can't Tell

Passage IV: question 14

It is ethically acceptable to segregate the mentally ill from general society for the protection of both.

A   True

B   False

C   Can't Tell

Passage IV: question 15

According to teleological ethical theories, the rightness of an action is determined by its consequences.

A True

B False

C Can't Tell

Passage IV: question 16

Psychiatrists belong to the school of teleological ethics as opposed to the school of deontological ethics.

A True

B False

C Can't Tell

Passage V: medical sociology – the macro level

At the macro level, medical sociologists study the patterns of disease found in societies and their possible causes. For example, 11.4 million working days were lost in 2008–09 in Britain as a result of 'stress'. Defined as 'the adverse reaction people have to excessive pressure or other types of demand placed on them' (UK Government Health & Safety Executive), stress is a relatively modern disease, unknown in wartime Britain, which nevertheless affects one in six of those in work, and has individual (e.g. poorer physical and mental health) and social consequences (work days lost, loss of productivity), and consequences in terms of healthcare usage (a significant proportion of patient GP visits are about work-related conditions). Stress at work can lead to lowered mental well-being, physical ill health and health-damaging behaviours (e.g. smoking, bad diet). Sociological studies have shown that factors such as lack of power and control in the workplace, job security, low pay, chequered work security (e.g. changing job frequently, multiple redundancies) are associated with work-related stress. Many sociological theories have been developed and applied to explore the relationship between work, stress and ill health ... it is of interest that work stress has been medicalised: people suffering from work stress (often poorly defined) are encouraged to see themselves as ill, in need of the ministrations of experts (e.g. doctors, stress management counsellors, alternative therapists, self-help materials) who are considered to know much more about their problems than they do. However, research suggests that organisational solutions which address the causes of stress such as workload, role clarity and organisational support (primary prevention) are more effective than those targeted at individual coping (secondary prevention) or counselling (tertiary prevention).

Source: Health, Behaviour and Society: Clinical Medicine in Context © Jennifer Cleland and Philip Cotton. Learning Matters, 2011.

Passage V: question 17

Employers are best placed to reduce work-related stress.

A True

B False

C Can't Tell

Passage V: question 18

People in wartime Britain were not subjected to work-related stress.

A True

B False

C Can't Tell

Passage V: question 19

The writer agrees with the medicalisation of work stress and the need to involve the ministration of experts to help in people's recovery.

A True

B False

C Can't Tell

Passage V: question 20

A health-damaging behaviour caused by stress at work might include people drinking excessive alcohol.

A True

B False

C Can't Tell

Passage VI: children at work

Child labour is a subject that still provides fierce debate and discussion, whether it concerns the exploitation of children in the developed world or the employment of children for a newspaper round. These debates are based upon what is harmful to a working child's development and what the nature of intervention should be, given a range of different social and economic circumstances. According to Woodhead (1998), our concern to protect children can easily become distorted by our modern Western sensibilities, leading to inappropriate responses that can make the problems faced by children worse rather than better. White (1996), for example, mentions the case of child workers in garment factories in Bangladesh being thrown out to satisfy consumer pressures for 'child-free' products. No attention had been given to the importance of work in the economic lives of these children and their families. The result was that the dismissed children continued to work, but in much more risky conditions in the informal and street economy. They had reduced earnings, worse nutrition and poorer health compared with the minority who had retained employment. The children themselves believed that light factory work combined with attending school for two or three hours a week was the best solution to their poverty. A new scheme was eventually introduced in which employers linked re-employment with schooling and future employment.

Source: Early Childhood Studies © Jenny Willan, Rod Parker-Rees and Jan Savage. Learning Matters, 2004.

Passage VI: question 21
Employers of children in garment factories in Bangladesh provide education for the children and offer employment when they are post-school age.

A True

B False

C Can't Tell

Passage VI: question 22
There is concern about the exploitation of children across both developed and developing countries.

A True

B False

C Can't Tell

Passage VI: question 23
Consumer pressure for 'child-free' products has been harmful to the well-being of children working in Asian garment factories.

A True

B False

C Can't Tell

Passage VI: question 24
Families with children working in the informal economy were better off economically than families with children working in the formal economy.

A True

B False

C Can't Tell

Passage VII: poverty and education

Even by 2002 three out of every ten Romanians were poor; one out of ten were extremely poor. At the same time, there is a strong positive association between economic growth and poverty reduction. Several variables predict poverty, but multivariate regressions show that the key correlate of poverty is education, with Roma ethnicity and being unemployed second and third in importance, respectively. Rural residents have more than double the probability of being poor than urban residents and rural areas account for 67 per cent of total poverty (Berryman et al., 2007).

Source: Primary practices and curriculum comparisons © Jackie Barbera and Deirdre Hewitt, *Global Issues and Comparative Education*. Learning Matters, 2009.

Passage VII: question 25

In Romania ethnicity tends to predict a person's socioeconomic standing in society.

A True

B False

C Can't Tell

Passage VII: question 26

Over 40 per cent of urban residents in Romania live in poverty.

A True

B False

C Can't Tell

Passage VII: question 27

The majority of the population residing in Romania's urban areas are not of Roma ethnicity.

A True

B False

C Can't Tell

Passage VII: question 28

Improving education in Romania is likely to help to reduce poverty in rural areas.

A True

B False

C Can't Tell

Passage VIII: education for citizenship

The Crick Report, *Education for Citizenship and the Teaching of Democracy in Schools*, was commissioned as a governmental response to fears of social disengagement and civic apathy among young people in Britain, and as an antidote to the perceived corrosive influence of much of contemporary culture. In 2002, citizenship education became a statutory requirement of all English secondary schools. It included three distinct strands: moral and social responsibility, *community involvement* and *political literacy*. In 2007 it was recommended that a fourth strand be developed, *Identity and diversity: living together in the UK*, intended specifically to address additional and growing concerns that British society was insufficiently 'cohesive' and did not adequately consider itself a united community.

Source: Learning in Contemporary Culture © Will Curtis and Alice Pettigrew. Learning Matters, 2009.

Passage VIII: question 29
Issues concerning race and equality are not contained in the citizenship curriculum.

A True

B False

C Can't Tell

Passage VIII: question 30
The curriculum for secondary schools in Wales, Scotland and Northern Ireland does not include citizenship as a statutory requirement.

A True

B False

C Can't Tell

Passage VIII: question 31
Citizenship has been included as part of the curriculum in England partly because of young people's lack of interest in their local communities.

A True

B False

C Can't Tell

Passage VIII: question 32
Britain has become a pluralist society where small groups maintain their unique cultural identities to the detriment of community cohesion.

A True

B False

C Can't Tell

Passage IX: origin of knowledge

The origin and acquisition of knowledge in humans has been a matter of intense philosophical debate, which can be traced back at least to Plato. Historically, views have tended to fall within one of three main camps: nativists considered all individuals to be born with the knowledge they needed and that anything else was acquired by some innate or inherited characteristic; empiricists considered all individuals to acquire knowledge out of experience; and rationalists considered all individuals to acquire knowledge by engaging in reasoning. Today, individuals are considered to be born at least partly 'hard-wired' with an architecture of the mind which facilitates cognition, rather than with a mind full of knowledge *per se*. Understanding that architecture is fundamental to understanding how we learn.

Source: The mystery of learning © John Sharp and Barbara Murphy, *Education Studies: An Issues-based Approach*, second edition. Learning Matters, 2009.

Passage IX: question 33

Historically, it was thought that humans acquire knowledge genetically, through experience, or by the use of reasoning.

A True

B False

C Can't Tell

Passage IX: question 34

Empiricists believed that humans only attained knowledge through experience and not through education.

A True

B False

C Can't Tell

Passage IX: question 35

Nativists believed that knowledge was not acquired from others or by training or education.

A True

B False

C Can't Tell

Passage IX: question 36

Understanding the mental processes inherited by children will improve the level of educational attainment.

A True

B False

C Can't Tell

Passage X: 'tweenies' and 'tweenagers'

The terms 'tweenies' and 'tweenagers' have emerged within the last ten years to explain recent cultural changes in pre-teenage childhood cohorts. Originally coined to term a marketing demographic, 'tweenagers' are 8- to 12-year-old children who appear to exhibit characteristics of teenagers more than those of children. The *branding* and *commercial appropriation* (Russell and Tyler, 2002) of childhood, and especially female childhood, has resulted in disturbing trends. The key characteristics of an emergent 'tweenager' age cohort include: *educational pressures*, especially national tests; *'pester power'* – parents with less time to spend with their children and increasing numbers of divorces might be more likely to consent to demands; *marketing and consumption patterns*, such as mobile phones, accessories, jewellery, make-up; *celebrity culture* – infantilisation of celebrity and especially young females; *peer pressure*, to look a certain way, to grow up fast, to try drugs and alcohol.

Source: *Learning in Contemporary Culture* © Will Curtis and Alice Pettigrew. Learning Matters, 2009.

Passage X: question 37

Young people are confronted with stresses and demands that they do not have the experience to cope with.

A True

B False

C Can't Tell

Passage X: question 38

Generally, 'tweenagers' have more commodities targeted at them and more power than this age group will have ever experienced before.

A True

B False

C Can't Tell

Passage X: question 39

Females are more likely to exhibit the characteristics of a 'tweenager' than males.

A True

B False

C Can't Tell

Passage X: question 40

Children aged 8 to 12 have exhibited the characteristics of 'tweenagers' only over the past ten years.

A True

B False

C Can't Tell

Passage XI: global studies

Every country in the world, with the exceptions of the USA and Somalia, is a signatory to the United Nations Convention on the Rights of the Child (UNCRC). The convention contains 54 articles (points) in which children's rights are recognised and obligations placed on states (governments) to recognise these rights in practice. The definition of a child under the convention is anyone under the age of 18. In their most recent report to the UN inspectors, the four Children's Commissioners for England, Scotland, Wales and Northern Ireland identified the following infringements of the UNCRC which they say deny hope and opportunity to many of Britain's 14 million children and adolescents: *a punitive juvenile justice system; public attitudes that demonise teenagers; lack of protection against physical punishment in the home and one of the highest levels of child poverty in Europe* (Carvel 2008).

Source: Education and social care: Friends or foes? © Sue K Flowers, *Global Issues and Comparative Education*. Learning Matters, 2009.

Passage XI: question 41

Students in full-time education in universities or colleges are not protected by the UNCRC.

A True

B False

C Can't Tell

Passage XI: question 42

The youth courts in Britain are more concerned with punishing children rather than rehabilitating them.

A   True

B   False

C   Can't Tell

Passage XI: question 43

More children in Britain are physically abused by a parent or guardian than in any other UNCRC signatory.

A   True

B   False

C   Can't Tell

Passage XI: question 44

There is a public perception in Britain today that adolescents are malevolent and evil.

A   True

B   False

C   Can't Tell

Verbal Reasoning practice subtest: answers

Question number	Correct response	Question number	Correct response
1	A – True	23	A – True
2	C – Can't Tell	24	B – False
3	B – False	25	A – True
4	C – Can't Tell	26	B – False
5	A – True	27	C – Can't Tell
6	C – Can't Tell	28	A – True
7	A – True	29	B – False
8	C – Can't Tell	30	C – Can't Tell
9	C – Can't Tell	31	A – True
10	A – True	32	C – Can't Tell
11	C – Can't Tell	33	A – True
12	B – False	34	B – False
13	B – False	35	A – True
14	C – Can't Tell	36	C – Can't Tell
15	A – True	37	C – Can't Tell
16	C – Can't Tell	38	A – True
17	A – True	39	A – True
18	C – Can't Tell	40	B – False
19	B – False	41	B – False
20	C – Can't Tell	42	C – Can't Tell
21	C – Can't Tell	43	C – Can't Tell
22	A – True	44	A – True

Verbal Reasoning practice subtest: explanation of answers

Passage 1: political and social influences on health

Passage 1: question 1

There is a very complex interaction of factors that contribute to health.

Answer: True

The answer to this question can be found in the first two sentences of the passage and specifically, 'health is determined by wider determinants, such as where we live, what our income is relative to other people and what level of education we have. Political and social factors which influence health are not isolated, but interplay in a complex way. From this extract it can be asserted that there is a very complex interaction of factors that contribute to health'.

Passage 1: question 2

In Tamil Nadu female contraception usage is greater than male contraception usage.

Answer: Can't Tell

Although the passage directly states, 'research shows that female contraception usage in developed Indian states (e.g. Tamil Nadu) is significantly higher than in less developed states', it provides no comparison of male contraception usage. In the reference to male contraception in the passage, 'Both socioeconomic status and husband's education are strongly associated with family planning in both states', there is no indication as to the extent of male contraception usage.

Passage 1: question 3

Unlike women in Tamil Nadu, those who live in the Bihar are not allowed to work outside their homes.

Answer: False

The passage states, 'women in northern states such as Bihar are strongly subject to traditional conservatism, are predominantly less educated and less likely to work outside their homes'. It does not say that they may not work outside their homes, only that they are 'less likely' to do so.

Passage 1: question 4

States that are misruled, and have inefficient governance structures and corrupt bureaucracies, are likely to be poorly associated with family planning.

Answer: Can't Tell

Although from the information contained in the passage, this statement might apply to the state of Bihar, it could not be accepted as a general rule without further research and relevant information.

Passage II: the funding debate

Passage II: question 5

Students who are seeking a career as a teacher, in any subject, receive government funding if undertaking a teacher training degree programme.

Answer: True

The passage quite clearly states that students undertaking 'professional courses also receive grants from the relevant professional funding bodies (for example, teacher training degrees are funded by the Teacher Development Agency)'. The 'subject' the student selects is irrelevant to the answer.

Passage II: question 6

Higher education students from lower socioeconomic backgrounds pay lower tuition fees than the better off.

Answer: Can't Tell

In reality, students from lower socioeconomic backgrounds may receive financial support and pay lower tuition fees than the better off – certainly, the passage states that 'Previously the state subsidised higher education for many students, depending on their family's financial income. However, there is no information in the passage about the current situation with regard to subsidies or means-tested grants for students, and further details would be required'.

Passage II: question 7

Generally, students in England pay higher tuition fees than their counterparts in Wales or Scotland.

Answer: True

The passage states that 'Welsh students are effectively exempt from top-up fees if they stay in Wales, because they receive a non-means tested grant from the Welsh Government', and 'In Scotland, students have to make no personal contribution to fees except when studying for a second degree or postgraduate award.' Generally, in England students have to pay tuition fees even though these may vary between educational institutions.

Passage II: question 8

Students undertaking a first degree in Scotland pay no tuition fees as long as they stay in Scotland for the duration of their degree programme.

Answer: Can't Tell

The passage states that 'In Scotland, students have to make no personal contribution to fees except when studying for a second degree or postgraduate award.' It might be assumed that, similarly to Welsh students, Scottish students pay no personal contribution to fees for first degrees if they stay in Scotland. However, this is not stated categorically. Also, it is not made clear whether the 'no personal contribution' applies only to Scottish students or also to students from other countries studying in Scotland. Further information would be required to determine a True or False answer.

Passage III: can adult learners be confrontational too?

Passage III: question 9

Two-thirds of teachers surveyed have not experienced or observed difficult or negative behaviour from learners aged over 21.

Answer: Can't Tell

The passage states that of 100 teachers who were asked about the relationship between learners' age and negative behaviour, one third who responded to this question replied that they had experienced or observed difficult or negative behaviour from adult learners (that is, those over 21). At first glance it might be assumed, therefore, that the remaining two-thirds of teachers had not experienced negative behaviour in adult learners. However, the passage actually states that 'one third of the teachers who responded to this question', which might suggest that not all of the 100 teachers actually responded to the question. Consequently, further details would be required to confirm this or otherwise before a definitive answer to this statement could be made.

Passage III: question 10

The behaviour of adult learners can be as challenging as that of learners in their teens.

Answer: True

This statement is True as the passage states, 'one third of the teachers ... experienced or observed difficult or negative behaviour from adult learners (that is, those over 21) as well as from the younger (14–19) age group'.

Passage III: question 11

Due to the added pressures experienced by adults, teaching adult learners is far more difficult than teaching learners in their teens.

Answer: Can't Tell

The passage says that difficult or negative behaviour is displayed by both adults and young learners and goes on to identify some pressures experienced by adult learners (e.g. time, family, financial responsibilities). Pressures experienced by young learners are not mentioned. However, we cannot be sure that problematic adult behaviour is directly related to the added pressures described – the passage suggests these may be a factor affecting the behaviour of adult learners, but no evidence for this conjecture is given. The passage does say that 'for the teacher, the idea of issuing rules to an adult learner, or challenging their behaviour or pulling them up on their language or attitude, may somehow be more complicated than if the learner was a 16 year old'. It goes on to say that the teacher 'may feel as though challenging behaviour from an adult is more difficult to deal with than challenging behaviour from a young learner, particularly if the adult in question is older than you are'. So we can assume that some teachers, at least, might feel that teaching adults is more difficult than teaching learners in their teens, but we cannot assume, without further information, that such teaching is 'far more difficult', so the answer must be Can't Tell.

Passage III: question 12

Policies and practices in relation to dealing with the negative behaviour of young learners are different from those for dealing with adult learners' negative behaviour.

Answer: False

The passage clearly states that 'The policies and practices which impact on adult learners are much the same as those which affect learners in their teens.' In any case, the passage does not state that these policies and practices relate to dealing with negative behaviour. Therefore the statement is False.

Passage IV: ethics and mental health law

Passage IV: question 13

Due to the establishment of the civil rights and user movements, the personal freedom of the mentally ill now takes precedence over the previous overarching moral system.

Answer: False

Although the civil rights and user movements helped in the development of social welfare and more humanistic approaches to the mentally ill, the passage actually states, 'a paternalistic theme persists that emphasises protection of the individual and a degree of control which is teleological in nature'.

Passage IV: question 14

It is ethically acceptable to segregate the mentally ill from general society for the protection of both.

Answer: Can't Tell

This statement essentially repeats the second sentence of the passage, i.e. 'it was ethically acceptable to segregate the mentally ill from general society for the protection of both'. The passage statement is in the past tense (was) whereas the question statement is in the present tense and may lead to a False answer being considered. There may well be occasions where a mentally ill person may be deemed such a danger to him/herself or others that it is morally correct for that person to be segregated from general society, and this may lead to a True answer being considered. However, this is not contained within the passage and the answer must therefore be Can't Tell as the statement itself is unclear and would need further clarification for a False or True answer to be given.

Passage IV: question 15

According to teleological ethical theories, the rightness of an action is determined by its consequences.

Answer: True

Teleology is defined at the beginning of the passage, 'The end justifies the means, and although mental health issues were perceived socially as moral conditions, it was ethically acceptable to segregate the mentally ill from general society for the protection of both.' It advocated paternalistic policies with an overarching moral system overriding personal freedom in some circumstances.

Passage IV: question 16

Psychiatrists belong to the school of teleological ethics as opposed to the school of deontological ethics.

Answer: Can't Tell

The reference to psychiatry is contained in the fourth sentence of the passage: 'As treatment and understanding of mental health conditions developed, so did the ethics of psychiatric intervention, and whereas teleology remained the dominant school of thought, there was more consideration of the individual as a person, rather than a problem.' From this reference it is not possible to determine whether psychiatrists belonged to the school of teleological ethics or deontological ethics, or both.

Passage V: medical sociology – the macro level

Passage V: question 17

Employers are best placed to reduce work-related stress.

Answer: True

The passage states, 'However, research suggests that organisational solutions which address the causes of stress such as workload, role clarity and organisational support (primary prevention) are more effective than those targeted at individual coping (secondary prevention) or counselling (tertiary prevention).' It therefore follows that employers appear to hold the key to reducing stress in the workplace.

Passage V: question 18

People in wartime Britain were not subjected to work-related stress.

Answer: Can't Tell

The passage states: 'stress is a relatively modern disease, unknown in wartime Britain'. Although not mentioned in the passage, there is little doubt that work-related stress has been with us since time immemorial or at least since employment began. However, more information would have been required in the passage to make a definitive statement.

Passage V: question 19

The writer agrees with the medicalisation of work stress and the need to involve the ministration of experts to help in people's recovery.

Answer: False

This answer is supported by the passage which states: 'it is of interest that work stress has been medicalised: people suffering from work stress (often poorly defined) are encouraged to see themselves as ill, in need of the ministrations of experts (e.g. doctors, stress management counsellors, alternative therapists, self-help materials) who are considered to know much more about their problems than they do'. This displays a degree of cynicism by the writer who appears to question the medicalisation of work stress and the use of experts.

Passage V: question 20

A health-damaging behaviour caused by stress at work might include people drinking excessive alcohol.

Answer: Can't Tell

The passage states, 'Stress at work can lead to lowered mental well-being, physical ill health and health-damaging behaviours (e.g. smoking, bad diet).' Although it might be assumed that 'drinking excessive alcohol' is undoubtedly a health-damaging behaviour that may be caused by stress at work, it does not specifically state this in the passage. More information would be required to confirm this.

Passage VI: children at work

Passage VI: question 21

Employers of children in garment factories in Bangladesh provide education for the children and offer employment when they are post-school age.

Answer: Can't Tell

Although the passage states that 'A new scheme was eventually introduced in which employers linked re-employment with schooling and future employment', it is not clear that the employers actually *provide* education and future employment. The 'link' could be less direct than this. It is also not clear whether or not this scheme applies to all garment factories in Bangladesh. Further information would be required, so the answer must be Can't Tell.

Passage VI: question 22

There is concern about the exploitation of children across both developed and developing countries.

Answer: True

The passage states explicitly that there is 'fierce debate and discussion, whether it concerns the exploitation of children in the developed world or the employment of children for a newspaper round'.

Passage VI: question 23

Consumer pressure for 'child-free' products has been harmful to the well-being of children working in Asian garment factories.

Answer: True

The passage clearly states: 'child workers in garment factories in Bangladesh being thrown out to satisfy consumer pressures for "child-free" products. No attention had been given to the importance of work in the economic lives of these children and their families. The result was that the dismissed children continued to work, but in much more risky conditions in the informal and street economy. They had reduced earnings, worse nutrition and poorer health compared with the minority who had retained employment.'

Passage VI: question 24

Families with children working in the informal economy were better off economically than families with children working in the formal economy.

Answer: False

The passage states that 'the dismissed children continued to work, but in much more risky conditions in the informal and street economy. They had reduced earnings … compared with the minority who had retained employment.' In this context the 'formal' economy relates to those children employed in garment factories.

Passage VII: poverty and education

Passage VII: question 25

In Romania ethnicity tends to predict a person's socioeconomic standing in society.

Answer: True

The passage clearly states that Roma ethnicity is the second most important factor in predicting poverty.

Passage VII: question 26

Over 40 per cent of urban residents in Romania live in poverty.

Answer: False

The passage states 'rural areas account for 67 per cent of total poverty'. Therefore urban areas must account for 33 per cent of total poverty and not 'over 40 per cent' as posed in the statement.

Passage VII: question 27

The majority of the population residing in Romania's urban areas are not of Roma ethnicity.

Answer: Can't Tell

No information is provided in the passage in relation to the ethnic distribution of the population in Romania.

Passage VII: question 28
Improving education in Romania is likely to help to reduce poverty in rural areas.

Answer: True

The passage states: 'Several variables predict poverty, but multivariate regressions show that the key correlate of poverty is education' and therefore education is likely to help to reduce poverty.

Passage VIII: education for citizenship

Passage VIII: question 29
Issues concerning race and equality are not contained in the citizenship curriculum.

Answer: False

The passage states: 'In 2007 it was recommended that a fourth strand be developed, *Identity and diversity: living together in the UK.*' From this it can be assumed that 'race' is part of the curriculum. Equality may also stem from this addition to the curriculum but would certainly be included within the strand *moral and social responsibility.*

Passage VIII: question 30
The curriculum for secondary schools in Wales, Scotland and Northern Ireland does not include citizenship as a statutory requirement.

Answer: Can't Tell

The Crick Report dealt with issues of citizenship across Britain and the development of a fourth strand to the curriculum specifically mentions the UK and British society. However, the passage states: 'In 2002, citizenship education became a statutory requirement of all English secondary schools.' There is no mention of it being a statutory requirement in Wales, Scotland and Northern Ireland.

Passage VIII: question 31
Citizenship has been included as part of the curriculum in England partly because of young people's disinterest in their local communities.

Answer: True

The passage refers to concerns about people's disinterest in their communities on three occasions. Specifically in relation to young people the passage states 'fears of social disengagement and civic apathy among young people in Britain'. One of the three distinct strands is *community involvement* and the fourth strand refers to *Identity and diversity: living together in the UK.*

Passage VIII: question 32

Britain has become a pluralist society where small groups maintain their unique cultural identities to the detriment of community cohesion.

Answer: Can't Tell

Although this may in part be true, the passage does not contain sufficient information to justify this response. It does not mention pluralism as a cause for the breakdown in community involvement.

Passage IX: origin of knowledge

Passage IX: question 33

Historically, it was thought that humans acquire knowledge genetically, through experience, or by the use of reasoning.

Answer: True

Nativists believe that humans acquire knowledge genetically: 'all individuals to be born with the knowledge they needed and that anything else was acquired by some innate or inherited characteristic; empiricists considered all individuals to acquire knowledge out of experience, and rationalists considered all individuals to acquire knowledge by engaging in reasoning'.

Passage IX: question 34

Empiricists believed that humans only attained knowledge through experience and not through education.

Answer: False

The passage states: 'empiricists considered all individuals to acquire knowledge out of experience'. It does not mention 'education' specifically but it can be defined as any act or experience that has a formative effect on the individual.

Passage IX: question 35

Nativists believed that knowledge was not acquired from others or by training or education.

Answer: True

The passage states: 'nativists considered all individuals to be born with the knowledge they needed and that anything else was acquired by some innate or inherited characteristic'. In this sense nativists did not believe knowledge to be acquired by training or education.

Passage IX: question 36

Understanding the mental processes inherited by children will improve the level of educational attainment.

Answer: Can't Tell

The passage states: 'Today, individuals are considered to be born at least partly "hard-wired" with an architecture of the mind which facilitates cognition, rather than with a mind full of knowledge *per se*. Understanding that architecture is fundamental to understanding how we learn.' Although understanding how we learn may improve the level of educational attainment, this is not mentioned in the passage and further information would be required.

Passage X: 'tweenies' and 'tweenagers'

Passage X: question 37

Young people are confronted with stresses and demands that they do not have the experience to cope with.

Answer: Can't Tell

This is a very generalised statement and although the passage clearly indicates the pressures to which young people are exposed, and although it may be the case, the passage does not elicit any information on their abilities to cope with these pressures.

Passage X: question 38

Generally, 'tweenagers' have more commodities targeted at them and more power than this age group will have ever experienced before.

Answer: True

In relation to commodities the passage clearly states: 'marketing and consumption patterns, such as mobile phones, accessories, jewellery, make up', etc. In relation to 'more power' the passage states: 'parents with less time to spend with their children and increasing numbers of divorces might be more likely to consent to demands'.

Passage X: question 39

Females are more likely to exhibit the characteristics of a 'tweenager' than males.

Answer: True

This is made quite clear in the passage: 'The branding and commercial appropriation (Russell and Tyler, 2002) of childhood, and especially female childhood' and later in the passage 'infantilisation of celebrity and especially young females'.

Passage X: question 40

Children aged 8 to 12 have exhibited the characteristics of 'tweenagers' only over the past ten years.

Answer: False

The passage states: 'The terms "tweenies" and "tweenagers" have emerged within the last ten years to explain recent cultural changes in pre-teenage childhood cohort.' This does not mean that the characteristics of 'tweenagers' have emerged within the last ten years.

Passage XI: *global studies*

Passage XI: question 41

Students in full-time education in universities or colleges are not protected by the UNCRC.

Answer: False

The passage states: 'The definition of a child under the convention is anyone under the age of 18.' It does not mention whether or not a child is in full-time education either at university or college. It is simply an age limitation and children under 18 may well be attending university or college.

Passage XI: question 42

The youth courts in Britain are more concerned with punishing children rather than rehabilitating them.

Answer: Can't Tell

The recent report to the UN inspectors claimed that Britain had a 'punitive juvenile justice system'. However, to make a more informed judgement about the statement, more information would be required as the report by the four Children's Commissioners is not elaborated on.

Passage XI: question 43

More children in Britain are physically abused by a parent or guardian than in any other UNCRC signatory.

Answer: Can't Tell

The passage states that the report to the UN inspectors stated: 'public attitudes that demonise teenagers; lack of protection against physical punishment in the home and one of the highest levels of child poverty in Europe'. The passage does not provide comparative statistics of child abuse across the Convention's signatories.

Passage XI: question 44

There is a public perception in Britain today that adolescents are malevolent and evil.

Answer: True

The report to the UN inspectors relates to 'children and adolescents' and mentions the 'public attitudes that demonise teenagers'. Therefore, there is a public perception that adolescents are malevolent and evil.

Chapter 2
The Quantitative
Reasoning subtest

This chapter will help you to:

- understand the purpose and the format of quantitative reasoning tests;
- prepare for the Quantitative Reasoning subtest using general numerical aptitude questions;
- test your knowledge and understanding of numerical-type questions;
- identify those numerical skills where development is required.

Introduction

Pearson VUE describes the purpose of this subtest as follows:

> The Quantitative Reasoning subtest assesses a candidate's ability to solve numerical problems. This subtest requires the candidate to solve problems by extracting relevant information from tables and other numerical presentations. It assumes familiarity with numbers to a good pass at GCSE but the problems to be solved are less to do with numerical facility and more to do with problem solving (i.e. knowing what information to use and how to manipulate it using simple calculations and ratios). Hence it measures reasoning using numbers as a vehicle rather than measuring a facility with numbers.

As outlined in the introduction to this part of the book, commercially produced numerical aptitude tests have been in existence for many years, mainly for use in the selection and assessment of staff. There have been numerous books written on how to pass or how to master psychometric tests, and what follows is a précis of what you need to consider specifically in approaching the Quantitative Reasoning subtest. Essentially, the advice on preparation for any aptitude test, contained in the first chapter, holds true for numerical tests.

Quite simply, numerical tests are designed to measure your ability to understand numbers. This relates to the four basic arithmetic operations of addition, subtraction, multiplication and division, as well as number sequences and simple mathematics. Therefore, in preparing for such tests, you need to be able to perform simple calculations without the use of a calculator.

This chapter provides you with an opportunity to test your understanding and knowledge of the range of questions you are likely to be presented with in the UKCAT. By taking this opportunity you should be able to identify any numerical areas which you may need to develop. Obviously, as with any other type of examination, numerical questions can be presented in a variety of ways. However, the basic computations used will always be the same. So learn or remind yourself of the basics. The section following the subtest provides the answers to the questions. This includes not only the correct answer and rationale but also the reasons why the other options are incorrect. In addition, this section also provides the 'mathematical rule' for each question. All this is designed to reinforce or build on your understanding and knowledge of the syllabus areas.

Quantitative Reasoning subtest

For the purposes of this chapter, a range of questions has been designed to cover relevant areas of the Level 2 and Level 3 Adult Numeracy Core Curriculum produced by the Qualifications and Curriculum Development Agency. Level 3 is equivalent to GCSE standard, and a score of 27 or above (out of 36) on the practice test below equates to a Grade C or above at GCSE. This should be sufficient to deal with the scope of questions contained within the subtest. In reality, at this level, you should be getting all the questions correct.

The curriculum areas covered in the practice test are as follows.

- Basic arithmetic operations of addition, subtraction, multiplication and division.
- Powers and roots.
- Proportional change and ratios.
- Measurement of average and range to compare distributions, and estimate mean, median and range of grouped data.
- Conversion between fractions, decimals and percentages.
- Formulae, equations and expressions.
- Conversion of measurements between systems.

Response formats and example question

The type of format used in the Quantitative Reasoning subtest is the same as the one used as an example of multiple-choice questions in the introduction to this part of the book. That is, a *stem* in the form of a table, chart or graph, followed by a *lead-in question* and then five possible *choices* – A, B, C, D or E.

Example question

The following example requires you to select the correct answer from the five options provided. The rationale for the correct and incorrect answers is provided after the question.

The table below shows the miles travelled by a sales representative.

	Mon	Tue	Wed	Thu	Fri	Sat
WEEK 1	197.5	189	213.5	231	190	437
WEEK 2	116.5	145	202	173	52	

You want to find her median mileage over the 11 days. Which of these would you do?

A   Find the sixth number and divide this by 2.

B   Add all the numbers together and divide by 11.

C   Rearrange the numbers into numerical order and then find the sixth number.

D   Find the average for each week and divide this by 2.

E   Add the two middle numbers together and divide this by 2.

Median: rule

The **median** of a distribution is the middle value when the values are arranged in order. When there are two middle values (i.e. for an even number of values), you add the two middle numbers and divide by 2.

Answer C is correct: Rearrange the numbers into numerical order and then find the sixth number.

Rationale

There are 11 values, an odd number, so arrange the values into numerical order and then find the middle value, which is the sixth number, and this is the median.

A is incorrect: Find the sixth number and divide this by 2. Here there is an odd number of values so there is no need to divide anything by 2, only find the middle value.

B is incorrect: Add all the numbers together and divide by 11. This is the method for finding the mean, not the median.

D is incorrect: Find the average for each week and divide this by 2. This is not a method for finding any type of average.

E is incorrect: Add the two middle numbers together and divide this by 2. This is the method for finding the median when there is an even number of values.

Quantitative Reasoning practice subtest

The Quantitative Reasoning subtest consists of 36 items associated with tables, charts and/ or graphs. A period of 25 minutes is allowed for the test, with one minute for instruction and 24 minutes for items.

If you want to simulate 'test conditions', you are advised to use rough paper to mark down your choice for each of the questions (i.e. A, B, C, D or E). The answers can then be checked against the 'answers' in the following section. Obviously, incorrect answers may identify a development need in a particular area of the curriculum. A simple on-screen calculator is available during the test.

Remember that each of the questions is always accompanied by five possible answers (A, B, C, D and E), and that only **one** answer is correct.

Also remember to read through all five competing answers before selecting what you consider to be the correct answer. By reading the four 'incorrect' answers you should confirm that your choice is, in fact, correct.

Questions 1 to 4 are about skyscrapers. Below are examples of the tallest skyscrapers across the USA with the height in metres shown in parenthesis.

Trump International Chicago (423)	Transamerica San Francisco (258)
Bank of America Atlanta (312)	Hancock Place Boston (241)
Devon Energy Oklahoma City (258)	Republic Plaza Denver (218)
Detroit Marriott Detroit (222)	JP Morgan Chase Houston (305)
Key Tower Cleveland (289)	Empire State Building New York (381)
IDS Tower Minneapolis (241)	Bank of America Houston (238)
RSA Battle House Mobile (227)	Columbia Centre Seattle (284)
Aon Centre Chicago (346)	John Hancock Centre Chicago (344)
30 Hudson Street Jersey City (238)	U.S. Steel Tower Pittsburgh (256)
Southeast Financial Centre Miami (233)	U.S. Bank Los Angeles (310)
Comcast Centre Philadelphia (297)	Chase Tower Indianapolis (253)
Bank of America Charlotte (265)	Bank of America Dallas (281)

1. What fraction of the skyscrapers are over 300 metres but less than 400 metres in height?

    A $\dfrac{1}{2}$

    B $\dfrac{1}{3}$

    C $\dfrac{1}{4}$

    D $\dfrac{1}{5}$

    E $\dfrac{1}{6}$

2. What is the ratio of skyscrapers that are greater than 258 metres high but less than 290 metres compared with skyscrapers that are less than 258 metres but greater than 220 metres?

    A 1:2

    B 2:3

    C 2:5

 D 3:7

 E 4:9

3. How many of the skyscrapers are less than 850 feet in height (1 metre = 3.3 feet)?

 A 4

 B 6

 C 8

 D 10

 E 12

4. What can you say that 25% of the skyscrapers are?

 A Less than 250 metres high.

 B At least 230 metres but less than 250 metres high.

 C More than 300 metres high.

 D At least 290 metres but less than 350 metres high.

 E At least 245 metres high.

Questions 5 to 8 are about the following table, which shows the average A-level raw score pass rates per subject area for students entering both redbrick universities and other universities.

Redbrick universities	Pass rate	Other universities	Pass rate
English language	82	English language	78
English literature	75	English literature	63
Mathematics	88	Mathematics	76
History	69	History	72
Geography	72	Geography	65
Law	79	Law	58
Economics	66	Economics	71
French	87	French	67
German	82	German	71
Latin	64	Latin*	0

* Latin does not apply to other universities.

5. To the nearest round number, what is the mean average pass rate across all subjects for other universities?

    A 9

    B 69

    C 78

    D 138

    E 621

6. What is the median average pass rate for redbrick universities?

    A 71

    B 75

    C 77

    D 79

    E 88

7. What can you say about the range of the redbrick universities' average pass rates compared with the range of average pass rates of students entering the other universities?

    A The mode for the other universities is lower.

    B They are the same.

    C It is lower.

    D The median for the redbrick universities is higher.

    E It is higher.

8. What is the mode average pass rate of the redbrick universities?

    A 71

    B 72

    C 82

    D 85

    E 88

Questions 9 to 12 refer to the pie chart below, which groups the level of turnover of a number of organisations included in a business sector survey.

The number of organisations per group is shown in parentheses.

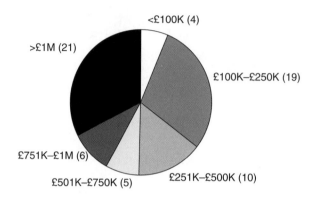

9. What percentage, to two decimal places, of organisations has a turnover in excess of £1m?

A 49.53%

B 46.34%

C 32.31%

D 57.89%

E 62.16%

10. What is the ratio of the number of organisations with a turnover of £501k–£750k compared with the rest of the organisations?

A 1:5

B 4:9

C 1:10

D 1:12

E 1:15

11. The Learning and Skills Council has asked the publishers of this business sector information also to produce the turnover of the organisations in euros. In converting pounds sterling to euros, where £1 = €1.45, what would be the lower limit of the range for those organisations with a turnover of £251k–£500k, in euros?

A €145,000

B €362,500

   C €363,950

   D €725,000

   E €726,450

12. The 65 organisations in this survey employ a total of 850 people, of whom about 63% are employed by those organisations with a turnover in excess of £1m. The remaining employees are spread pro rata across the other organisations. How many employees, to the nearest round number, work for a company with a turnover of £251k–£500k?

   A 7

   B 12

   C 15

   D 19

   E 26

Questions 13 to 16 relate to the table below that shows the average gross weekly earnings by UK country.

Year	United Kingdom	England	Wales	Scotland	Northern Ireland
1999	407.8	414.9	358.7	377.0	352.4
2000	425.1	433.3	372.8	388.6	367.6
2001	449.7	459.2	385.8	411.1	381.5
2002	472.1	482.0	405.2	434.6	396.8
2003	487.1	497.2	421.8	447.0	411.5
2004	498.2	508.1	438.3	455.5	430.9
2005	516.4	525.5	454.8	479.0	450.7
2006	534.9	544.3	466.2	499.7	469.4
2007	550.3	560.8	472.0	514.6	471.7
2008	575.6	586.7	498.2	536.3	487.0
2009	587.2	597.4	506.3	555.1	509.1
2010	598.3	608.6	516.0	570.1	511.6

13. Which country, including the United Kingdom, had the highest range of average gross weekly earnings between 1999 and 2010?

   A Wales

   B Northern Ireland

C United Kingdom

D Scotland

E England

14. Which one of the following statements is supported by the information contained in the table?

A In 2002 Wales's average gross weekly earnings were approximately 10% less than those in England.

B Scotland has the third highest average gross weekly earnings in the country.

C In 2010 Northern Ireland's average gross annual earnings will be over $\frac{1}{10}$ less than the average UK earnings.

D Compared to 1999, in 2010 the difference in average gross weekly earnings between England and Scotland has decreased.

E Northern Ireland's average gross weekly earnings exceeded those of Wales in three separate years.

15. What is the percentage increase (to one decimal place) of the average gross weekly earnings in the United Kingdom between 1999 and 2010?

A 28.9%

B 31.8%

C 40.7%

D 46.7%

E 71.2%

16. What is the approximate ratio of the average gross weekly earnings of Northern Ireland in 2004 compared to the country's earnings in 2010?

A 1:2

B 1:3

C 2:3

D 3:4

E 4:5

Questions 17 to 20 are about the table on page 59, which is being used by a group of 12 people forming a diet club. They have agreed to use a calorie count method and have produced the table showing the serving size, calorie count and grams of fat for bread, biscuits, cakes, eggs and dairy products.

Item	Serving size (grams)	Calorie count	Grams of fat
Bagel	85	216	1.4
Baguette	150	360	1.8
Chocolate cake	34	180	10.4
Biscuit	15	74	3.3
Danish pastry	67	287	17.4
Doughnut	49	140	2.0
Hot cross bun	70	205	3.9
Jaffa cake	12	46	1.0
Scone	70	225	17.6
White crusty roll	50	140	1.2
Brown bread	25	74	0.7
Granary bread	25	59	0.7
Pitta bread	25	147	1.1
White bread	37	84	0.6
Wholemeal bread	36	79	1.0
Toast	33	88	0.6
Butter	10	74	8.2
Cheddar cheese	40	172	14.8
Cream cheese	34	58	4.8
Eggs size 3	57	84	6.2

17. The estimated average requirements are a daily calorie intake of 1,940 calories per day for women and 2,550 for men. The group agrees to follow the same daily menu that provides for an intake of 1,940 calories. The men then select items to take them up to their recommended calorie intake. One of the men decides he will achieve this by eating just one serving size bagel and butter and as much toast as he is allowed where a serving of 33 grams equates to one slice of toast. What is the maximum number of slices of toast the man may have to stay under the recommended calorie limit?

A 3 slices

B 4 slices

C 7 slices

D 9 slices

E 11 slices

The group categorises the items of food into low- to high-calorie content and produces the following table.

Calorie count per serving	Number of items
<80	7
>80 but <109	3
>109 but <149	3
>149 but <189	2
189 and over	6

The group then checks its table.

18. Is there anything wrong with the total number of items in the table?

   A One too few of calorie count >149 but <189.

   B Two too many of calorie count <80.

   C One too many of calorie count 189 and over.

   D Total number of calorie count correct.

   E One too few of calorie count >109 but <149.

19. A group member wants to ascertain the median calorie count for all the items in the table. Which one of the following should he do?

   A Rearrange the numbers into numerical order, find the tenth number and divide by 2.

   B Add all the numbers together and divide by 20.

   C Find the average of all the numbers and divide by 2.

   D Find the calorie count number that occurs most frequently.

   E Rearrange the numbers into numerical order, add the tenth and eleventh numbers and divide by 2.

20. It is the birthday of one of the group and another member wants to buy a chocolate cake, large enough for each member to have one serving size. However, before going shopping she wants to know what weight of cake she will need for the group, measured in ounces. Grams are converted to ounces by dividing grams by 28.3.

If X is the weight of the required cake in ounces, and G is the weight of one serving size in grams, which one of the following options is the correct formula?

A $\quad X = 12\left(\dfrac{G}{28.3}\right)$

B $\quad G = \dfrac{12X}{28.3}$

C $\quad G = \dfrac{12}{28.3X}$

D $\quad X = 28.3\left(\dfrac{G}{12}\right)$

E $\quad X = \dfrac{28.3}{12G}$

Questions 21 to 24 relate to the following information about the Links View Golf and Country Club, which provides tailor-made stays for those wishing to use the facilities of either their two 18-hole championship golf courses or the spa complex and treatment centre.

The table below shows the golf packages currently being offered.

Packages	Cost	Breakfast	Dinner	Offer includes
Stay & Play 1 night (Mon–Thurs)	£129*	YES	YES	2 rounds of golf on either course
Stay & Play 1 night (Fri–Sat)	£139*	YES	YES	2 rounds of golf on either course
Stay & Play Sunday Special 1 night only	£129*	YES	YES	All-day golf pass for 2 days
Stay & Play 2 nights (Mon–Thurs)	£209*	YES	YES	3 rounds of golf on either course
Stay & Play 2 nights (Fri–Sat)	£229*	YES	YES	3 rounds of golf on either course
Stay & Play 3 nights (Mon–Thurs)	£259*	YES	YES	4 rounds of golf on either course
Stay & Play 3 nights (Fri–Sun)	£289*	YES	YES	4 rounds of golf on either course
*Price per person based on two sharing – add £20 supplement for single room occupancy *Deduct £5 per person per night for Fairways & Bunkers lodge rooms				

21. A golf society comprising three couples and two single people (not sharing) has decided to stay at the Golf and Country Club, arriving at lunchtime on a Friday. One of the couples and one of the singles plan to stay one night only and the remainder will stay for two nights. Those staying one night wish to be accommodated in the lodge rooms.

What would be the total cost for the golf society?

A £1,607.00

B £1,587.00

C £1,602.00

D £1,507.00

E £1,547.00

22. Discounting the supplements, what is the range of prices of the packages offered by the Golf and Country Club?

A £129.00

B £139.00

C £160.00

D £198.00

E £209.00

23. From January to April the Golf and Country Club has a special winter deal offering a discount on its golf packages if combined with a spa and treatments package. For a three-night stay (Fri–Sun) the spa package, which is normally £75 per couple, has been discounted by 5%, and there is a 15% discount on the golf package. Two couples decide to take advantage of this offer. How much would the special winter deal cost them, per person, to the nearest whole number?

A £281.00

B £283.00

C £246.00

D £317.00

E £327.00

24. The spa complex offers the following treatments: facials and skin treatments; health massage; *cellulite and body contouring; pedicure and manicure; facial thread vein treatment; *reiki; crystal therapy; reflexology; and aromatherapy. All treatments cost £37.95, and – apart from those marked with an asterisk – all are currently available on a 3-for-2 basis.

Two women decide to use the spa complex facilities. One woman decides to have the pedicure, crystal therapy and reflexology, and the other woman decides to have the health massage, reiki and crystal therapy. It is one woman's birthday and the other woman decides to pay for her treatments as a gift, as well as paying for her own.

If she set aside £250.00, how much money would she have left after paying for all the treatments?

A £174.10

B £136.15

C £98.20

D £60.25

E £22.30

Questions 25 to 28 relate to the chart below, which shows the results of the final of the pole vault competition at an athletics meeting. The heights shown are in metres; S = successful vault and F = failed vault. Competitors who have three failed attempts at a height are eliminated.

	4.2	4.4	4.6	4.8	5.0	5.2	5.4	5.6	5.8	6.0
Tully	S	S	S	S	S	S	S	FS	FS	FFF
Roberts	S	FS	FFS	FFF	–	–	–	–	–	–
Abada	S	S	FS	FFS	FFF	–	–	–	–	–
Walker	S	FS	S	FS	FFS	FS	FFS	FFF	–	–
Burgess	S	S	FS	S	FS	FS	FFF	–	–	–
Bubka	S	S	S	S	S	S	S	S	S	FS
Hartwig	FS	FS	FS	FS	FS	FFS	FS	FFS	FFF	–
Mack	S	FS	FFF	–	–	–		–		–
Mesnil	S	S	S	FS	FS	FFS	FFS	FFF	–	–
Markov	S	S	FS	FS	FFS	S	FS	FFS	FFF	–
Smith	S	S	FS	S	FS	FFS	FFF	–	–	–
Seagren	S	S	S	FS	S	FS	FFS	FS	FFS	FFF

25. What percentage of competitors, to the nearest whole number, had a failed vault when the bar was set at 4.6 metres?

   A 33%

   B 42%

   C 50%

   D 58%

   E 67%

26. Before the bar was raised to 4.8 metres what number of failed vaults had occurred compared to the total number of vaults, expressed as a fraction?

   A $\dfrac{1}{4}$

   B $\dfrac{1}{3}$

   C $\dfrac{1}{2}$

   D $\dfrac{2}{9}$

   E $\dfrac{3}{10}$

27. When the bar was set at 5.2 metres, what ratio of competitors had more than one failed vault compared to those remaining in the competition?

   A 1:2

   B 1:3

   C 1:4

   D 2:3

   E 3:4

28. For all the competitors in this final, what is the average greatest height successfully vaulted, to one decimal place?

   A 5.0 metres

   B 5.1 metres

   C 5.2 metres

   D 5.3 metres

   E 5.4 metres

Questions 29 to 32 are based on the table below that details the deals available from broadband providers.

Provider	Speed	Downloads	Contract	Cost (monthly)
Chat-Chat	20MB	20GB	12 months	£12.00
Yellow	24MB	unlimited	12 months	£12.50
E20	24MB	40GB	18 months	£7.50
Pure Media	24MB	unlimited	12 months	£12.00
DTT	20MB	40GB	18 months	£15.00

All the providers except **E20** have 'special' offers for new customers: **Chat-Chat** – 40% reduction for 6 months; **Yellow** – first 3 months free; **Pure Media** – £40.00 off; **DTT** – £1.00 a month for first 3 months.

29. Irrespective of the speed, downloads and contract period, which one of the providers would be the cheapest over the first 6 months?

    A Chat-Chat

    B Yellow

    C E20

    D Pure Media

    E DTT

30. Ignoring special offers, which one of the following statements is true?

    A Only providers with unlimited downloads have 24MB speed.

    B The mean average monthly contract cost of the five providers to the nearest £ is £12.00.

    C There is a 50% cost difference in the providers who only offer an 18 months' contract.

    D The monthly contract cost of providers with 20GB downloads is less than those having 40GB downloads.

    E Providers who offer 20MB speeds require an 18 months' contract.

31. When considering an 18 months' contract with either E20 or DTT, expressed as a percentage (to the nearest whole number), how much more would it cost to use DTT instead of E20?

    A 47%

    B 60%

C 69%

D 77%

E 85%

32. Where a person wants a minimum 24MB speed, 40GB for downloads and a 12 months' contract, taking into account the special offers for new customers, what would be the actual price of the cheapest provider over the 12 months?

A £104.00

B £112.50

C £138.00

D £144.00

E £150.00

Questions 33 to 36 relate to merchant ships and boats. When travelling on the water, distance is measured in nautical miles (nm) and speed in knots (kts).

33. A merchant vessel leaves Liverpool port (UK) at 0900 hours on Monday, 1 March en route to Bilbao port (Spain). The distance between the two ports is 1,138 miles. The average cruising speed of the merchant vessel on this journey is 15 knots.

   What time, day and date does the vessel arrive at Bilbao port to the nearest hour? (1 knot = 1.15 miles per hour; Bilbao port is UK time + 1 hour.)

   A 1800 hours, Wednesday, 3 March.

   B 0200 hours, Thursday, 4 March.

   C 0300 hours, Thursday, 4 March.

   D 0400 hours, Thursday, 4 March.

   E 1400 hours, Thursday, 4 March.

34. Johnson has entered her 'firebrand' dinghy in a race being held in her twin town of La Rochelle in France organised by the local yacht club. The race consists of completing a course measuring 3 kilometres marked out by a series of orange buoys. She decides to practise the course the day before the race. The wind is difficult with gusts and calms in almost equal measure. In sailing the course Johnson manages an average speed of 3 knots for 10 minutes, 10 knots for 20 minutes and 7 knots for 30 minutes.

   How many laps of the marked course did Johnson complete, to one decimal place? (1 knot = 1.852 kilometres per hour (km/h))

   A 3.5 laps

   B 4.5 laps

C 6.0 laps

D 6.7 laps

E 12.3 laps

35. A cruise ship is powered by an oil turbine with an average oil usage of 10 litres of oil per 4 nautical miles (nm) travelled. The capacity of oil that can be stored on the ship is 7,500 litres. The ship is currently 42% of the way through its cruise round the Caribbean islands. The distance back to the ship's home quay is 768 nm. What percentage of oil will be in the ship's storage tank when it arrives at its home quay if the oil tank was 68% full at the time of departure?

A 7%

B 14%

C 15%

D 18%

E 24%

36. A French ferry travels between Dunkirk and Dover, making four return trips each weekday, and five on each day of the weekend. The distance between Dunkirk and Dover is 70 miles. The ferry has a fuel capacity of 1,200 litres and on average travels 5 miles for each litre of fuel. Fuel costs in the UK are 54p per litre. In France the cost of one litre of fuel is 2.5% cheaper than in the UK due to less VAT being paid.

What is the value, in euros, of the fuel remaining in the tank at the end of one week where the tank was full at the outset? (£1 = €1.16)

A €164.97

B €169.20

C €221.13

D €226.80

E €232.47

Quantitative Reasoning practice subtest: answers

Question number	Correct response	Question number	Correct response
1	C	19	E
2	B	20	A
3	D	21	B
4	D	22	C
5	B	23	A
6	C	24	D
7	E	25	D
8	C	26	E
9	C	27	B
10	D	28	D
11	C	29	D
12	A	30	B
13	E	31	C
14	C	32	A
15	D	33	D
16	E	34	B
17	A	35	E
18	C	36	C

Quantitative Reasoning practice subtest: explanation of answers

Question 1

Fractions: rule

To find one number as a **fraction** of the other, you write the numbers as a fraction, with the first number on the top and the second number on the bottom. The top line of a fraction is called the numerator and the bottom line of a fraction is called the denominator.

Answer C is correct: ¼.

Rationale

Step 1: there is a total of 24 skyscrapers, so this number goes on the bottom as the denominator.

Step 2: there are 6 skyscrapers between 300 and 400 metres, so this number goes on the top as the numerator.

Step 3: the fraction is therefore $\frac{6}{24}$.

Step 4: this fraction can be cancelled down as both the numerator and denominator are divisible by 6, so the fraction is $\frac{1}{4}$.

Answer A is incorrect: ½. For this answer to be correct, the number of skyscrapers between 300 and 400 metres would need to be 12, so $\frac{12}{24}$, which can be cancelled down to ½.

Answer B is incorrect: $\frac{1}{3}$. For this answer to be correct, the number of skyscrapers between 300 and 400 metres would need to be 8, so $\frac{8}{24}$, which can be cancelled down to $\frac{1}{3}$.

Answer D is incorrect: $\frac{1}{5}$. This answer could not be obtained from the parameters of the question. The only fraction possible where the number of skyscrapers between 300 and 400 metres was 5 would be $\frac{5}{24}$.

Answer E is incorrect: $\frac{1}{6}$. For this answer to be correct, the number of skyscrapers between 300 and 400 metres would need to be 4, so $\frac{4}{24}$, which can be cancelled down to $\frac{1}{6}$.

Question 2

Less than, less than or equal to, greater than, greater than or equal to: rule

Less than *n* does not include *n*.

Less than or equal to *n* does include *n*.

Greater than *n* does not include *n*.

Greater than or equal to *n* does include *n*.

Ratio: rule

A **ratio** allows one quantity to be compared with another quantity. Any two numbers can be compared by writing them alongside each other with the numbers separated by a ratio sign (:).

Answer B is correct: 2:3.

Rationale

Step 1: there are 6 skyscrapers 258 metres high but less than 290 metres.

Step 2: there are 9 skyscrapers less than 258 metres but higher than 220 metres.

Step 3: write the figures separated by a ratio sign (:) with the lower number being compared first, so here 6:9.

Step 4: cancel these figures down if possible, so both can be divided by 3 to give 2:3.

Answer A is incorrect: 1:2. We know the number of skyscrapers that are 258 metres high but less than 290 metres is 6, and 1 can be a factor of that number. However, the number of skyscrapers less than 258 metres but higher than 220 metres is 9, and since 2 cannot be a factor of 9, the ratio cannot be 1:2.

Answer C is incorrect: 2:5. We know the number of skyscrapers that are 258 metres high but less than 290 metres is 6, and 2 can be a factor of that number. However, the number of skyscrapers less than 258 metres but higher than 220 metres is 9, and since 5 cannot be a factor of 9, the ratio cannot be 2:5.

Answer D is incorrect: 3:7. We know the number of skyscrapers that are 258 metres high but less than 290 metres is 6, and 3 can be a factor of that number. However, the number of skyscrapers less than 258 metres but higher than 220 metres is 9, and since 7 cannot be a factor of 9, the ratio cannot be 3:7.

Answer E is incorrect: 4:9. We know the number of skyscrapers that are 258 metres high but less than 290 metres is 6, and 4 cannot be a factor of that number, therefore that ratio cannot be 4:9.

Question 3

Conversion: rule

The **conversion** is the equation for converting metres to feet (1 metre – 3.3 feet).

Answer D is correct: 10.

Rationale

Step 1: convert 850 feet to metres, $\dfrac{850}{3.3} = 257.58$ metres

Step 2: from the table, identify the number of skyscrapers below 257.58 metres = 10

Answer A is incorrect: 4. For this answer to be correct, the number of skyscrapers would have needed to be less than 770 feet in height.

Answer B is incorrect: 6. For this answer to be correct, the number of skyscrapers would have needed to be less than 786 feet in height.

Answer C is incorrect: 8. For this answer to be correct, the number of skyscrapers would have needed to be less than 796 feet in height.

Answer E is incorrect: 12. For this answer to be correct, the number of skyscrapers would have needed to be less than 852 feet in height.

Question 4

Percentages: rule
To express one number as a **percentage** of another, write the first number as a fraction of the second and convert the fraction to a percentage by multiplying by 100.

Answer D is correct: At least 290 metres but less than 350 metres high.

Rationale
Step 1: in this instance we are given a percentage, i.e. 25% of the total number of skyscrapers, so we can find the number of skyscrapers as a percentage of the whole.

Step 2: 25% of $24 = \dfrac{24}{100} \times 25 = 6$, there are 6 skyscrapers between 290 and 350 metres. Answer A is incorrect: Less than 250 metres high. There are 8 skyscrapers that are less than 250 metres high.

Answer B is incorrect: At least 230 metres but less than 250 metres high. There are 5 skyscrapers at least 230 metres but less than 250 metres.

Answer C is incorrect: More than 300 metres high. There are 7 skyscrapers that are more than 300 metres high.

Answer E is incorrect: At least 245 metres high. There are 8 skyscrapers that are at least 245 metres high.

Question 5

Mean: rule
The **mean** (or arithmetic mean) of a distribution is found by summing the values of the distribution and dividing by the number of values.

Answer B is correct: 69.

Rationale

Step 1: mean = sum of values ÷ number of values.

Step 2: $\dfrac{58 + 63 + 65 + 67 + 71 + 71 + 72 + 76 + 78}{9}$

Step 3: mean = $\dfrac{621}{9}$ = 69.

Answer A is incorrect: 9. This is the number of values in the distribution of the other universities and not the mean.

Answer C is incorrect: 78. This is the extreme upper value of the other universities, i.e. the highest subject average pass rate of the other universities, and not the mean.

Answer D is incorrect: 138. This is the sum of the value (621) divided by half the number of values (4.5) whereas the number of values is actually 9.

Answer E is incorrect: 621. This is the sum of the values; it needs to be divided by the number of values, which is 9, to find the mean.

Question 6

Median: rule

The **median** of a distribution is the middle value when the values are arranged in order. When there are two middle values (i.e. for an even number of values), then you add the two numbers and divide by 2.

Answer C is correct: 77.

Rationale

Step 1: arrange the values in order so 64, 66, 69, 72, 75, 79, 82, 82, 87, 88.

Step 2: there is an even number of values so the median is $\dfrac{75 + 79}{2}$ = 77, as 75 and 79 are the 'middle' values in the distribution.

Answer A is incorrect: 71. This is the middle value, the median average pass rate, of the other universities.

Answer B is incorrect: 75. This is the fifth value in the distribution and not the middle value; the median is halfway between 75 and 79.

Answer D is incorrect: 79. This is the sixth value in the distribution and not the middle value; the median is halfway between 75 and 79.

Answer E is incorrect: 88. This is simply the highest average pass rate.

Question 7

Range: rule
The **range** of a distribution is found by working out the difference between the highest value and the lowest value. The range should always be given as a single value.

Answer E is correct: It is higher.

Rationale
Step 1: redbrick universities' greatest value = 88. Lowest value = 64. The range = greatest value – lowest value = 88 – 64 = 24.

Step 2: other universities' greatest value = 78. Lowest value = 58. The range = greatest value – lowest value = 78 – 58 = 20.

Step 3: therefore the range of the redbrick universities' average pass rates is higher than that of the other universities.

Answer A is incorrect: The mode for the other universities is lower. This answer is incorrect as the mode is irrelevant to calculating the range.

Answer B is incorrect: They are the same. The range of the redbrick universities is 24 and the range of other universities is 20, therefore the ranges are not the same.

Answer C is incorrect: It is lower. The range of redbrick universities is greater than the range of other universities, therefore this option is incorrect.

Answer D is incorrect: The median for the redbrick universities is higher. This answer is incorrect as the median is irrelevant to calculating the range.

Question 8

Mode: rule
The **mode** is the number in a distribution that has the highest frequency; that is, it appears the most times in a collection of values.

Answer C is correct: 82.

Rationale
The value 82 appears the most times (twice) in the list of redbrick universities' average pass rates.

Answer A is incorrect: 71. This value is the mode for the other universities, appearing twice in the list of average pass rates.

Answer B is incorrect: 72. This value appears in the list of redbrick universities' average pass rates but it only appears once. 72 also appears once in the list of other universities but cannot be calculated within the rule as the two lists are separate.

Answer D is incorrect: 85. This value does not appear at all in the list of average pass rates for redbrick universities.

Answer E is incorrect: 88. This is simply the highest value in the list of average pass rates for redbrick universities but is not the mode.

Question 9

Percentages: rule

To express one number as a **percentage** of another, write the first number as a fraction of the second and convert the fraction to a percentage by multiplying it by 100.

Answer C is correct: 32.31%.

Rationale

Step 1: the number of organisations with a turnover in excess of £1m = 21. The number of organisations in the sample = 65.

Step 2: 21 as a fraction of 65 = $\dfrac{21}{65}$

Step 3: convert to a percentage, so $\dfrac{21}{65} \times 100 = 32.31\%$.

Step 4: therefore 32.31% of the organisations have a turnover in excess of £1m.

Answer A is incorrect: 49.53%. Using approximations, we know that 50% of something is half of it and half of 65 is approximately 33, so this cannot be the correct answer as we know the number of organisations with a turnover in excess of £1m is 21 and therefore a percentage figure considerably less than 50%.

Answer B is incorrect: 46.34%. Using approximations, we know that 50% of something is half of it and half of 65 is approximately 33, so this cannot be the correct answer as the number of organisations with a turnover in excess of £1m is 21 and therefore a percentage figure less than 50%. However, this option would have to be calculated to ensure the answer was incorrect.

Answer D is incorrect: 57.89%. Using approximations, we know that 50% of something is half of it and half of 65 is approximately 33. There are 21 organisations with a turnover in excess of £1m, so the answer must be under 50%.

Answer E is incorrect: 62.16%. Using approximations, we know that 50% of something is half of it and half of 65 is approximately 33, so this cannot be the correct answer as the number of organisations with a turnover in excess of £1m is 21 and therefore a percentage considerably under 50%.

Question 10

Ratios: rule

A **ratio** allows one quantity to be compared with another quantity. Any two numbers can be compared by writing them alongside each other with the numbers separated by a ratio sign (:).

Answer D is correct: 1:12.

Rationale

Step 1: five organisations have a turnover of £501k–£750k and therefore 65 – 5 = 60 organisations have a different turnover.

Step 2: write the figures separated by the ratio sign with the number being compared first, so here 5:60.

Step 3: cancel these figures down if possible. Both can be divided by 5 to give 1:12.

Step 4: the ratio of the number of organisations with a turnover of £501k–£750k compared with the rest of the organisations is 1:12.

Answer A is incorrect: 1:5. Multiplying both sides of this ratio by 5 gives 5:25 and so this option cannot be correct, as the ratio is 5:60.

Answer B is incorrect: 4:9. Multiplying both sides of this ratio by 5 gives 20:45 and so this option cannot be correct, as the ratio is 5:60.

Answer C is incorrect: 1:10. Multiplying both sides of this ratio by 5 gives 5:50 and so this option cannot be correct, as the ratio is 5:60.

Answer E is incorrect: 1:15. Multiplying both sides of this ratio by 5 gives 5:75 and so this option cannot be correct, as the ratio is 5:60.

Question 11

Conversion: rule

The equation for **converting** pounds to euros is € = £ × 1.45.

Answer C is correct: €363,950.

Rationale

Step 1: € = £ × 1.45.

Step 2: substitute £ with 251,000, so € = 251,000 × 1.45.

Step 3: € = 363,950.

Answer A is incorrect: €145,000. This conversion is from £100k (i.e. € = 100,000 × 1.45 = €145,000).

Answer B is incorrect: €362,500. This conversion is from £250k (i.e. € = 250,000 × 1.45 = €362,500).

Answer D is incorrect: €725,000. This conversion is from £500k (i.e. € = 500,000 × 1.45 = €725,000).

Answer E is incorrect: €726,450. This conversion is from £501k (i.e. € = 501,000 × 1.45 = €726,450).

Question 12

Percentage and proportion: rule

To find the **percentage** of an amount, find 1% of the amount and then multiply to get the required amount. This question also contains **subtraction** and **division**.

Answer A is correct: 7.

Rationale

Step 1: find 1% of the amount $\left(\dfrac{850}{100} = 8.5\right)$.

Step 2: multiply by the percentage required (8.5 × 63 = 535.5).

Step 3: find the remaining number of employees (850 − 535.5 = 314.5).

Step 4: divide the remaining employees by the number of other organisations $\left(\dfrac{314.5}{44} = 7.14\right)$ which, to the nearest round number, is 7.

Answer B is incorrect: 12. This answer is incorrect as the number of employees working for organisations with a turnover in excess of £1m (535.5) has been divided by the number of other organisations (44), instead of dividing the remaining number of employees (314.5) by 44.

Answer C is incorrect: 15. This answer is incorrect as the number of remaining employees (314.5) has been divided by the number of organisations with a turnover in excess of £1m (21).

Answer D is incorrect: 19. This answer is incorrect as it has taken the total number of employees (850) and divided by the number of other organisations (44).

Answer E is incorrect: 26. This answer is incorrect as the number of employees working for organisations with a turnover in excess of £1m (535.5) has been divided by the number of those organisations (21).

Question 13

Range: rule

The **range** of a distribution is found by working out the difference between the highest value and the lowest value. The range should always be given as a single value.

Answer E is correct: England.

Rationale

Step 1: in relation to England, the highest value in the distribution is 608.6 and the lowest value is 414.9.

Step 2: the difference between the highest and lowest value is 608.6 − 414.9 = 193.7.

Answer A is incorrect: Wales. The highest value is 516.0 and the lowest value is 358.7, so 516.0 − 358.7 = 157.3. The range for Wales could have been discounted early on due to the obvious difference in the highest and lowest values compared to the three 'highest' answers.

Answer B is incorrect: Northern Ireland. The highest value is 511.6 and the lowest value is 352.4, so 511.6 − 352.4 = 159.2. Similar to Wales, Northern Ireland could have been discounted early on due to the obvious difference in the highest and lowest values compared to the three 'highest' answers.

Answer C is incorrect: United Kingdom. The highest value is 598.3 and the lowest value is 407.8, so 598.3 − 407.8 = 190.5.

Answer D is incorrect: Scotland. The highest value is 570.1 and the lowest value is 377.0, so 570.1 − 377.0 = 193.1.

Question 14

Interpreting data: rule
When **interpreting data**, this may involve identifying information presented in some form of pictorial or visual display.

Answer C is correct: In 2010 Northern Ireland's average gross annual earnings will be over $\frac{1}{10}$ less than the average UK earnings.

Rationale
Step 1: in 2010 the average gross weekly earnings were 598.3 (UK) and 511.6 (Northern Ireland).

Step 2: find the percentage difference, 598.3 − 511.6 − 86.7, so $\frac{86.7}{598.3} \times 100 = 14.19\%$ (14.5%).

Step 3: 14.5% as a fraction is $\frac{14.5}{100}$; $\frac{1}{10}$ is $\frac{10}{100}$, so the earnings will be over $\frac{1}{10}$ less than the average UK earnings. The word 'annual' is a distracter in the statement.

Answer A is incorrect: In 2002 Wales's average gross weekly earnings were approximately 10% less than those in England. In 2002 average gross weekly earnings in England were 482.0 and in Wales were 405.8. 10% of 482.0 = $\frac{482.0}{100} \times 10 = 48.2$; 482.0 − 48.2 = 433.8.

Answer B is incorrect: Scotland has the third highest average gross weekly earnings in the country. The table shows that England with 608.6 is the highest and that Scotland with 570.1 is the second highest. Obviously, the UK figures can be discounted.

Answer D is incorrect: Compared to 1999, in 2010 the difference in average gross weekly earnings between England and Scotland has decreased. The earnings gap in 1999 was 414.9 (England) − 377.0 (Scotland) = 37.9 and in 2010 was 608.6 (England) − 570.1 (Scotland) = 38.5, so the gap has increased by 0.6.

Answer E is incorrect: Northern Ireland's average gross weekly earnings exceeded those of Wales in three separate years. The table indicates that Northern Ireland's average gross weekly earnings only exceeded Wales in two separate years, i.e. 2006 and 2009.

Question 15

Percentage change: rule

To work out the **percentage change**, work out the increase or decrease and divide it by the original amount, then multiply by 100. Percentage change = (change ÷ original amount) x 100, where the change may be an increase, decrease, profit, loss, error, etc.

Answer D is correct: 46.7%.

Rationale

Step 1: gather the information. In 1999 the average gross weekly earnings in the UK were 407.8 and in 2010 were 598.3.

Step 2: the increase between 1999 and 2010 is 598.3 − 407.8 = 190.5.

Step 3: the percentage increase is $\frac{190.5}{407.8} \times 100 = 46.71$, to one decimal place 46.7.

Answer A is incorrect: 28.9%. This answer has taken the increase of the 2000 and 2010 averages instead of the 1999 and 2010 averages, and also divided the increase by the 2010 figure. This gives a calculation of 598.3 − 425.1 = 173.2, and shows the percentage increase as $\frac{173.2}{598.3} \times 100 = 28.9\%$.

Answer B is incorrect: 31.8%. This answer has divided the increase by the 2010 figure instead of the 1999 figure. This gives a calculation of 598.3 − 407.8 = 190.5 and shows the percentage increase as $\frac{190.5}{598.3} \times 100 = 31.8\%$.

Answer C is incorrect: 40.7%. This answer has taken the increase of the 2000 and 2010 averages instead of the 1999 and 2010 averages. This gives a calculation of 598.3 − 425.1 = 173.2, so that the percentage increase is $\frac{173.2}{425.1} \times 100 = 40.7\%$.

Answer E is incorrect: 71.2%. This answer has incorrectly transposed the UK 2010 figure as 698.3 instead of 598.3. This gives a calculation of 698.3 − 407.8 = 290.5, so that the percentage increase is $\frac{290.5}{407.8} \times 100 = 71.2\%$.

Question 16

Ratio: rule

A **ratio** allows one quantity to be compared with another quantity. Any two numbers can be compared by writing them alongside each other with the numbers separated by a ratio sign (:).

Answer E is correct: 4:5.

Rationale

Step 1: in 2004 the average gross weekly earnings in Northern Ireland were 430.9 and in 2010 were 511.6.

Step 2: write the figures separated by a ratio sign (:) with the lower number being compared first, so here 430.9:511.6.

Step 3: use approximation so the ratio is 430.9:511.6 or 43:51 or 40:50.

Step 4: cancel these figures down if possible; both are divisible by 10 to give an approximate ratio of 4:5.

Answer A is incorrect: 1:2. The figures provided in the table for Northern Ireland would not allow a ratio of 1:2.

Answer B is incorrect: 1:3. The figures provided in the table for Northern Ireland would not allow a ratio of 1:3.

Answer C is incorrect: 2:3. The figures provided in the table for Northern Ireland would not allow a ratio of 2:3.

Answer D is incorrect: 3:4. The figures provided in the table for Northern Ireland would not allow a ratio of 3:4.

Question 17

Interpreting data: rule
When **interpreting data**, this may involve identifying information presented in some form of pictorial or visual display.

Answer A is correct: 3 slices.

Rationale
Step 1: calculate the maximum number of calories the man can use, i.e. 2,550 − 1,940 = 610.

Step 2: calculate the calorie intake of one serving size bagel and butter, i.e. 216 + 74 = 290.

Step 3: calculate the number of calories the man can use after the bagel and butter are subtracted from his allowance, i.e. 610 − 290 = 320.

Step 4: therefore the maximum number of slices the man will be allowed is 320 divided by 88 (calorie count for toast), i.e. $\dfrac{320}{88} = 3.6\,\text{slices}$.

Answer B is incorrect: 4 slices. This answer has only subtracted the calorie count for the bagel in Step 2 above and then divided by 88, i.e. $\dfrac{394}{88} = 4.5\,\text{slices}$.

Answer C is incorrect: 7 slices. This is a purely random answer and has no basis in any calculations.

Answer D is incorrect: 9 slices. This has correctly calculated the calorie count in Step 3 above but has then divided this by 33, the serving size in grams, and not the calorie count, i.e. $\dfrac{320}{33} = 9.7\,\text{slices}$.

Answer E is incorrect: 11 slices. As with answer B, this has subtracted the calorie count for the bagel only but in addition has divided the remainder by 33 (serving size in grams) and not the calorie count, i.e. $\dfrac{394}{33} = 11.9$ slices.

Question 18

Interpreting data: rule
When **interpreting data**, this may involve identifying information presented in some form of pictorial or visual display.

Answer C is correct: One too many of calorie count 189 and over.

Rationale
Step 1: sum the number of items in the first table, which is 20.

Step 2: sum the number of items in the second table, which is 7 + 3 + 3 + 2 + 6 = 21.

Step 3: 21 − 20 = +1, therefore there is one too many in the second table. Checking against each category reveals that calorie count 189 and over has 6 instead of 5 items.

Answer A is incorrect: One too few of calorie count >149 but <189. There is one too many items in the second table and not one too few.

Answer B is incorrect: Two too many of calorie count <80. There is only one too many items in the second table, not two too many.

Answer D is incorrect: Total number of calorie count correct. There is one too many items in the second table, therefore this statement is incorrect.

Answer E is incorrect: One too few of calorie count >109 but <149. There is one too many items missing from the second table and not one too few.

Question 19

Median: rule
The **median** of a distribution is the middle value when the values are arranged in order. When there are two middle values (i.e. for an even number of values), then you add the two middle numbers and divide by 2.

Answer E is correct: Rearrange the numbers into numerical order, add the tenth and eleventh numbers and divide by 2.

Rationale
The median of a distribution is the middle value when the values are arranged in order. In the table there are 20 separate values and therefore the sum of the tenth and eleventh numbers, divided by 2, is the median.

Answer A is incorrect: Rearrange the numbers into numerical order, find the tenth number and divide by 2. Here there is an even number of values so you need to find the two middle numbers (tenth and eleventh), add them together and divide them by 2.

Answer B is incorrect: Add all the numbers together and divide by 20. This is the method for finding the mean, not the median.

Answer C is incorrect: Find the average of all the numbers and divide by 2. This is not a method for finding any type of average.

Answer D is incorrect: Find the calorie count number that occurs most frequently. This is the method for finding the mode, not the median.

Question 20

Substitution: rule
Substitution means that you replace the letters in a formula or expression with the given number.

Answer A is correct: $X = 12\left(\dfrac{G}{28.3}\right)$.

Rationale
Step 1: we are looking for the weight of the cake in ounces (X), so X must be on the left of the equals sign.

Step 2: we are given the serving size in grams, but we are looking for a weight in ounces, so we need to convert grams to ounces. We are told that grams are converted to ounces by dividing by 28.3, so one serving size in ounces $= \dfrac{G}{28.3}$.

Step 3: we are looking for the weight of a cake providing 12 servings (one for each member of the group), so $\dfrac{G}{28.3}$. must be multiplied by 12. So the correct formula is $X = 12\ \dfrac{G}{28.3}$.

Answer B is incorrect: $G = \dfrac{12}{28.3X}$. This is incorrect as it has the G on the left side but it is not grams that are being calculated. We do not need to check the remainder of the equation.

Answer C is incorrect: $G = \dfrac{12}{28.3X}$. Again, this is not correct as it has the G on the left side so we do not have to check the remainder of the equation.

Answer D is incorrect: $X = 28.3\left(\dfrac{G}{12}\right)$. Here the 28.3 and the 12 are the wrong way round as we must divide G by 28.3 and then multiply the result by 12.

Answer E is incorrect: $X = \dfrac{28.3}{12G}$. This is incorrect as G must be divided by 28.3, and the result must be multiplied by 12 rather than divided by it.

Question 21

Addition and subtraction: rule

Performing **addition** is one of the simplest numerical tasks – it is a mathematical operation that represents combining collections of objects (in this case numbers) together into a larger collection. It is signified by the plus sign (+). To **subtract**, take one value from another.

Answer B is correct: £1,587.00.

Rationale

Step 1: identify the costs.

2 couples for 2 nights (Fri–Sat): £229 × 4 = £916

1 single for 2 nights (Fri–Sat) + single occupancy supplement: £229 × 1 + £20 = £249.

1 couple for 1 night (Fri) – lodge room deductions: (£139 × 2) – (£5 × 2) = £268.

1 single for 1 night (Fri) + single occupancy supplement – lodge room deductions: (£139 × 1) + £20 – £5 = £154.

Step 2: sum the costs: £916 + £249 + £268 + £154 = £1,587.

Step 3: the total cost for the golf society is £1,587.00.

Answer A is incorrect: £1,607.00. This figure includes a further £20 single supplement for the single person staying two nights whereas the £20 supplement includes both nights.

Answer C is incorrect: £1,602.00. This figure does not include the three £5 deductions for the couple and single person staying in the lodge rooms.

Answer D is incorrect: £1,507.00. This figure results from using the Mon–Thurs rate of £209 for the two couples staying two nights, and not the Fri–Sat rate of £229.

Answer E is incorrect: £1,547.00. This figure results from failing to add on total room supplements of £40 for the two single occupancies.

Question 22

Range: rule

The **range** of a distribution is found by working out the difference between the highest value and the lowest value. The range should always be given as a single value.

Answer C is correct: £160.00.

Rationale

Step 1: the highest value package offered is £289.00.

Step 2: the lowest value package offered is £129.00.

Step 3: the range of prices of the packages is £289.00 – £129.00 = £160.00.

Answer A is incorrect: £129.00. This is the mode of the distribution, i.e. the number that has the highest frequency in the distribution.

Answer B is incorrect: £139.00. Although this is one of the values of the packages, it has no relevance to this question.

Answer D is incorrect: £198.00. This is the mean of the distribution, i.e. the costs of the packages have been summed and divided by the number of values: $\frac{1383}{7} = £197.57$ (£198.00 to the nearest whole number).

Answer E is incorrect: £209.00. This is the median of the distribution, i.e. the middle value when all the values are arranged in order.

Question 23

Percentage: rule
A **percentage** is a way of expressing a number as a fraction of 100 (per cent meaning 'per hundred'), denoted using the % sign. Percentages are used to express how large/small one quantity is relevant to another quantity. The first quantity usually represents a part of, or a change in, the second quantity, which should be greater than zero.

Answer A is correct: £281.00.

Rationale
Step 1: 3 nights (Fri–Sun) for 2 couples: £289 × 4 = £1,156.

Step 2: special winter deal, 15% reduction: $\frac{1156}{100} \times 85 = £982.60$.

Step 3: spa package for 2 couples: £75 × 2 = £150.

Step 4: special winter deal, 5% reduction = $\frac{150}{100} \times 95 = £142.50$.

Step 5: total cost for 2 couples, with reductions = £1,125.10.

Step 6: total cost per person = $\frac{1125.10}{4} = £281.275$, or £281.00 to the nearest whole number.

Answer B is incorrect: £283.00. This is the answer where the spa package has not been discounted by 5% = £283.15; i.e. £283.00 to the nearest whole number.

Answer C is incorrect: £246.00. This is the answer where only the 15% reduction on the golf package has been used and no account has been taken of the spa package = £245.65; i.e. £246.00 to the nearest whole number.

Answer D is incorrect: £317.00. This is the answer where the cost of the spa package has been taken as £75 per person discounted at 5% = £316.90; i.e. £317.00 to the nearest whole number.

Answer E is incorrect: £327.00. This is the answer where no discounts have been calculated for either the golf or spa = £326.50; i.e. £327.00 to the nearest whole number.

Question 24

Addition and subtraction: rule

Performing **addition** is one of the simplest numerical tasks – it is a mathematical operation that represents combining collections of objects (in this case numbers) together into a larger collection. It is signified by the plus sign (+). To **subtract**, take one value from another.

Answer D is correct: £60.25.

Rationale

Step 1: woman A has three treatments, none of which is marked with an asterisk so she gets three treatments for the price of two, i.e. £37.95 × 2 = £75.90.

Step 2: woman B has three treatments but one of these (reiki) is not part of the 3-for-2 offer, therefore the cost of her treatments is £37.95 × 3 = £113.85.

Step 3: total cost of treatments for the two women is £75.90 + £113.85 = £189.75.

Step 4: the amount of money the woman paying has left is £250.00 – £189.75 = £60.25.

Answer A is incorrect: £174.10. To arrive at this answer, only the costs relating to woman A (£75.90) have been deducted, i.e. £250.00 – £75.90 = £174.10.

Answer B is incorrect: £136.15. To arrive at this answer, only the costs relating to woman B (£113.85) have been deducted, i.e. £250.00 – £113.85 = £136.15.

Answer C is incorrect: £98.20. To arrive at this answer, the costs of treatments for both women have been calculated on a 3-for-2 basis (£151.80) and then deducted, i.e. £250.00 – £151.80 = £98.20.

Answer E is incorrect: £22.30. To arrive at this answer, no 3-for-2 discount has been taken into account and the full cost of six treatments used (£227.70) and then deducted, i.e. £250.00 – £227.70 = £22.30.

Question 25

Percentages (fraction): rule

To change a **fraction** to a **percentage** multiply by 100.

Answer D is correct: 58%.

Rationale

Step 1: find the number of competitors who had a failed vault when the bar was set at 4.6 metres; this is 7.

Step 2: the fraction of competitors who had a failed vault is therefore $\frac{7}{12}$ where 12 is the number of competitors.

Step 3: to change the fraction to a percentage, multiply by 100%, i.e. $\frac{7}{12} \times 100\% = 58.33\%$.

Step 4: therefore 58% of competitors, to the nearest whole number, had a failed vault when the bar was set at 4.6 metres.

Answer A is incorrect: 33%. To arrive at this answer, the number of competitors who had a failed vault at 4.6 metres would need to be 4, i.e. $\frac{4}{12} \times 100\% = 33.33\%$, or 33% to the nearest whole number.

Answer B is incorrect: 42%. To arrive at this answer, the number of competitors who had a failed vault at 4.6 metres would need to be 5, i.e. $\frac{5}{12} \times 100\% = 41.66\%$, or 42% to the nearest whole number.

Answer C is incorrect: 50%. To arrive at this answer, the number of competitors who had a failed vault at 4.6 metres would need to be 6, i.e. $\frac{6}{12} \times 100\% = 50\%$.

Answer E is incorrect: 67%. To arrive at this answer, the number of competitors who had a failed vault at 4.6 metres would need to be 8, i.e. $\frac{8}{12} \times 100\% = 66.66\%$, or 67% to the nearest whole number.

Question 26

Fractions: rule
To find one number as a **fraction** of another, you write the numbers as a fraction, with the first number on the top and the second number on the bottom. The top line of a fraction is called the numerator and the bottom line of a fraction is called the denominator.

Answer E is correct: $\frac{3}{10}$.

Rationale
Step 1: the number of failed vaults = 15 (numerator).

Step 2: the total number of vaults = 50 (denominator).

Step 3: write the number as a fraction, i.e. $\frac{15}{50}$. Both the numerator and denominator are divisible by 5, so the fraction can be simplified to $\frac{3}{10}$.

Step 4: the number of failed vaults that occurred compared to the total number of vaults, expressed as a fraction, is $\frac{3}{10}$.

Answer A is incorrect: $\frac{1}{4}$. For this answer to be correct, the number of failed vaults would need to be 12 and the successful vaults 48, i.e. $\frac{12}{48} = \frac{1}{4}$.

Answer B is incorrect: $\frac{1}{3}$. For this answer to be correct, the number of failed vaults would need to be 16 and the successful vaults 48, i.e. $\frac{16}{48} = \frac{1}{3}$.

Answer C is incorrect: $\frac{1}{2}$. For this answer to be correct, the number of failed vaults would need to be 25 and the successful vaults 50, i.e. $\frac{25}{50} = \frac{1}{2}$.

Answer D is incorrect: $\frac{2}{9}$. For this answer to be correct, the number of failed vaults would need to be 12 and the successful vaults 54, i.e. $\frac{12}{54} = \frac{2}{9}$.

Question 27

Ratios: rule

A **ratio** allows one quantity to be compared to another quantity. Any two numbers can be compared by writing them alongside each other with the numbers being separated by a ratio sign (:).

Answer B is correct: 1:3.

Rationale

Step 1: three competitors failed more than one vault when the bar was set at 5.2 metres and a total of nine competitors remained in the competition.

Step 2: write these figures separated by the ratio sign, i.e. 3:9.

Step 3: cancel these numbers if possible; on this occasion both numbers are divisible by 3, to give a ratio of 1:3.

Answer A is incorrect: 1:2. This answer results from counting all those competitors failing the vault at this height (i.e. 6) and comparing this to all those in the competition, ignoring those eliminated (12), giving a ratio of 6:12; both numbers are divisible by 6, which leaves 1:2.

Answer C is incorrect: 1:4. This answer results from comparing the number of competitors with more than one failed vault with all those in the competition, i.e. 3:12; both numbers are divisible by 3, giving a ratio of 1:4.

Answer D is incorrect: 2:3. As in answer A above, this results from counting 6 competitors with a failed vault, but this time comparing with the number of competitors remaining, i.e. 6:9; both numbers are divisible by 3, giving a ratio of 2:3.

Answer E is incorrect: 3:4. This answer results from comparing the number of competitors remaining with the original number in the competition, i.e. 9:12; both numbers are divisible by 3, giving a ratio of 3:4.

Question 28

Mean: rule

The **mean** or average of a distribution is found by summing the values of the distribution and dividing by the number of values.

Answer D is correct: 5.3 metres.

Rationale

Step 1: identify from the chart the greatest height that each competitor successfully vaulted: 4.4, 4.6, 4.8, 5.2, 5.2, 5.4, 5.4, 5.6, 5.6, 5.8, 5.8, 6.0.

Step 2: sum the heights identified, i.e. 4.4 + 4.6 + 4.8 + 5.2 + 5.2 + 5.4 + 5.4 + 5.6 + 5.6 + 5.8 + 5.8 + 6.0 = 63.8.

Step 3: to obtain the average, divide the sum of the numbers by the number of competitors, i.e. $\dfrac{63.8}{12} = 5.3$ metres , to one decimal place.

Answer A is incorrect: 5.0 metres. This would be the mean if the sum of the values was 60, i.e. $\dfrac{60}{12} = 5.0$ metres.

Answer B is incorrect: 5.1 metres. This would be the mean if the sum of the values was 61.4, i.e. $\dfrac{61.4}{12} = 5.1$ metres.

Answer C is incorrect: 5.2 metres. This would be the mean if the sum of the values was 62.4, i.e. $\dfrac{62.4}{12} = 5.2$ metres.

Answer E is incorrect: 5.4 metres. This would be the mean if the sum of the values was 64.9, i.e. $\dfrac{64.9}{12} = 5.4$ metres.

Question 29

Multi-stage calculations: rule
This question contains **addition, subtraction, multiplication** and **percentages**.

Answer D is correct: Pure Media.

Rationale
Step 1: calculate the cost of each broadband provider to ascertain the cheapest.

Step 2: Pure Media: £40.00 off; 6 months at £12.00 = £72.00 – £40.00 = £32.00.

Answer A is incorrect: Chat-Chat. 40% reduction for 6 months; 60% of £12.00 = $\dfrac{60}{100} \times 12 = £7.20 \times 6$ months = £43.20.

Answer B is incorrect: Yellow. 3 months free = 3 months at £12.50 = £37.50.

Answer C is incorrect: E20. No special offers; 6 months at £7.50 = £45.00.

Answer E is incorrect: DTT. £1.00 for the first 3 months = £3.00; 3 months at £15.00 = £45.00 + £3.00 = £48.00.

Question 30

Mean: rule
The **mean** (or arithmetic mean) of a distribution is found by summing the values of the distribution and dividing by the number of values.

Answer B is correct: The mean average monthly contract cost of the five providers to the nearest £ is £12.00.

Rationale

Step 1: the mean monthly contract cost is the sum of the values divided by the number of values.

Step 2: the sum of the values is 59 and the number of values is 5. Therefore $\frac{59}{5} = 11.8$, which to the nearest £ is £12.00.

Answer A is incorrect: Only providers with unlimited downloads have 24MB speed. Yellow and Pure Media are the only two providers with unlimited downloads and 24MB speed but E20 with 40GB downloads also has 24MB speed.

Answer C is incorrect: There is a 50% cost difference in the providers who only offer an 18 months' contract. The two providers are E20 at £7.50 and DTT at £15.00; the cost difference is actually 100%.

Answer D is incorrect: The monthly contract cost of providers with 20GB downloads is less than those having 40GB downloads. Chat-Chat has 20GB downloads and costs £12 per month. However, E20 with 40GB downloads only costs £7.50 per month.

Answer E is incorrect: Providers who offer 20MB speeds require an 18 months' contract. DTT offers 20MB speeds and requires an 18 months' contract. However, Chat-Chat, which also offers 20MB speeds, only requires a 12 months' contract.

Question 31

Percentage change: rule

To work out the **percentage change**, work out the increase or decrease and divide it by the original amount, then multiply by 100. Percentage change = (change ÷ original amount) × 100, where the change may be an increase, decrease, profit, loss, error, etc.

Answer C is correct: 69%.

Rationale

Step 1: gather all the relevant information required for the calculations. E20 has no special offers and costs £7.50 per month for 18 months; DTT has a special offer of £1.00 per month for the first 3 months and then £15.00 per month for 15 months.

Step 2: calculate the cost for 18 months for E20; £7.50 per month for 18 months = £135.00.

Step 3: calculate the cost for 18 months for DTT; £1.00 per month for the first 3 months = £3 + 15 months at £15.00 = £228.00.

Step 4: difference in cost = £228.00 − £135.00 = £93.00.

Step 5: percentage difference (increase ÷ original amount) x 100 = $\frac{93}{135} \times 100 = 68.88 = 69\%$ (to the nearest whole number).

Answer A is incorrect: 47%. A 47% increase can quickly be discounted as £93.00 and is well over 50% of the £135.

Answer B is incorrect: 60%. You would have to do the full calculations to disregard this option.

Answer D is incorrect: 77%. You would have to do the full calculations to disregard this option.

Answer E is incorrect: 85%. An 85% increase can quickly be discounted as £93.00 and could not be over 80% of £135.00.

Question 32

Multi-stage calculations: rule
This question contains **addition**, **subtraction** and **multiplication**.

Answer A is correct: £104.00.

Rationale
Step 1: identify the broadband providers that fit the criteria 'minimum 24MB speed, 40GB for downloads and a 12 months' contract'.

Step 2: only Yellow and Pure Media fit the criteria.

Step 3: the cheapest is Pure Media; £40.00 off; 12 months at £12.00 = £144.00 − £40.00 = £104.00.

Answer B is incorrect: £112.50. This is the cost of Yellow. First 3 months free; 9 months at £12.50 = £112.50.

Answer C is incorrect: £138.00. This is the cost of DTT; £1.00 a month for first 3 months = £3.00; 9 months at £15.00 = £135.00 + 3 = £138.00. Also DTT does not meet the criteria as it has an 18 months' contract where 12 months was specified.

Answer D is incorrect: £144.00. This is the cost of Pure Media over 12 months without taking account of the £40.00 off special offer; 12 months at £12.00 = £144.00.

Answer E is incorrect: £150.00. This is the cost of Yellow over 12 months without taking account of the first 3 months being free; 12 months at £12.50 = £150.00.

Question 33

Multi-stage calculations and conversion: rule
This question contains **multiplication**, **addition** and **division**. The equation for **converting** knots to miles per hour is 1 knot = 1.15mph.

Answer D is correct: 0400 hours, Thursday, 4 March.

Rationale
Step 1: convert knots to miles per hour: 15 × 1.15 = 17.25mph.

Step 2: calculate time at sea: $\frac{1138}{17.25} = 65.97$ hours, i.e. $\frac{65.97}{24} = 2.748$ days − approximate to 2.75 days = 2 days 18 hours + 1 hour for time difference = 2 days 19 hours.

Step 3: 0900 hours Monday, 1 March + 2 days 19 hours = 0400 hours Thursday, 4 March.

Answer A is incorrect: 1800 hours, Wednesday, 3 March. This answer is random, i.e. it has not been obtained by using any of the figures provided in the question.

Answer B is incorrect: 0200 hours, Thursday, 4 March. This answer has in fact deducted one hour for the time difference between Liverpool and Bilbao instead of adding it.

Answer C is incorrect: 0300 hours, Thursday, 4 March. This answer has simply failed to add on the extra hour for the time difference between Liverpool and Bilbao.

Answer E is incorrect: 1400 hours, Thursday, 4 March. This answer has used knots only in the calculations, failing to convert them to miles per hour.

Question 34

Multi-stage calculations and conversion: rule
This question contains **multiplication, addition** and **division**. The equation for **converting** knots to kilometres per hour is 1 knot = 1.852 kilometres per hour.

Answer B is correct: 4.5 laps.

Rationale
Step 1: 3 knots for 10 minutes: $3 \times 1.852 = 5.6$ km/h: $\dfrac{10}{60} \times 5.6 = 0.9$ kilometres.

Step 2: 10 knots for 20 minutes: $10 \times 1.852 = 18.5$ km/h: $\dfrac{20}{60} \times 18.5 = 6.2$ kilometres.

Step 3: 7 knots for 30 minutes: $7 \times 1.852 = 13.0$ km/h: $\dfrac{30}{60} \times 13.0 = 6.5$ kilometres.

Step 4: sum number of kilometres: $0.9 + 6.2 + 6.5 = 13.6$ kilometres.

Step 5: divide distance travelled by course size: $\dfrac{13.6}{3} = 4.5$ laps.

Answer A is incorrect: 3.5 laps. This answer has miscalculated Step 2 where it has not converted the 10 knots to km/h, providing a figure of 3.3 kilometres instead of 6.2 kilometres.

Answer C is incorrect: 6.0 laps. The answer has incorrectly calculated Step 4 using the figure 5.6 instead of 0.9 from Step 1, thereby arriving at a sum of 18 kilometres instead of 13.6.

Answer D is incorrect: 6.7 laps. The answer has incorrectly calculated Step 4 using the figure 13.0 instead of 6.5 from Step 3, thereby arriving at a sum of 20.1 kilometres instead of 13.6.

Answer E is incorrect: 12.3 laps. This answer has summed the speed in knots, i.e. $3 + 10 + 7 = 20$, converted this to kilometres and divided the answer by the length of the course.

Question 35

Percentage change: rule

To work out the **percentage change**, work out the increase or decrease and divide it by the original amount, then multiply by 100. Percentage change = (change ÷ original amount) × 100, where the change may be an increase, decrease, profit, loss, error, etc.

Answer E is correct: 24%.

Rationale

Step 1: distance left to travel: 58% = 768 nm, therefore 100% of journey = $\frac{768}{58} \times 100 = 1,324$ nm.

Step 2: total oil used: $\frac{1,324}{4} \times 10 = 3,310$ litres.

Step 3: oil remaining: 68% of $\frac{7,500}{100} \times 68 = 5,100 - 3,310 = 1,790$ litres.

Step 4: 1,790 litres as a percentage of 7,500 litres: $\frac{1,790}{7,500} \times 100 = 24\%$.

Answer A is incorrect: 7%. At Step 1, 42% was used in the calculation instead of 58%.

Answer B is incorrect: 14%. At Step 3, 58% was used in the calculation instead of 68%.

Answer C is incorrect: 15%. At Step 1, 68% was used in the calculation instead of 58%.

Answer D is incorrect: 18%. At Step 4, 1,324 nm was used in the calculation instead of 1,790 litres.

Question 36

Multi-stage calculations and conversion: rule

This question contains **multiplication, addition** and **division**. The equation for **converting** sterling to euros is £1 = €1.16.

Answer C is correct: €221.13.

Rationale

Step 1: convert 54p to euros = £0.54 x 1.16 = €0.63.

Step 2: 30 return journeys at 140 miles = 4,200 miles.

Step 3: 4,200 miles divided by 5 miles per litre of fuel = $\frac{4200}{5} = 840$ litres.

Step 4: fuel remaining = 1,200 − 840 = 360 litres.

Step 5: 360 litres @ €0.63 per litre = €226.80.

Step 6: deduct 2.5% = $\frac{226.80}{100} \times 2.5 = €5.67$

Step 7: the value of the fuel remaining in the tank is €226.80 − €5.67 = €221.13.

Note: The calculations can be done differently to arrive at the correct answer. For example, at Step 1 the cost in euros of one litre of fuel could be obtained or the conversion to euros could be left until Step 7.

Answer A is incorrect: €164.97. This answer has miscalculated Step 1 in converting pounds to euros. Instead of multiplying, it has divided 54p by €1.16. Therefore, at Step 5 it has multiplied 360 by €0.47 (€169.20) and not €0.63 and then deducted 2.5% to arrive at this answer.

Answer B is incorrect: €169.20. This answer has miscalculated Step 1 in converting pounds to euros. Instead of multiplying, it has divided 54p by €1.16. Therefore at Step 5 it has multiplied 360 by €0.47 (€169.20) and not €0.63, and has failed to deduct the 2.5%.

Answer D is incorrect: €226.80. The answer has failed to complete Step 6, i.e. it has failed to deduct the 2.5%.

Answer E is incorrect: €232.47. At Step 6 and 7 this answer has calculated the 2.5% but then added it to the value of the fuel remaining in the tank rather than deducting it.

Chapter 3
The Abstract Reasoning subtest

This chapter will help you to:

- understand the purpose and format of abstract reasoning tests;
- prepare for the Abstract Reasoning subtest using general abstract reasoning questions;
- test your knowledge and understanding of abstract reasoning-type questions;
- identify those abstract reasoning skills where development is required.

Introduction

Pearson VUE describes the purpose of this subtest as follows: 'The Abstract Reasoning subtest assesses candidates' ability to infer relationships from information by convergent and divergent thinking.'

First, we will clarify what is generally meant by convergent and divergent thinking. These styles of thinking, or cognitive styles, were first identified and named by J.P. Guilford in the 1950s and have been extensively researched since. The following is a brief description of the two styles.

Convergent thinking

The problem-solving skills associated with convergent thinking are characterised by the tendency to focus on the one correct, or single best, solution to a problem. Therefore, problems that have unique solutions lend themselves well to convergent thinking.

Divergent thinking

The problem-solving skills associated with divergent thinking are characterised by the ability to produce a number of novel ideas that are relevant to a particular problem. Therefore open-ended problems that do not have unique solutions lend themselves well to divergent thinking.

How are convergent and divergent thinking usually measured?

Convergent thinking is usually measured by conventional multiple-choice questions that have unique correct answers (as in the Abstract Reasoning subtest). The measurement of divergent thinking attempts to tap more creative approaches by asking for more solutions to the problem, of which more than one answer could be correct.

The UKCAT claims for the Abstract Reasoning subtest are as follows.

> The items include irrelevant and distracting material which can lead the individual to unsatisfactory solutions. The non-critical person may remain satisfied with such solutions. The test therefore measures both an ability to change track, critically evaluate and to generate hypotheses which can be relevant in the development of new ideas and systems.

However, the format of the subtest does appear to be based on convergent thinking as each question has a unique correct answer.

You may be interested to know that research has found that convergers usually specialise in physical sciences, mathematics or classics, hold conventional attitudes and opinions, pursue technical or mechanical interests, and tend to be emotionally inhibited. Divergers, on the other hand, usually specialise in the arts or biology, hold unconventional attitudes and opinions, pursue interests involving interaction with others, and tend to be emotionally uninhibited. It has been suggested that divergent thinking is an essential prerequisite of exceptional intellectual performance. However, candidates for higher education have usually been selected on the basis of exam results, which generally tap convergent thinking, and the UKCAT appears to be the same.

What are abstract reasoning tests?

Abstract reasoning tests purport to measure 'general intelligence' or 'general intellectual reasoning ability'. General intelligence is supposedly our innate capacity to reason as opposed to our socially and educationally developed verbal and numerical reasoning capacity. Some argue that verbal and numerical reasoning tests can probe innate skills (as does the UKCAT), but there is a strong correlation between the results from GCSEs and A-levels with tests of aptitude. The arguments about intelligence theories are vast and, to some extent, have never been resolved. However, increasingly employers and educational institutions are using reasoning tests as selection measures. Therefore we need to attempt to 'level the playing field'.

Abstract reasoning tests attempt to measure how well you can solve problems from basic principles. To answer these types of questions, you need to identify the underlying logic. Abstract reasoning questions are usually presented in sequences of symbols, patterns or shapes arranged in squares or rows. Examples of these types of questions are in the 'Example questions' section of this chapter.

Typically, to answer these types of questions, you have to work through three stages.

Stage one

The identification of the symbols or shapes used and what they have in common. For example, the things to look for will be as follows.

- *Number*: the number of symbols or shapes.
- *Size*: do the shapes or symbols vary in size – small to large?
- *Shape*: various symbols, circles, squares, triangles or other multi-sided or faceted shapes.

- *Characteristics*: curved lines, straight lines, dotted lines, number or type of angles or points, open sides to shapes, divided shapes, shapes that can be drawn with or without removing the pencil from the paper or backtracking (for example, an X or a square).

- *Colour*: colour may be used, but not usually; could be negative to positive (e.g. black to white or vice versa).

Stage two

The identification of the pattern that the symbols or shapes form.

- *Repeating patterns*: the symbols repeated in twos, threes, fours, etc.

- *Rotation*: the symbol or shape rotated clockwise or anti-clockwise.

- *Mirror images*: are the symbols or shapes mirror images (e.g. flipped left to right or top to bottom)?

- *Direction*: do the symbols or shapes move from top left, to top right, to bottom right, to bottom left, or do they move diagonally?

Stage three

Generally, this would be the identification of which symbol(s), shape(s), etc. form the next part of the sequence. In the case of the UKCAT Abstract Reasoning subtest, it is the identification of whether the 'test shape' belongs with 'Set A', 'Set B' or 'Neither Set'. Therefore, you will need to use the processes described in stage one and stage two above to determine whether the test shape has the same characteristics as Set A, Set B or Neither Set.

Abstract Reasoning subtest

The Abstract Reasoning subtest is an on-screen test that consists of 55 items associated with 13 pairs of Set A and Set B shapes. Five test shapes are presented with each pair of Set A and Set B shapes, and there are three answer options for each test shape: Set A, Set B or Neither Set. Only ONE of the three answer options is correct. Each test shape is presented with the pair of Set A and Set B shapes on a separate screen with the three answer options below. A period of 16 minutes is allowed for the test, with one minute for instruction and the remaining 15 minutes for items.

Before attempting the practice questions based on the approach taken in the UKCAT, you should find it beneficial to work through the following example questions.

The first three examples based on classic abstract reasoning items have just one question. Examples 4 and 5 relate to two sets of shapes (four boxes in each set) but with the same response format of the UKCAT. The final examples (6 and 7) are based on the UKCAT format and will serve as a 'trial run' prior to attempting the abstract reasoning practice test. This staged approach should develop your understanding of how this type of reasoning test is structured and should also develop your confidence and ability when answering the questions.

Sets of shapes and response formats

The sets of shapes are normally regular or irregular shapes and symbols which are usually black and white, but colour may be used. For the purpose of the UKCAT, the two sets of shapes (Set A and Set B) each contain six boxes. Each pair of sets will be followed by five test shapes which have to be matched to the response format of Set A, Set B or Neither Set. The example questions will clarify this.

Example questions

The following three examples require you to select the correct answer from the six options provided.

Example 1

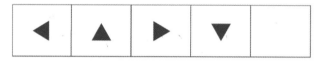

What comes next?

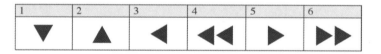

Rationale

Stage 1: the shapes in the question are all single, same-size, black triangles.

Stage 2: the triangles rotate clockwise by 90° each time.

Stage 3: the solution must be a single, black triangle; the triangle must be rotated clockwise by a further 90°.

Distracters: options 1, 2 and 5 could be considered but can be eliminated, as there is not a logical pattern.

Irrelevant: options 4 and 6 can be eliminated immediately as logic points to a single black triangle.

The answer to Example 1 is 3. The triangle will be back in the original position, as at the start of the sequence.

Example 2

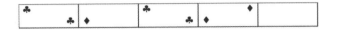

What comes next?

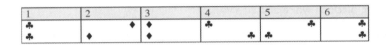

Rationale

Stage 1: the shapes in the question are all black, same-size clubs or diamonds; there are three groups of two shapes and one single shape.

Stage 2: the shapes are sequenced 2, 1, 2 and 2; the only repeat is the alternating two clubs in the same position.

Stage 3: the solution must be two clubs.

Distracters: options 1, 5 and 6 could be considered but can be eliminated, as there is no logical pattern.

Irrelevant: options 2 and 3 are diamonds and can be eliminated immediately as logic points to clubs.

The answer to Example 2 is 4. The two clubs are in the same position.

Example 3

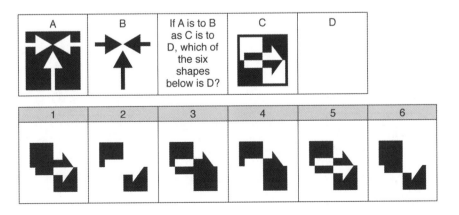

Rationale

Stage 1: the shapes in boxes A and B of the question are the same but B is the negative of A (e.g. white to black and black to white); the shape in box C is different from A and B.

Stage 2: the shape in box C must relate to box D using the same criteria as the relationship between A and B.

Stage 3: the solution must be a negative of C.

Distracters: all the other options are distracters but can be easily discounted when examined for change from black to white and vice versa.

Irrelevant: all options could have been relevant on the basis of shape. The answer to Example 3 is 5. This is the negative of item C.

The following two examples use a format very similar to the UKCAT in that you have to match a test shape to Set A, Set B or Neither Set. However, in this staged approach we are using only four boxes in Set A and B as opposed to the six used in the UKCAT. The key point is, first, to determine what distinguishes each set to arrive at the rationale.

Answering the associated questions should then be a relatively quick process as the test shapes will contain the key characteristics identified as belonging to Set A, Set B or Neither Set.

Examples 4 and 5

Set A

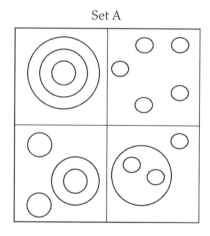

Set B

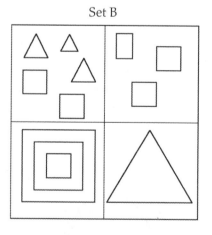

Example 4 Test Shape

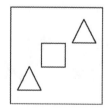

Example 5 Test Shape

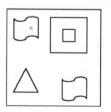

Rationale

Stage 1: the shapes in Set A are all circles, the shapes in Set B are triangles and/or squares; the size and number of the shapes vary in both sets; the shapes are all white in both sets; shapes can be within others in both sets; the shapes in Set A are all circular (curved lines), the shapes in Set B have straight lines only.

Stage 2: both sets contain no logical repeats, rotations, mirror images or direction changes.

Stage 3: therefore, the solution must be the Stage 1 characteristic of shapes with curved lines in Set A and shapes with straight lines in Set B. Any test shape containing both will belong with Neither Set.

Distracters: shapes, numbers of shapes and position of shapes (including shapes within others).

Irrelevant: two different shapes in Set B.

The answer to Example 4 is Set B. The test shape belongs to Set B as all the shapes have straight lines.

The answer to Example 5 is Neither Set. The test shape belongs to Neither Set as two of the shapes have both straight and curved lines.

The following examples are based on the UKCAT format.

Examples 6 and 7

Set A

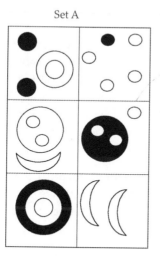

Set B

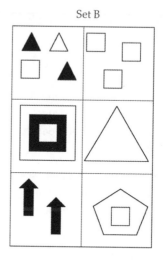

Example 6 Test Shape

Example 7 Test Shape

Rationale

Stage 1: the shapes in Set A include circles, ovals and crescents; the shapes in Set B include triangles, squares, rectangles and arrows; the size and number of the shapes vary in both sets; the shapes are white, black or black and white in both sets; shapes can be within others in both sets; the shapes in Set A all have curved lines, the shapes in Set B all have straight lines.

Stage 2: both sets contain no logical repeats, rotations, mirror images or direction changes.

Stage 3: therefore, the solution must be the Stage 1 characteristic of shapes with curved lines in Set A and shapes with straight lines in Set B. Any test shape containing both will belong with Neither Set.

Distracters: shapes, numbers of shapes, position of shapes and shapes within others.

Irrelevant: different shapes in both sets and use of black.

The answer to Example 6 is Neither Set. The test shape belongs to Neither Set as the shapes have both straight and curved lines.

The answer to Example 7 is Set B. The test shape belongs to Set B as the shapes all have straight lines.

Abstract Reasoning practice subtest

The Abstract Reasoning practice subtest provided below is a full test comprising 55 items associated with 11 pairs of Set A and Set B shapes. These questions do not replicate those used in the UKCAT but are of the same format. The shapes in Set A are related in some way, as are the shapes in Set B, but the sets are not related to each other. Following each pair of sets there are five test shapes (questions). Examine Set A and Set B using the stages described in the introductory section, and decide whether each individual test shape belongs to Set A, Set B or Neither Set.

If you want to simulate 'test conditions', you are advised to use rough paper to mark down your choice for each of the questions (i.e. Set A, Set B or Neither Set). A period of 14 minutes is allowed for the subtest, with one minute for administration and the remaining 13 minutes to answer the questions.

The correct answer and rationale to each of the questions are produced in the section following the practice subtest.

Questions 1 to 5

Set A   Set B

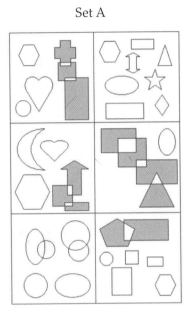   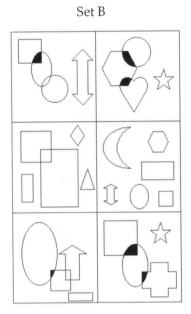

Test shapes

Question 1   Question 2   Question 3   Question 4   Question 5

Questions 6 to 10

Set A   Set B

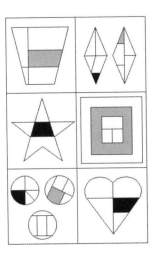   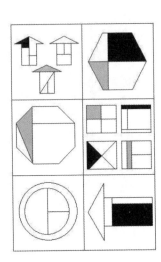

Test shapes

Question 6   Question 7   Question 8   Question 9   Question 10

Questions 11 to 15

Set A

Set B

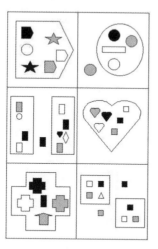

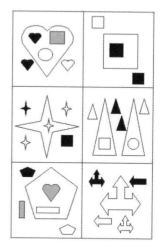

Test shapes

Question 11   Question 12   Question 13   Question 14   Question 15

Questions 16 to 20

Set A

Set B

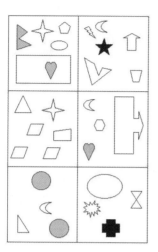
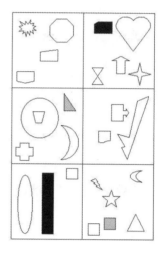

Test shapes

Question 16   Question 17   Question 18   Question 19   Question 20

Questions 21 to 25

Set A

Set B

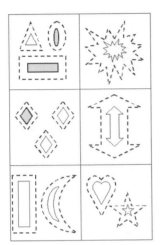

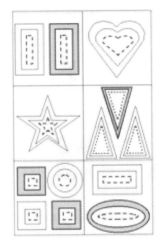

Test shapes

Question 21   Question 22   Question 23   Question 24   Question 25

Questions 26 to 30

Set A

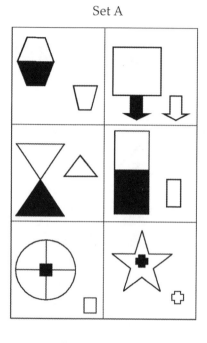

Set B

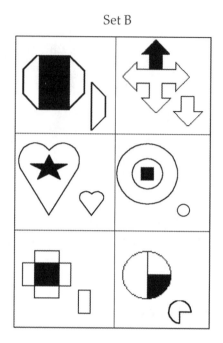

Test shapes

Question 26	Question 27	Question 28	Question 29	Question 30

Questions 31 to 35

Set A

Set B

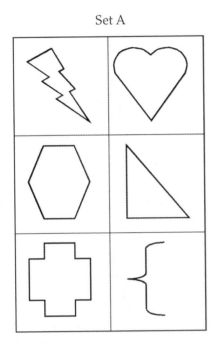
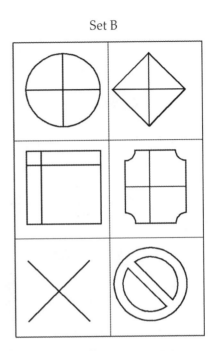

Test shapes

Question 31 Question 32 Question 33 Question 34 Question 35

Questions 36 to 40

Set A

Set B

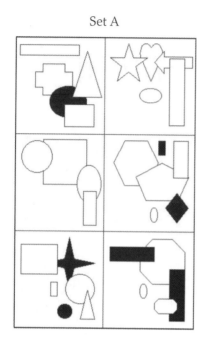

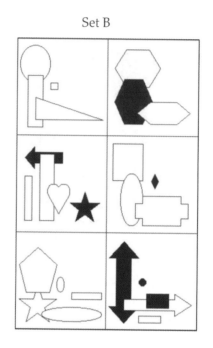

Test shapes

Question 36   Question 37   Question 38   Question 39   Question 40

Questions 41 to 45

Set A   Set B

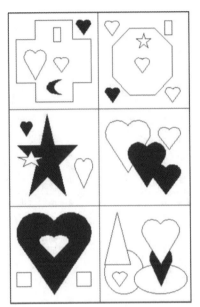

Test shapes

Question 41   Question 42   Question 43   Question 44   Question 45

Questions 46 to 50

Set A   Set B

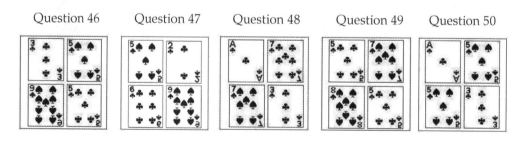

Test shapes

| Question 46 | Question 47 | Question 48 | Question 49 | Question 50 |

Questions 51 to 55

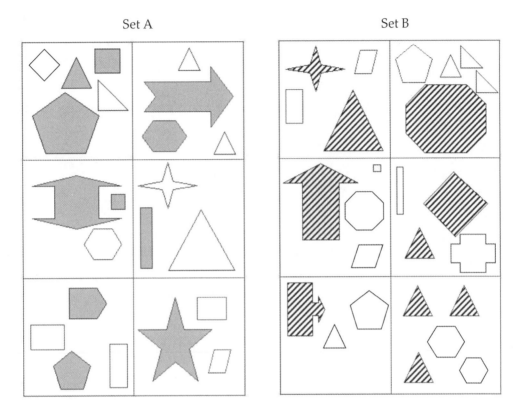

Set A   Set B

Test shapes

Question 51	Question 52	Question 53	Question 54	Question 55

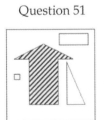 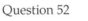 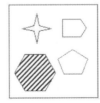 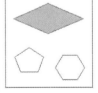

Abstract Reasoning practice subtest: answers

Question number	Correct response	Question number	Correct response
1	Neither Set	34	Set B
2	Set B	35	Set A
3	Neither Set	36	Set B
4	Neither Set	37	Neither Set
5	Set A	38	Set B
6	Neither Set	39	Set A
7	Set B	40	Neither Set
8	Neither Set	41	Neither Set
9	Neither Set	42	Set B
10	Set A	43	Neither Set
11	Set B	44	Set B
12	Neither Set	45	Set A
13	Set B	46	Set A
14	Set A	47	Set B
15	Neither Set	48	Neither Set
16	Set B	49	Neither Set
17	Neither Set	50	Set A
18	Set B	51	Neither Set
19	Set A	52	Neither Set
20	Neither Set	53	Set B
21	Set B	54	Set A
22	Neither Set	55	Set A
23	Set B		
24	Set A		
25	Neither Set		
26	Neither Set		
27	Set B		
28	Set A		
29	Neither Set		
30	Set A		
31	Set A		
32	Set B		
33	Set A		

Abstract Reasoning practice subtest: explanation of answers

Questions 1 to 5

Rationale

Stage 1: the shapes in Set A include a cross, diamond, star, crescent and a pentagon, and hexagons, hearts, squares, rectangles, circles, arrows, triangles and ovals; the shapes in Set B include a heart, hexagon, diamond, triangle, crescent and a cross, and squares, ovals, circles, arrows, stars and rectangles; the sizes of the shapes differ in both sets; the numbers of the different shapes vary in both sets; the shapes are white and grey in Set A and white and black in Set B but there is more grey in Set A than black in Set B.

Stage 2: both sets contain no rotations, mirror images or direction changes; however, both sets contain a logical repeat: in Set A all the boxes contain shapes with eight enclosed areas (including the overlaps); if straight-sided shapes overlap, then the remainder of the shape is grey. In Set B all the boxes contain shapes with six enclosed areas (including the overlaps); if a shape with a curved side overlaps one with a straight side, then the overlap is black.

Stage 3: therefore, the solution must lie in the Stage 2 characteristic of each box in Set A containing shapes with eight enclosed areas where the remaining part of overlapping straight-sided shapes is grey, and each box in Set B containing shapes with six enclosed areas where the overlap between a curved-sided shape and a straight-sided shape is black. Any test shape not meeting these criteria belongs to Neither Set.

Distracters: shapes, numbers of shapes, size of shapes, position of shapes and boxes containing no shading.

Irrelevant: different shapes in both sets.

Answer to question 1 is Neither Set: the test shape belongs to Neither Set as the remaining parts of the overlapping straight-sided shapes need to be grey to meet the Set A criteria, and there are too many enclosed areas for Set B.

Answer to question 2 is Set B: the test shape belongs to Set B as there are six enclosed areas and no overlaps between curved-sided and straight-sided shapes.

Answer to question 3 is Neither Set: the test shape belongs to Neither Set as the remaining parts of the overlapping straight-sided shapes need to be grey to meet the Set A criteria, and there are too many enclosed areas for Set B.

Answer to question 4 is Neither Set: the test shape belongs to Neither Set as the overlap between the square and the circle should be black in order to belong to Set B.

Answer to question 5 is Set A: the test shape belongs to Set A as there are eight enclosed areas and the remaining parts of the overlapping straight-sided shapes are grey.

Questions 6 to 10

Rationale

Stage 1: the shapes in Set A include a rhomboid, star and a heart, and diamonds, squares and circles; the shapes in Set B include a hexagon and an octagon, and arrows, squares and circles; the sizes of the shapes differ in both sets; the numbers of shapes vary in both sets; the shapes are white, grey and black in both sets; the individual shapes within the boxes are divided into five in Set A and into four in Set B.

Stage 2: both sets contain no rotations, mirror images or direction changes.

Stage 3: therefore, the solution must be the Stage 1 characteristic of individual shapes being divided into five and four in Set A and Set B, respectively. Any test shape not meeting the criteria belongs to Neither Set.

Distracters: shapes, numbers of shapes, size of shapes, position of shapes, black and grey shading and shapes within shapes.

Irrelevant: different shapes in both sets.

Answer to question 6 is Neither Set: the test shape belongs to Neither Set as the shape has been divided into six.

Answer to question 7 is Set B: the test shape belongs to Set B as the shapes have been divided into four.

Answer to question 8 is Neither Set: the test shape belongs to Neither Set as one of the shapes has been divided into five and the other four, therefore this test shape has the characteristics of both sets.

Answer to question 9 is Neither Set: the test shape belongs to Neither Set as it has only been divided into three.

Answer to question 10 is Set A: the test shape belongs to Set A as the shape has been divided into five.

Questions 11 to 15

Rationale

Stage 1: the shapes in Set A include a diamond and a triangle, and arrows, stars, circles, rectangles, hearts, squares and crosses; the shapes in Set B include hearts, squares, circles, stars, triangles, pentagons, rectangles and arrows; the sizes of the shapes differ in both sets; the numbers of shapes vary in both sets; the shapes are white, grey and black in both sets; the shapes have curved and straight lines in both sets.

Stage 2: both sets contain no rotations, mirror images or direction changes; there is a logical repeat in each set: the larger outline shapes in Set A are reflected three times as smaller images within the shape and are shaded white, grey and black; the larger outline shapes in Set B are reflected at least twice as smaller images on the outside of the shape and at least one must be white and one black.

Stage 3: therefore, the solution must be the Stage 2 characteristic of the large shape being reflected as three smaller white, grey and black images within the shape in Set A and the large shape being reflected as two smaller black and white images on the outside of the shape in Set B. Any test shape not meeting the criteria belongs to Neither Set.

Distracters: smaller shapes outside larger shapes in Set A; more than two smaller shapes outside larger shapes in Set B; smaller shapes within larger shapes in Set B and number of shapes.

Irrelevant: different shapes in both sets.

Answer to question 11 is Set B: the test shape belongs to Set B as the large shape is reflected as both a black and a white smaller image on the outside of the shape. The additional images outside and within the shape are distracters.

Answer to question 12 is Neither Set: the test shape belongs to Neither Set as the shape is reflected as three smaller white, grey and black images within the shape and is also reflected by smaller black and white images on the outside of the shape, therefore it has the characteristics of both sets.

Answer to question 13 is Set B: the test shape belongs to Set B as the large shape is reflected as both a black and a white smaller image on the outside of the shape.

Answer to question 14 is Set A: the test shape belongs to Set A as the large shape is reflected as three smaller white, grey and black images within the shape. The additional images outside the shape are distracters and are incorrectly coloured for Set B.

Answer to question 15 is Neither Set: the test shape belongs to Neither Set as the larger shape is not repeated against the criteria for either Set A or Set B in terms of shading.

Questions 16 to 20

Rationale
Stage 1: the shapes in Set A include a rectangle, pentagon, rhomboid and hexagon, and stars, ovals, irregular shapes, hearts, parallelograms, moons, arrows, triangles and circles; the shapes in Set B include an octagon, heart, circle, rhomboid, cross, oval and rectangle, and irregular shapes, arrows, stars, triangles, moons and squares; the sizes of the shapes differ in both sets; the numbers of shapes vary in both sets; the shapes are white, grey and black in both sets; the shapes have curved and straight lines in both sets; the shapes in Set A contain one shape which has at least one right angle; the shapes in Set B contain two shapes which have at least one right angle each.

Stage 2: both sets contain no rotations, mirror images or direction changes.

Stage 3: therefore, the solution must be the Stage 1 characteristic of shapes that contain one shape which has at least one right angle in Set A and shapes that contain two shapes which have at least one right angle each in Set B. Any test shape not meeting the criteria belongs to Neither Set.

Distracters: shapes, numbers and sizes of shapes, shapes within others, duplicate shapes, grey and black shading, and the position of shapes.

Irrelevant: the use of other angles.

Answer to question 16 is Set B: the test shape belongs to Set B as it contains two shapes which have at least one right angle each and any shading is a distracter.

Answer to question 17 is Neither Set: the test shape belongs to Neither Set as it contains three shapes which have at least one right angle and this does not meet the criteria for either Set A or Set B.

Answer to question 18 is Set B: the test shape belongs to Set B as it contains two shapes which have at least one right angle each and any shading or shapes within others are distracters.

Answer to question 19 is Set A: the test shape belongs to Set A as it contains one shape which has at least one right angle.

Answer to question 20 is Neither Set: the test shape belongs to Neither Set as it does not contain any shapes with right angles.

Questions 21 to 25

Rationale

Stage 1: the shapes in Set A include triangles, ovals, rectangles, irregular shapes, diamonds, arrows, moons, hearts and stars; the shapes in Set B include rectangles, hearts, stars, triangles, squares, circles and ovals; the sizes of the shapes differ in both sets; the numbers of shapes vary in both sets; the shapes are white, grey and black in both sets; the shapes have curved and straight lines in both sets; the outlines of all the shapes in Set A are broken and the shape is reflected within with a solid outline, and the outlines of Set B are solid with the shape reflected within twice, the inner of which has a broken outline.

Stage 2: both sets contain no rotations, mirror images or direction changes.

Stage 3: therefore, the solution must be the Stage 1 characteristic of shapes with broken outlines with the shape reflected within with a solid outline in Set A; and shapes with solid outlines with the shape reflected twice within, the inner of which has a broken outline, in Set B. Any test shape not meeting the criteria belongs to Neither Set.

Distracters: shapes, numbers of shapes, size of shapes, position of shapes and shading.

Irrelevant: different shapes in both sets.

Answer to question 21 is Set B: the test shape belongs to Set B as the shape has a solid outline with the shape reflected twice within, the inner of which has a broken outline.

Answer to question 22 is Neither Set: the test shape belongs to Neither Set as the shape has a solid outline with the shape reflected twice within; however, the middle shape has a broken line which would need to be the inner shape if it was to belong to Set B.

Answer to question 23 is Set B: the test shape belongs to Set B as the shape has a solid outline with the shape reflected twice within, the inner of which has a broken outline. The number of shapes is a distracter.

Answer to question 24 is Set A: the test shape belongs to Set A as the shape has a broken outline with the shape reflected within with a solid outline.

Answer to question 25 is Neither Set: the test shape belongs to Neither Set as the shape has a circle instead of a solid outlined heart inside the broken outlined heart, therefore it does not have the correct characteristics for Set A.

Questions 26 to 30

Rationale

Stage 1: the shapes in Set A include a hexagon, trapezium, circle and star, and squares, arrows, triangles, rectangles and crosses; the shapes in Set B include an octagon, trapezium, star and three-quarters of a circle, and rectangles, arrows, hearts, circles and squares; the sizes and numbers of the shapes vary in both sets; the shapes are white, black or black and white in both sets; shapes can be within others in both sets.

Stage 2: both sets contain no rotations, mirror images or direction changes; both sets contain logical repeats: in Set A the black part of the large shape is reflected separately as a white shape which may differ in size; in Set B the separate shape does not reflect the black part of the large shape but it is still white.

Stage 3: therefore, the solution must be the Stage 2 characteristic of the black part of the larger shape being reflected as a separate white shape in Set A and the black part of the larger shape not being reflected in the smaller white shape in Set B. Any test shape not meeting the criteria belongs to Neither Set.

Distracters: shapes, numbers of shapes, position of shapes, shapes within others and the repeat of part of the shapes in Set B.

Irrelevant: differing shapes in both sets.

Answer to question 26 is Neither Set: the test shape belongs to Neither Set as there is not a smaller white shape.

Answer to question 27 is Set B: the test shape belongs to Set B as the black rectangular part of the large shape is not reflected in the smaller white shape.

Answer to question 28 is Set A: the test shape belongs to Set A as the black arrow within the larger shape is reflected in the smaller white shape.

Answer to question 29 is Neither Set: the test shape belongs to Neither Set as the black triangle from the larger shape is reflected as a smaller black image, not white.

Answer to question 30 is Set A: the test shape belongs to Set A as the black circle within the star is reflected in the smaller white shape.

Questions 31 to 35

Rationale

Stage 1: the shapes and symbols in Set A include a lightning flash, heart, hexagon, triangle, cross and bracket; the shapes and symbols in Set B include a circle, diamond, square, plaque, 'X' and 'no entry' symbol; the sizes and numbers of the shapes are equal in both sets; the shapes are white or lines only in both sets; the shapes in Set A can all be drawn without lifting the pen or pencil off the paper; the shapes in Set B have intersecting lines or lines within, which means they cannot be drawn without backtracking or lifting the pen or pencil off the paper.

Stage 2: both sets contain no logical repeats, rotations, mirror images or direction changes.

Stage 3: therefore, the solution must be the Stage 1 characteristic of shapes that can be drawn without lifting the pen or pencil off the paper, as in Set A; or shapes that cannot be drawn without backtracking or lifting the pen or pencil off the paper, as in Set B. Therefore, by definition, all test shapes will meet the criteria for either Set A or Set B.

Distracters: shapes, and single intersecting lines when within shapes as in question 35.

Irrelevant: differing shapes in both sets.

Answer to question 31 is Set A: the test shape belongs to Set A as it can be drawn from any point without lifting the pen or pencil off the paper.

Answer to question 32 is Set B: the test shape belongs to Set B as the two adjoining brackets cannot be drawn from any point without lifting the pen or pencil off the paper.

Answer to question 33 is Set A: the test shape belongs to Set A as it can be drawn from any point without lifting the pen or pencil off the paper.

Answer to question 34 is Set B: the test shape belongs to Set B as the addition of two lines (or legs) to the trapezium means it cannot be drawn from any point without lifting the pen or pencil off the paper.

Answer to question 35 is Set A: the test shape belongs to Set A as it can be drawn without lifting the pen or pencil off the paper, provided you start from either end of the middle or intersecting line.

Questions 36 to 40

Rationale

Stage 1: the shapes in Set A include a cross, heart, arrow, hexagon, pentagon and diamond, and rectangles, triangles, ovals, squares, stars, circles and octagons; the shapes in Set B include a triangle, heart, diamond, cross, square, circle and pentagon, and rectangles, hexagons, arrows, stars and ovals; the sizes of the shapes differ in both sets; the numbers of shapes vary in both sets; the shapes are white and black in both sets.

Stage 2: both sets contain no rotations, mirror images or direction changes; however, both sets contain a logical repeat: in Set A all the boxes contain four shapes that create three overlaps and the bottom left-hand corner is always blank, and in Set B all the boxes contain three shapes that create two overlaps and the top right-hand corner is always blank.

Stage 3: therefore, the solution must be the Stage 2 characteristic of each box containing four shapes that create three overlaps with the bottom left-hand corner always blank in Set A, and each box containing three shapes that create two overlaps with the top right-hand corner always blank in Set B. Any test shape not meeting the criteria belongs to Neither Set.

Distracters: shapes, numbers of shapes, sizes of shapes and black shading.

Irrelevant: different shapes in both sets.

Answer to question 36 is Set B: the test shape belongs to Set B as there are three shapes that create two overlaps and the top right-hand corner is blank.

Answer to question 37 is Neither Set: the test shape belongs to Neither Set as there are five shapes that create four overlaps which is not a requirement for either set.

Answer to question 38 is Set B: the test shape belongs to Set B as there are three shapes that create two overlaps and the top right-hand corner is blank.

Answer to question 39 is Set A: the test shape belongs to Set A as there are four shapes that create three overlaps and the bottom left-hand corner is blank.

Answer to question 40 is Neither Set: the test shape belongs to Neither Set as it does not contain any overlapping shapes and there are no blank corners.

Questions 41 to 45

Rationale

Stage 1: the shapes in Set A include a cross, crescent, octagon, triangle, circle and oval, and hearts, rectangles, stars and squares; the shapes in Set B include a hexagon, rectangle and diamond, and stars, crescents, circles, squares, hearts and ovals; the sizes of the shapes differ in both sets; the numbers of shapes vary in both sets; the shapes are black and white in both sets.

Stage 2: both sets contain no rotations, mirror images or direction changes; however, both sets contain a logical repeat: in Set A all the boxes contain at least one black and one white heart, and in Set B all the boxes contain at least two black stars and one white star.

Stage 3: therefore, the solution must be the Stage 2 characteristic of each box containing at least one black and one white heart in Set A, and each box containing at least two black stars and one white star in Set B. Note, the emphasis is on 'at least' – any test shape containing more than the required number of hearts or stars still meets the criteria for that set. Any test shape not meeting the criteria belongs to Neither Set.

Distracters: shapes, numbers of shapes, sizes of shapes and positions of shapes.

Irrelevant: overlapping or touching shapes and the use of the same shape in some boxes.

Answer to question 41 is Neither Set: the test shape belongs to Neither Set as the shape includes at least one black and one white heart, *and* at least two black stars and one white star, so it has the characteristics of both sets (and therefore belongs exclusively to neither).

Answer to question 42 is Set B: the test shape belongs to Set B as there are at least two black stars and one white star.

Answer to question 43 is Neither Set: the test shape belongs to Neither Set as it does not meet the minimum requirement of appropriately coloured hearts or stars for either set.

Answer to question 44 is Set B: the test shape belongs to Set B as there are at least two black stars and one white star.

Answer to question 45 is Set A: the test shape belongs to Set A as there is at least one black and one white heart.

Questions 46 to 50

Rationale

Stage 1: the shapes in Set A contain four playing cards, of which two are spades and two are clubs; Set B also contains four playing cards, of which two are spades and two are clubs. As no picture playing cards are used, the 'ace' is always low, i.e. value of 'one'.

Stage 2: in Set A the two clubs are diagonally opposite from top left to bottom right and the two spades are diagonally opposite from top right to bottom left; the cards are all odd numbers and total to an even number; the highest value card in each row of the box is always a spade and always top right and bottom left: in Set B the two clubs are diagonally opposite from top right to bottom left, and the two spades are diagonally opposite from top left to bottom right; the spades are all odd numbers and the clubs are all even numbers, and total to an even number; the highest value card in each row of the box is always a spade and always top left and bottom right.

Stage 3: therefore, the solution must be the Stage 2 characteristic as detailed above for each set. Any test shape not meeting the criteria belongs to Neither Set.

Distracters: repeats of the same card in any one box.

Irrelevant: repeats of the same cards in both sets.

Answer to question 46 is Set A: the test shape belongs to Set A as the two clubs are diagonally opposite from top left to bottom right and the two spades are diagonally opposite from top right to bottom left; the cards are all odd numbers and total to an even number; the highest value card in each row of the square is always a spade and always top right and bottom left.

Answer to question 47 is Set B: the test shape belongs to Set B as the two clubs are diagonally opposite from top right to bottom left and the two spades are diagonally opposite from top left to bottom right; the spades are all odd numbers and the clubs are all even numbers, and total to an even number; the highest value card in each row of the box is a spade.

Answer to question 48 is Neither Set: the test shape belongs to Neither Set as it contains three club cards and, therefore, can be eliminated immediately.

Answer to question 49 is Neither Set: the test shape belongs to Neither Set as the cards total to an odd number which is the only part of the criteria missing in order to belong to Set A.

Answer to question 50 is Set A: the test shape belongs to Set A as the two clubs are diagonally opposite from top left to bottom right, and the two spades are diagonally opposite from top right to bottom left; the cards are all odd numbers and total to an even number; the highest value card in each row of the box is a spade. The repeat of the five of spades is a distracter.

Questions 51 to 55

Rationale

Stage 1: the shapes and symbols in Set A include a rhomboid and triangles, squares, pentagons, arrows and stars; Set B includes a star, cross, rhomboid, diamond and hexagon, and squares, pentagons, triangles, octagons and arrows; the sizes of the shapes vary in both sets; the numbers of shapes vary in both sets; the shapes are grey and white in Set A and shaded and white in Set B.

Stage 2: both sets contain no rotations, mirror images or direction changes; however, both sets contain a logical repeat: in all the boxes in Set A, double the total number of sides of the white shapes added to the total number of sides of the grey shapes equals 26 sides; in all the boxes in Set B, double the total number of sides of the shaded shapes added to the total number of sides of the white shapes equals 30 sides.

Stage 3: therefore, the solution must be the Stage 2 characteristic of the total number of sides, where grey shapes are counted singly and white shapes are doubled in Set A and where shaded shapes are doubled and white shapes are counted singly in Set B. Any test shape not meeting the criteria belongs to Neither Set.

Distracters: shapes, sizes of shapes and the numbers of shapes.

Irrelevant: different shapes in both sets.

Answer to question 51 is Neither Set: the test shape belongs to Neither Set as the only possibility could be Set B and looking at the criteria for Set B the total number of sides adds to 25, not 30.

Answer to question 52 is Neither Set: the test shape belongs to Neither Set as the only possibility could be Set A and looking at the criteria for Set A the total number of sides adds to 36, not 26.

Answer to question 53 is Set B: the test shape belongs to Set B as the sides of the shaded hexagon (6) doubled equals 12, added to the 8 sides of the white star, the 5 sides of the arrow and the 5 sides of the pentagon totals 30.

Answer to question 54 is Set A: the test shape belongs to Set A as the sides of the white rhomboid (4) and arrow (5) doubled equals 18, added to the 5 sides of the grey arrow and the 3 sides of the triangle totals 26.

Answer to question 55 is Set A: the test shape belongs to Set A as the sides of the white pentagon (5) and the hexagon (6) doubled equals 22, added to the 4 sides of the grey diamond totals 26.

Chapter 4
The Decision Analysis subtest

This chapter will help you to:

- understand the purpose and the format of the Decision Analysis subtest;
- prepare for the Decision Analysis subtest using general decision analysis questions;
- test your knowledge and understanding of decision analysis-type questions;
- identify those decision analysis skills where development is required.

Introduction

Pearson VUE describes the purpose of this subtest as follows:

> The Decision Analysis subtest assesses candidates' ability to decipher and make sense of coded information. You will be presented with a scenario and a significant amount of information together with items that become progressively more complex and ambiguous. The judgements that are required cannot be based on logical deduction alone and this simulates the realities of real-world decision-making where decisions cannot always be made with all the information neatly accessible in one place.

What are decision analysis tests?

Decision analysis tests are, as their name suggests, a measure of an individual's quality of decision-making, in respect of both the adequacy of the decision and the promptness with which the decision has been taken. The behavioural indicators implicit within decision analysis include the ability to identify the relevant information, analyse the facts and consider all the issues, promptness in making the decisions and basing decisions on a reasoned consideration of the evidence.

Decision analysis often forms part of a number of dimensions being assessed in the recruitment process and in other types of selection and, in particular, for situations requiring managerial skills. The dimensions can be assessed either through a series of exercises and scenarios or by the use of psychometric tests. However, the use of such tests specifically to determine an individual's ability to make decisions is unusual.

Decision Analysis subtest

Before attempting the practice questions based on the approach taken in the UKCAT, you should find it beneficial to work through the following questions. The scenario and items have been formatted along the lines to be used in the UKCAT, and the answers and the rationales for the correct answers follow each question.

Scenarios, response formats and example questions

The scenario for a decision analysis test can contain information in a variety of formats. However, in view of the time constraints imposed for this subtest, it is probable that the information contained in the scenario will be reasonably short and specific, and is likely to include an initial paragraph of explanatory text, a list of codes in tabular or similar format and a couple of worked examples. New information will be added at some stage during the test to add to the complexity of the items. This will be in the form of additional codes with a brief explanation. The information and examples will be accessible throughout the test.

The scenario provided by the Pearson VUE website, in their practice test, has an explanatory paragraph followed by information in a tabular format to which new information is added for the final example. The practice test information consists of a series of codes from which the items have been taken. Essentially, this requires the respondent to identify the words contained within part of the code and to see which answer options best fit those particular words.

The explanatory paragraph directs the respondent to make 'your best judgement' in selecting the correct option or options. 'Best judgement' means your judgement based solely on the codes themselves and not on what you might consider to be reasonable. This is not dissimilar to the Verbal Reasoning subtest in that you need to focus on the information provided and not use your knowledge or experience in answering any of the items.

Codes may be combined to produce a new but related concept (for example, the codes of 'air' and 'ice' could combine to become 'snow'). In addition, you will be asked to make more subtle judgements, particularly when the ordering of the codes is not obvious or when some codes appear to be missing.

In line with the Pearson VUE format for the Decision Analysis subtest, the scenarios used both in the example below and in the following practice test are in the style of coded information. Where appropriate, the requirement of selecting more than one option is clearly identified.

Example questions

The following examples are intended to go from the simple to the complex, commencing with a simple code and building into codes with both specific and additional information, increasing the level of complexity.

Example scenario 1

A group of explorers in the Amazon rain forest stumble upon what appears to be the ruined site of an ancient civilisation. In exploring one of the ruined buildings, they find a tablet of stone with what appears to be a coded message. What does it mean?

100504E   5OO5ES   65050A

This coded message can be answered by changing the numbers to roman numerals to reveal the meaning:

CLIVE LOVES VILLA

This example is used to introduce you to the world of cryptography (codes and ciphers) where use is often made of cryptograms (i.e. coded messages). However, you will be pleased to hear that the UKCAT does not require you to break a code or cipher. The scenario will provide you with both the code and its meaning. Although this sounds simple, it is not necessarily so, particularly when you are under time pressure to make prompt decisions. We'll therefore look at a scenario and items similar to those used in the UKCAT.

Example scenario 2

Counter-intelligence codes

In the secret world of counter-intelligence it is not unusual for messages between agencies and agents to be encrypted. In the modern era this encryption can be extremely sophisticated but, for the purposes of this scenario, a method of letter, number and symbol substitution is used. The codes used by one counter-intelligence agency within Europe are presented in the table below. The information from the codes may not always be complete, but you are asked to make your best judgement based on this information and not on what you might consider to be reasonable.

Table: counter-intelligence codes

Operating codes	Routine codes
α = delay	01 = explosive
β = previous	02 = today
γ = cancel	03 = sun
δ = negative	04 = rain
ε = increase	05 = agent
ζ = hot	06 = public
η = opposite	07 = smoke
υ = include	08 = safe
	09 = building
	10 = drop
	11 = tonight
	12 = dark
	13 = weapon
	14 = abort
	15 = secret
	16 = operation

Overleaf are two examples of how the codes work.

Example item 1

Examine the following coded message:

α, 16, 03, 04

The code combines the words 'delay', 'operation', 'sun', 'rain'.

Now examine the following sentences and try to determine which is the most likely interpretation of the code.

A The operation is delayed due to sun and rain.

B The operation is delayed due to sun.

C The operation is delayed due to rain.

D Delay the operation until it is dry.

E Delay operation rainbow.

All the options contain elements of the codes. However, a decision has to be made as to which of the options provides the most likely interpretation.

Answer and rationale

Option E, 'Delay operation rainbow', is the correct answer as it uses all the codes. Note 'sun' and 'rain' combine to make 'rainbow'.

Option A uses all the codes but it is not likely that the operation would be delayed for 'sun' and 'rain'. Look for a better option.

Option B does not use the code 'rain'. Option C does not use the code 'sun'.

Option D introduces the word 'dry', which could relate to 'sun', but it does not use the code 'rain'.

Example item 2

Examine the following coded message.

06, 09, ε(08η), 11

The code combines the words 'public', 'building', 'increase (safe opposite)', 'tonight'.

Now examine the following sentences and try to determine which is the most likely interpretation of the code.

A The public building is safe tonight.

B The public building is dangerous.

C People in the cinema are very safe tonight.

D People in the building are in extreme danger today.

E People in the cinema are in extreme danger tonight.

All the options contain elements of the codes. However, a decision has to be made as to which of the options provides the most likely interpretation.

Answer and rationale
Option E, 'People in the cinema are in extreme danger tonight', is the correct answer as it uses all the codes. 'Public' can be 'people', a 'cinema' is a 'building', 'extreme danger' is an 'increase of the opposite of safe'.

Option A does not 'increase the opposite of safe'.

Option B does not use the word 'tonight' and it does not increase 'danger'.

Option C increases 'safe' rather than the 'opposite of safe'.

Option D introduces the code 'today', which is not used.

The following two examples will include new information, as detailed below.

New information added – codes for specialisms and personality traits
The Head of Counter-intelligence has appointed new agents and they use a more sophisticated coding system that will impact on the previous codes.

Table: counter-intelligence codes including codes for specialisms and personality

Operating codes	Routine codes	Specialist codes	Personality codes
α = delay	01 = explosive	A = full	101 = emotional
β = previous	02 = today	B = wound	102 = assertive
γ = cancel	03 = sun	C = mortal	103 = trusting
δ = negative	04 = rain	D = fast	104 = confident
ε = increase	05 = agent	E = enjoyable	105 = practical
ζ = hot	06 = public		106 = volatile
η = opposite	07 = smoke		
υ = include	08 = safe		
	09 = building		
	10 = drop		
	11 = tonight		
	12 = dark		
	13 = weapon		
	14 = abort		
	15 = secret		
	16 = operation		

The following example has the codes in a different order from the solution.

Example item 3

Examine the following coded message.

101η, 101, 05, 102, 06, 106

The code combines the words 'emotional opposite', 'emotional', 'agent', 'assertive', 'public', 'volatile'.

Now examine the following sentences and try to determine which is the most likely interpretation of the code.

A   Agents are assertive and volatile with the public.

B   The public are calm in volatile situations.

C   People react in an emotionally volatile way with assertive agents.

D   Agents need to be assertive and emotional when dealing with calm people.

E   Agents need to be assertive and calm when dealing with emotionally volatile people.

All the options contain elements of the codes. However, a decision has to be made as to which of the options provides the most likely interpretation.

Answer and rationale

Option E, 'Agents need to be assertive and calm when dealing with emotionally volatile people', is the correct answer as it uses all the codes. 'Public' can be 'people', 'calm' is the 'opposite of emotional'.

Option A does not use 'emotional opposite' (calm) or 'emotional'.

Option B does not use the words 'agent' and 'assertive'.

Option C does not use 'emotional opposite' (calm).

Option D is possible as it uses all the codes, but it is not the most likely solution. Look for a better option.

The following example has two options that could be correct and also has some information missing. When you sit the UKCAT you may not be aware that information is missing, but an analysis of the options should make this obvious. You are required to make a logical decision as to what the missing information is.

Example item 4

Examine the following coded message.

$D\varepsilon$, 16, 15, 05, 08, 11

The code combines the words 'fast increase', 'operation', 'secret', 'agent', 'safe', 'tonight'.

Now examine the following sentences and try to determine which is the most likely interpretation of the code.

A   A fast operation will ensure the safety of the public.

B   The secret agent will operate faster.

C   The secret agent is safe tonight following the operation.

D   The agent will have to carry out tonight's secret mission very quickly to ensure the safety of the public.

E   The agent will have to carry out tonight's secret operation very fast to ensure the building is safe.

All the options contain elements of the codes. However, a decision has to be made as to which of the options provides the most likely interpretation.

Answer and rationale

Options D and E could both be correct. Option D, 'The agent will have to carry out tonight's secret mission very quickly to ensure the safety of the public', uses all the codes with the addition of the missing information 'public'. The word 'operation' can be 'mission' and 'very fast' can be 'very quickly'. Option E, 'The agent will have to carry out tonight's secret operation very fast to ensure the building is safe', uses all the codes with the addition of the missing information 'building'.

Option A includes the addition of the missing information 'public' but it does not increase 'fast' and it does not use the words 'agent' and 'tonight'.

Option B cannot be discounted because it does not add in any missing information, but it can be discounted because it does not use the words 'safe' and 'tonight'.

Option C cannot be discounted because it does not add in any missing information, but it can be discounted because it does not use the word 'fast'.

Decision Analysis practice subtest

The Decision Analysis subtest is an on-screen test that consists of one scenario and 28 associated items. The scenario may contain text, tables and other types of information. The 28 items have five response options and for some items more than one of the options may be correct. Where more than one of the response options is correct this is clearly identified within the item. A period of 32 minutes is allowed for the test, with one minute for instruction and the remaining 31 minutes for items.

If you want to simulate 'test conditions', you are advised to use rough paper to mark down your choice for each of the questions (i.e. A, B, C, D or E). For questions with more than one answer option you will need to note all the appropriate options.

The correct answer and rationale for each of the questions are produced in the section following the practice subtest.

Decision Analysis practice subtest: questions

Intergalactic Space Agency codes

The Intergalactic Space Agency (ISA) is a highly expert team of code breakers. Their main remit is the interception of alien communications in the interests of universal security within the known universe. In order to meet their undertakings, they are required to identify and decipher all intergalactic communications. The ISA is recruiting new agents and has set the following codes as its application test. To pass this test you will be required to interpret the coded questions and select the best option or options from those listed. The information from the codes may not always be complete, but you are asked to make your 'best judgement' based on this information and not on what you might consider to be reasonable.

Table: Intergalactic Space Agency codes

Operating codes	Basic codes
T = opposite	♦ = me
U = negative	☆ = others
V = unite	◆ = oxygen
W = hot	♣ = hydrogen
X = enlarge	♥ = fire
Y = slow	▲ = Mars
Z = similar	☽ = Moon
	☀ = Sun
	✚ = tonight
	❑ = home
	👁 = see
	→ = ship
	■ = heavy
	? = hard
	✔ = prefer

Below are two examples of how the codes work.

Example item 1

Examine the following coded message.

☀, XW, ♦, ?, 👁

The code combines the words 'Sun', 'enlarge hot', 'me', 'hard', 'see'.

Now examine the following sentences and try to determine which is the most likely interpretation of the code.

A   The Sun is very large and is blinding me.

B   The very hot Sun is burning me.

C   I like to see hot sunny weather.

D   The hot Sun makes me squint.

E   The Sun is very hot and I find it hard to see.

All the options contain elements of the codes. However, a decision has to be made as to which of the options provides the most likely interpretation.

Answer and rationale

Option E, 'The Sun is very hot and I find it hard to see', is the correct answer as it uses all the codes. Note 'me' can be 'I' and 'enlarge hot' is 'very hot'.

Option A uses 'hard' and 'see', which could combine to make 'blinding', but this option enlarges 'Sun' and does not use the word 'hot'.

Option B introduces the word 'burning' and, although there is a code for 'fire', this is not included. In addition, the code 'see' is missing.

Option C uses 'like' and 'weather', which are not code words. 'Sun' could become 'weather' but the code is not used twice.

Option D is almost possible, but 'hot' is not enlarged.

Example item 2

Examine the following coded message.

⚥ , X(U✓), ♥

The code combines the words 'me', 'enlarge (negative prefer)', 'fire'.

Now examine the following sentences and try to determine which is the most likely interpretation of the code.

A   I really like a fire.

B   I dislike sitting by the fire at home.

C   I am really fiery.

D   A big fire suits me.

E   I really dislike fire.

All the options contain elements of the codes. However, a decision has to be made as to which of the options provides the most likely interpretation.

Answer and rationale

Option E, 'I really dislike fire', is the correct answer as it uses all the codes. 'Me' becomes 'I' and 'enlarge (negative prefer)' becomes 'really dislike'.

Option A uses 'enlarge prefer' instead of 'enlarge (negative prefer)' (dislike).

Option B introduces 'sitting', which is not a code, and 'home', which is not included.

Option C increases 'fire' and does not use 'negative prefer' (dislike).

Option D introduces the word 'big', which could be 'enlarge', but 'suits' is not the opposite of 'prefer'.

New information added – codes for technical aspects and personality traits

The ISA team has identified new codes that will impact on the previous codes.

Table: Intergalactic Space Agency codes including codes for technical aspects and personality traits

Operating codes	Basic codes	Technical codes	Characteristic codes
T = opposite	♦ = me	501 = warp	901 = warm
U = negative	✶ = others	502 = damage	902 = sociable
V = unite	◆ = oxygen	503 = capacity	903 = aggression
W = hot	♣ = hydrogen	504 = vacuum	904 = tense
X = enlarge	♥ = fire	505 = boost	905 = cynical
Y = slow	▲ = Mars	506 = aliens	
Z = similar	◖ = Moon		
	☀ = Sun		
	✚ = tonight		
	❏ = home		
	👁 = see		
	→ = ship		
	■ = heavy		
	? = hard		
	✓ = prefer		

Question 1

What is the best interpretation of the following coded message?

V(♦ ✶), TY, ▲ ◖ ☀ →, ❏, ✚

A We are going home by spacecraft.

B Fly me to the Moon tonight.

C We need a fast spacecraft to get home tonight.

D A fast spacecraft will get us home.

E Tonight the spaceship is going to Mars.

Question 2

What is the best interpretation of the following coded message?

♣, ♦, ♦ ♣, ■T

A Hydrogen and oxygen are heavy gases.

B Oxygen is lighter than hydrogen.

C Oxygen and hydrogen are floating gases.

D Hydrogen and oxygen are light gases.

E Hydrogen is lighter than oxygen.

Question 3

What would be the best way to encode the following message?

The atmosphere on the Moon makes me light and slow.

A ◆♣, ◖, ♦ , ■T, Y

B ◆♣, ◖, ♦ V✲, ■T, Y

C ◆♣, ◖, ✫ , ■T, Y

D ◆♣, ◖, ♦ , ■, Y

E ◆♣, ◖, ♦ , ■T, YT

Question 4

What is the best interpretation of the following coded message?

❑, ✳X, XT👁, ◆♣

A The sunshine at home is blinding.

B The atmosphere on Earth is good when the Sun shines.

C Oxygen and hydrogen levels are the opposite on the Sun and Earth.

D   The atmosphere totally obscured the sunshine on Earth.

E   Sunshine is greater at home when the atmosphere is clear.

Question 5

What is the best interpretation of the following coded message?

TW, W, ⚲ V ✶□, 901, ◖, ▲

A   Earth is warm, the Moon is cold and Mars is hot.

B   Our home is cold and the Moon and Mars are hot.

C   Earth and the Moon are cold and Mars is hot.

D   Our planet is warm and Mars is hot.

E   Earth and Mars are hot and the Moon is cold.

Question 6

What is the best interpretation of the following coded message?

□, ⚲ , T□, 901T, U904, ✓

A   I am anxious when not at home.

B   Home is where I chill out.

C   I like to relax and chill out at home.

D   I prefer to be in a warm home.

E   A warm home is where I like to be.

Question 7

What is the best interpretation of the following coded message?

U♥, 504, 501, →

A   The ship's engines fail to fire in a vacuum.

B   The ship's warp drive is in a vacuum.

C   Firing the ship's engines creates a vacuum.

D   A vacuum is required to fire the ship's engines.

E   The ship's engines only fire in a vacuum.

Question 8

What is the best interpretation of the following coded message?

903, ╫ ✳, 502, 902, V✳

(NB: **Two** options are correct.)

A   Aggressive people do not join social groups.

B   Social groups are marred by aggressive people.

C   Aggression breaks up social groups.

D   Social groups can contain aggressive people.

E   Aggressive people damage social groups.

Question 9

What is the best interpretation of the following coded message?

(901, 902, 903, 904, 905), 506, 506T, UT

A   Humans have positive personalities but aliens are negative.

B   Humans and aliens both have negative personalities.

C   Aliens are warm and sociable, while humans are cynical.

D   Humans and aliens both have positive personalities.

E   Aliens have opposite personalities to humans.

Question 10

What is the best interpretation of the following coded message?

905X, 506T, 👁X, WT, ▲ 506

A   Martians are cold and cynical.

B   Earthlings are cold and cynical compared to Martians.

C   Martians are viewed with cold cynicism by earthlings.

D   Martians are seen as cynical.

E   Earthlings and Martians are cold and cynical.

Question 11

What is the best interpretation of the following coded message?

501, Z→, 505X, XX

A   The ship's warp has been increased.

B   The craft is boosted by the warp drive.

C   Increased power is what the ship needs.

D   Extra warp would increase the ship's speed.

E   The craft's drive and boosters have been increased.

Question 12

What is the best interpretation of the following coded message?

⚡ ✻, →, X502, ◆♣, ✳(T■)

A   Oxygen, hydrogen and sunlight damage our spaceship.

B   Hydrogen is lighter than oxygen on our Sun.

C   Our ship to the Sun runs on oxygen and hydrogen.

D   The sunlight and elements destroy our spaceship.

E   Oxygen and hydrogen are destructive elements.

Question 13

What is the best interpretation of the following coded message?

✓, ⚡ ✻, ◆, T◆, U✓, T506

A   Humans prefer oxygen.

B   Humans do not like carbon dioxide, as they prefer oxygen.

C   Aliens prefer carbon dioxide to oxygen.

D   Humans like carbon dioxide and oxygen.

E   Aliens do not like oxygen, as they prefer carbon dioxide.

Question 14

What is the best interpretation of the following coded message?

506, 902, 503, ⚡

A   I am sociable with aliens.

B   I have the capacity to be aggressive in dealing with aliens.

C   I have the ability to be sociable and aggressive in dealing with aliens.

D   Aliens do not have the capacity to be sociable and aggressive with me.

E   I have the same capacity of character as aliens.

Question 15

What is the best interpretation of the following coded message?

⋆, 506, T903

(NB: **Two** options are correct.)

A   Other people make aliens aggressive.

B   Aliens are peace-loving people.

C   Aliens are gentle unlike other people.

D   Aliens are a non-aggressive race.

E   Others are aggressive to aliens.

Question 16

What is the best interpretation of the following coded message?

?TU, VT, 506, 506T

(NB: **Two** options are correct.)

A   It's not very easy to separate aliens from non-aliens.

B   Aliens are hard and should be kept separate.

C   It's quite hard to separate aliens from non-aliens.

D   It's easy to unite aliens and non-aliens.

E   Aliens and non-aliens cannot be separated.

Question 17

What is the best interpretation of the following coded message?

V, 905T, →, ⋆ U

A   Trust the others with the ship.

B   The others are cynical about uniting with the ship.

C   The others on the ship cannot be trusted.

D   Trust nobody with the ship.

E   The others will not be joining the ship.

Question 18

What is the best interpretation of the following coded message?

◆U, ▲, ◖, ✳, Z, XZT, WTW

(NB: **Two** options are correct.)

A   Oxygen levels and temperatures on Mars, the Sun and the Moon are similar.

B   Oxygen levels are similarly low on Mars, the Sun and the Moon but the temperatures vary greatly.

C   The lack of oxygen on Mars, the Sun and the Moon makes the temperatures vary.

D   Mars, the Sun and the Moon are very hot and devoid of oxygen.

E   The lack of oxygen on Mars, the Sun and the Moon is similar but the temperatures are very different.

Question 19

What is the best interpretation of the following coded message?

506T, 901, 902, 903, 904, 905, U, UT, YTY, ▲X

A   The moods of humans are influenced by Mars.

B   Negative and positive characteristics can be found in humans and aliens alike.

C   The movement of the planets has a positive or negative impact on human characteristics.

D   Human characteristics are opposite to aliens from Mars.

E   Fast-moving planets influence human personality traits.

Question 20

Which **two** of the following would be the most useful additions to the codes when attempting to convey the following message?

The cold, thin air on Jupiter makes me very sleepy.

A   planet

B   tired

C   chilly

D   narrow

E   atmosphere

Question 21

What is the best interpretation of the following coded message?

X V(903, 904), ⚲ , 506, V(⚲ ✶), 502, ❑

A   We get very tense when aliens attack our planet.

B   I get very angry when people break into my house.

C   It makes me very hostile when aliens attack our planet.

D   The planet is being damaged by hostile aliens.

E   Aliens are aggressive and damage my house.

Question 22

What would be the best way to encode the following message?

The fire damage to the warp drive is a very tense situation for us.

A   ♥, 502, 904X, 506, ⚲ V✶

B   ⚲ V✶, ♥, 502, 904X, 506

C   ⚲ V✶, ♥, 502, 904, 501

D   ♥, 502, 904X, 501, ⚲ ✶

E   ⚲ V✶, ♥, 502, 904X, 501

Question 23

What is the best interpretation of the following coded message?

→, X♥, XT902, 506, V(⚲ ✶)

A   The aliens were very unfriendly and fired at our ship.

B   The fire on our ship was started by aliens.

C   We fired at the unfriendly alien ship.

D   The alien ship was subjected to unfriendly fire.

E   Firing at our ship was not very sociable.

Question 24

What would be the best way to encode the following message?

Martians have the capacity to be both friendly and aggressive just like us.

A   503, ▲506, 902, 903, V(♦ ✶), Z

B   ▲, 506, 503, V(902 903), ✶, Z

C   ▲506, V(902 903), V(♦ ✶), Z

D   503, ▲506, V(902 903), V(♦ ✶), Z

E   ✓, ▲506, V(902 903), V(♦ ✶), Z

Question 25

What is the best interpretation of the following coded message?

V(Z♣◆), ✶, →, ◆X, 501

A   Hydrogen is heavier than oxygen and warps the ship.

B   Some gases are heavier than others and affect the ship's speed.

C   The warp speed of the ship is affected by gases.

D   Gases like oxygen and hydrogen affect the ship's speed.

E   The ship's warp drive runs on gas.

Question 26

Which **two** of the following would be the most useful additions to the codes when attempting to convey the following message?

The red and orange glow from Mars reflects off our ship.

A   mirror

B   ember

C   bounces

D   shine

E   colours

Question 27

What would be the best way to encode the following message?

Earthlings and Martians may be dissimilar but their spacecrafts use the same fuel.

A   ♥, Z, □X, ZT, ▲X, ◆◖✳→

B   ♥, Z, □, ZT, ▲X, ◆◖✳→

C   ʊ, Z, □X, ZT, ▲, ◆◖✳→

D   ʊ, Z, □X, ZT, ▲X, ◆◖✳→

E   ♥, Z, □X, ZT, ▲X, ◆◖✳

Question 28

What is the best interpretation of the following coded message?

502, V ╪ ✷506, ✳♥, WTX

A   Aliens suffer from sunburn and frostbite.

B   All of us prefer hot to cold climates.

C   The Sun and the frost cause damage.

D   Sunburn and frostbite afflict all of us.

E   Sunburn afflicts some and frostbite others.

Decision Analysis practice subtest: answers

Question number	Correct response
1	Option C
2	Option D
3	Option A
4	Option D
5	Option A
6	Option C
7	Option A
8	Options B & E
9	Option D
10	Option C
11	Option E
12	Option D
13	Option B
14	Option C
15	Options B & D
16	Options A & C
17	Option D
18	Options B & E
19	Option C
20	Options B & D
21	Option C
22	Option E
23	Option A
24	Option D
25	Option B
26	Options C & E
27	Option A
28	Option D

Decision Analysis practice subtest: explanation of answers

Question 1

Answer and rationale

V[✝ ✱], TY, ▲ ◀ ✳ →, ▢, +

The code combines the words 'unite me others', 'opposite slow', 'Mars Moon Sun ship', 'home', 'tonight'.

Option C, 'We need a fast spacecraft to get home tonight', is the correct answer as it uses all the codes, with 'unite me others' being used as 'we', 'opposite slow' being used as 'fast', 'Mars Moon Sun ship' being used as 'spacecraft'.

Option A has failed to use the code 'opposite slow' as 'fast' and has omitted the code 'tonight'.

Option B has not used the code 'unite me others' as 'we' or the code 'home', and 'Mars Moon Sun ship' has been poorly interpreted as 'fly me to the Moon'.

Option D has interpreted 'unite me others' as 'us', which is plausible; however, the code 'tonight' has not been used.

Option E has used the code 'Mars' twice and has failed to use the code 'home'.

Question 2

Answer and rationale

♣, ♦, ♦ ♣, ■T

The code combines the words 'hydrogen', 'oxygen', 'oxygen hydrogen', 'heavy opposite'.

Option D, 'Hydrogen and oxygen are light gases', is the correct answer as it uses all the codes, with 'oxygen hydrogen' being used as 'gases' and 'heavy opposite' being used as 'light'.

Option A has failed to use 'opposite' with 'heavy'.

Option B has enlarged 'heavy opposite' to 'lighter' and has not used the code 'oxygen hydrogen'.

Option C has used the code 'heavy opposite' as 'floating', which is a poor interpretation.

Option E has enlarged 'heavy opposite' to 'lighter' and has not used the code 'oxygen hydrogen'.

Question 3

Answer and rationale

Option A would be the best way to encode the message 'The atmosphere on the Moon makes me light and slow': ♦ ♣, ◀, ✝, ■T,Y

This option has the correct codes by using ◆♣ 'oxygen hydrogen' as 'atmosphere' and ■T 'heavy opposite' as 'light'.

Option B has used the code for ⚡V✴ 'me unite others', instead of the code for 'me'.

Option C has used the code for 'others', instead of the code for 'me'.

Option D has not used the code 'opposite' with the code for 'heavy'.

Option E has used the code YT 'slow opposite', instead of just the code for 'slow'.

Question 4

Answer and rationale
❏, ✳X, XT👁, ◆♣

The code combines the words 'home', 'Sun enlarge', 'enlarge opposite see', 'oxygen hydrogen'.

Option D, 'The atmosphere totally obscured the sunshine on Earth', is the correct answer as it uses all the codes, with 'home' being used as 'Earth', 'Sun enlarge' being used as 'sunshine', 'enlarge opposite see' being used as 'totally obscured' and 'oxygen hydrogen' being used as 'atmosphere'.

Option A has not used the code 'oxygen hydrogen', otherwise it would have been a plausible interpretation with 'enlarge opposite see' being used as 'blinding'.

Option B has not used the code 'enlarge opposite see' and has added the word 'good'.

Option C has applied the code 'opposite' to levels of oxygen and hydrogen instead of to the code 'see'.

Option E has not used the code 'opposite' with 'see' and has therefore misinterpreted the code as 'clear'.

Question 5

Answer and rationale
TW, W, ⚡V✴❏, 901, ◖, ▲

The code combines the words 'opposite hot', 'hot', 'me unite others home', 'moon', 'Moon', 'Mars'.

Option A, 'Earth is warm, the Moon is cold and Mars is hot', is the correct answer as it uses all the codes, with 'opposite hot' being used as 'cold' and 'me unite others home' being used as 'our home', which in turn is interpreted as 'Earth'.

Option B has failed to interpret 'our home' as 'Earth' and has omitted the code 'warm'.

Option C has not used the code 'warm'.

Option D has interpreted 'our home' as 'our planet' and has not used the codes 'moon' or 'cold'.

Option E has not used the code 'warm'.

Question 6

Answer and rationale

❑, 🧍, T❑, 901T, U904, ✓

The code combines the words 'home', 'me', 'opposite home', 'warm opposite', 'negative tense', 'prefer'.

Option C, 'I like to relax and chill out at home', is the correct answer as it uses all the codes, with 'opposite home' being used as 'out', 'warm opposite' being used as 'chill', 'negative tense' being used as 'relax' and 'prefer' being used as 'like'.

Option A has used 'negative tense' as 'anxious', has not used 'home' twice and has not used the codes 'opposite warm' and 'prefer'.

Option B has not used the code 'opposite' with 'warm' and has not used the code 'opposite home'.

Option D has not used the code 'negative tense'.

Option E has not used the code 'opposite home'.

Question 7

Answer and rationale

U♥, 504, 501, →

The code combines the words 'negative fire', 'vacuum', 'warp', 'ship'.

Option A, 'The ship's engines fail to fire in a vacuum', is the correct answer as it uses all the codes, with 'negative fire' being used as 'fail to fire' and 'warp' being used as 'engines'.

Option B has failed to use the code 'negative fire'.

Option C has used the code 'negative fire' as 'firing', which is incorrect.

Option D has failed to make the code 'fire' into 'negative fire'.

Option E has also failed to make the code 'fire' into 'negative fire'.

Question 8

Answer and rationale

903, 🧍☆, 502, 902, V☆

(NB: **Two** options are correct.)

The code combines the words 'aggression', 'me others', 'damage', 'sociable', 'unite others'.

Option B, 'Social groups are marred by aggressive people', and Option E, 'Aggressive people damage social groups', are the correct answers as both contain all the codes. Both options have used 'aggression' as 'aggressive', 'me others' as 'people', 'sociable' as 'social' and 'unite others' as 'groups'. Option B has used the code 'damage' as 'marred', otherwise both options have the same interpretation.

Option A has failed to use the code 'damage' and has inserted 'do not join'.

Option C has used the code 'damage' as 'breaks up' and has omitted the code 'me others' as 'people'.

Option D has failed to use the code 'damage' and has inserted 'can contain'.

Question 9

Answer and rationale
(901, 902, 903, 904, 905), 506, 506T, UT

The code combines the words 'warm', 'sociable', 'aggression', 'tense', 'cynical', 'aliens', 'aliens opposite', 'negative opposite'.

Option D, 'Humans and aliens both have positive personalities', is the correct answer as it uses all the codes, with 'warm', 'sociable', 'aggression', 'tense', 'cynical' being combined as 'personalities', 'aliens opposite' being used as 'humans' and 'negative opposite' being used as 'positive'.

Option A has wrongly assigned positive and negative personalities to humans and aliens respectively, and has added an additional 'negative' code.

Option B has used the code 'negative' instead of 'negative opposite' as 'positive'.

Option C has wrongly assigned some characteristics to aliens and some to humans.

Option E has used the code 'opposite' in isolation and has also assigned opposite personalities to aliens and humans.

Question 10

Answer and rationale
905X, 506T, 👁X, WT, ▲506

The code combines the words 'cynical enlarge', 'aliens opposite', 'see enlarge', 'hot opposite', 'Mars aliens'.

Option C, 'Martians are viewed with cold cynicism by earthlings', is the correct answer as it uses all the codes with 'cynical enlarge' being used as 'cynicism', 'aliens opposite' being used as 'earthlings', 'see enlarge' being used as 'viewed', 'hot opposite' being used as 'cold' and 'Mars aliens' being used as 'Martians'.

Option A has not used the codes 'aliens opposite' and 'see enlarge' and has not enlarged 'cynical'.

Option B has not used the code 'see enlarge' and has not enlarged 'cynical'.

Option D has not used the codes 'aliens opposite' and 'hot opposite'.

Option E has not used the code 'see enlarge' and has not enlarged 'cynical'.

Question 11

Answer and rationale

501, Z→, 505X, XX

The code combines the words 'warp', 'similar ship', 'boost enlarge', 'enlarge enlarge'.

Option E, 'The craft's drive and boosters have been increased', is the correct answer as it uses all the codes, with 'warp' being used as 'drive', 'similar ship' being used as 'craft's', 'boost enlarge' being used as 'boosters' and 'enlarge enlarge' being used as 'increased'.

Option A has used the code 'ship' instead of 'similar ship' and has not used the code 'boost enlarge'.

Option B has not used the code 'enlarge enlarge' and has used the code 'warp' twice.

Option C has used the code 'ship' instead of 'similar ship' and has combined 'warp' and 'boost enlarge' as 'power'.

Option D has used the code 'enlarge enlarge' separately as 'extra' and 'increase', and has used the code 'boost enlarge' as 'speed'.

Question 12

Answer and rationale

⚲ ⁕, →, X502, ◆♣, ⁕(T▪)

The code combines the words 'me others', 'ship', 'enlarge damage', 'oxygen hydrogen', 'Sun opposite heavy'.

Option D, 'The sunlight and elements destroy our spaceship', is the correct answer as it uses all the codes, with 'me others' being used as 'our', 'ship' being used as 'spaceship', 'enlarge damage' being used as 'destroy', 'oxygen hydrogen' being used as 'elements' and 'Sun opposite heavy' being used as 'sunlight'.

Option A has not used the code 'enlarge damage' as 'destroy', and is therefore a misinterpretation of this code, otherwise it would be a plausible interpretation.

Option B has not used the code 'ship' or the code 'enlarge damage', and has split 'Sun opposite heavy' as 'lighter' and 'Sun'.

Option C has not used the code 'enlarge damage' and has used the code 'Sun' instead of 'Sun opposite heavy'.

Option E has not used the codes 'me others', 'ship' and 'Sun opposite heavy', and it has used the code 'oxygen hydrogen' as 'elements'.

Question 13

Answer and rationale
✓, ✦ ☆, ◆, T◆, U✓, T506

The code combines the words 'prefer', 'me others', 'oxygen', 'opposite oxygen', 'negative prefer', 'opposite aliens'.

Option B, 'Humans do not like carbon dioxide, as they prefer oxygen', is the correct answer as it uses all the codes, with 'me others' being used as 'they', 'opposite oxygen' being used as 'carbon dioxide', 'negative prefer' being used as 'do not like' and 'opposite aliens' being used as 'humans'.

Option A has not used the codes 'negative prefer' and 'opposite oxygen'.

Option C has not used the codes 'me others' and 'negative prefer', and has used the code 'aliens' instead of 'opposite aliens'.

Option D has not used the code 'me others' and 'negative prefer'.

Option E has not used the code 'opposite aliens', otherwise it could have been a possible interpretation.

Question 14

Answer and rationale
506, 902, 503, ✦

The code combines the words 'aliens', 'sociable', 'capacity', 'me'.

Option C, 'I have the ability to be sociable and aggressive in dealing with aliens', is the correct answer even though it contains the word 'aggressive', which is not shown in the codes. This is an instance where you are being asked to make a more subtle judgement when some code(s) appear to be missing. In this instance it is necessary to consider carefully all the options before determining that this is the correct one.

Option A does not contain the code 'capacity' and can therefore be eliminated.

Option B does not contain the code 'sociable', although it has introduced another code, 'aggression'. On the basis of it not containing one of the codes, it can be eliminated.

Option D contains all the codes but again has included another code, 'aggression'. In addition, the option states 'do not have' and for this there would need to be some other 'negative' code. Because two new codes would be required as opposed to the one in Option C, this answer can be eliminated.

Option E is incorrect as it mentions 'character', which would include all the 'characteristics' and not just 'sociable' or even 'aggression'.

Question 15

Answer and rationale
✷, 506, T903

(NB: **Two** options are correct.)

The code combines the words 'others', 'aliens', 'opposite aggression'.

Option B, 'Aliens are peace-loving people', and Option D, 'Aliens are a non-aggressive race', are the correct answers. Both options contain all the codes and use appropriate terms for the codes 'opposite aggression' and 'others' – namely, 'peace-loving people' and 'non-aggressive race' respectively.

Option A does not take into account the code 'opposite aggression'.

Option C uses all the codes but adds further information that is not contained in the combinations (i.e. 'unlike other people').

Option E does not take into account the code 'opposite aggression'.

Question 16

Answer and rationale
?TU, VT, 506, 506T

(NB: **Two** options are correct.)

The code combines the words 'hard opposite (negative)', 'unite opposite', 'aliens', 'aliens opposite'.

Option A, 'It's not very easy to separate aliens from non-aliens', and Option C, 'It's quite hard to separate aliens from non-aliens', are the correct answers as both contain all the codes. Option A and Option C have interpreted 'hard opposite (negative)' as 'not very easy' and 'quite hard' respectively, both of which could be correct.

Option B has not used the 'aliens opposite' code to become 'non-aliens'.

Option D has not used the 'hard opposite (negative)' code to become 'not very easy' or 'quite hard'. Instead, it has used this code as 'easy'.

Option E has not used the 'hard opposite (negative)' code to become 'not very easy' or 'quite hard'. Instead, it has introduced the word 'cannot'.

Question 17

Answer and rationale
V, 905T, →, ✷U

The code combines the words 'unite', 'cynical opposite', 'ship', 'others negative'.

Option D, 'Trust nobody with the ship', is the correct answer as it uses all the codes.

'Unite' becomes 'with', 'cynical opposite' becomes 'trust' and 'others negative' becomes 'nobody'. Note, the codes do not have to be in the same order as the most logical interpretation.

Option A has not used the 'others negative' code to become 'nobody'. Instead, it has used the 'others' code.

Option B has not used the 'others negative' code to become 'nobody'. Instead it has used the 'others' code. In addition, it has not used the 'cynical opposite' to become 'trust'. Instead it has used the 'cynical' code.

Option C has not used the 'others negative' code to become 'nobody'. Instead, it has used the 'others' code.

Option E has not used the 'others negative' code to become 'nobody'. Instead, it has used the 'others' code. In addition, it has used the 'unite' code as 'joining' instead of 'with'.

Question 18

Answer and rationale
◆U, ▲, ◖, ☀, Z, XZT, WTW

(NB: Two options are correct.)

The code combines the words 'oxygen negative', 'Mars', 'Moon', 'Sun', 'similar', '(enlarge) similar opposite', 'hot opposite hot '.

Option B, 'Oxygen levels are similarly low on Mars, the Sun and the Moon but the temperatures vary greatly', and Option E, 'The lack of oxygen on Mars, the Sun and the Moon is similar but the temperatures are very different' are the correct answers as both contain all the codes. Options B and E have interpreted the 'oxygen negative' code as low levels of oxygen or a lack of oxygen respectively, both of which could be correct. The code '(enlarge) similar opposite' has been interpreted as 'vary greatly' or 'very different', again both of which could be correct. Both options have used the code 'hot opposite hot' as 'hot and cold', which in turn is interpreted as temperatures.

Option A has not used the code '(enlarge) similar opposite' as 'vary greatly' or 'very different'. Instead, it has used the code 'similar'.

Option C has associated the 'oxygen negative' code with the '(enlarge) similar opposite' and the 'hot opposite hot' codes, which is a poor interpretation on the codes alone.

Option D has interpreted 'oxygen negative' as 'devoid of oxygen', which could be correct, but it has not used the code 'hot opposite hot' as 'hot and cold' and in turn 'temperatures'. Instead, it has used the code 'hot'.

Question 19

Answer and rationale

506T, 901, 902, 903, 904, 905, U, UT, YTY,▲X

The code combines the words 'aliens opposite', 'warm', 'sociable', 'aggression', 'tense', 'cynical', 'negative', 'negative opposite', 'slow opposite slow', 'Mars enlarge'.

Option C, 'The movement of the planets has a positive or negative impact on human characteristics', is the correct answer as it uses all the codes. 'Slow opposite' becomes 'fast' and when combined with 'slow' this becomes movement. 'Mars enlarge' becomes 'planets', 'negative opposite' becomes 'positive', and the codes 'warm', 'sociable', 'aggression', 'tense' and 'cynical' are combined to become 'characteristics'. The word 'impact' is added and this is an instance where you are being asked to make a more subtle judgement when a code appears to be missing. It is necessary to consider carefully all the options before determining that this is the correct one.

Option A has not used the combined codes of 'slow opposite' (fast) and 'slow' to become 'movement'. In addition, the code 'Mars enlarge' has not been applied, neither have the codes 'negative' and 'negative opposite'. The word 'influenced' has been introduced which cannot be correct due to the other missing codes.

Option B has not used the combined codes of 'slow opposite' (fast) and 'slow' to become 'movement'. In addition, the code 'Mars enlarge' has not been applied. The code 'aliens' has been introduced along with other words, which cannot be correct due to the other missing codes.

Option D has applied 'opposite' to characteristics and has also omitted the codes of 'movement', 'negative' and 'positive'. In addition, the code 'Mars enlarge' has not been applied.

Option E has not used the code 'slow' but would need to be considered carefully, as otherwise it could be a plausible interpretation.

Question 20

Answer and rationale

Options B and D, 'tired' and 'narrow', would be the **two** most useful additions to the codes when attempting to convey the message 'The cold, thin air on Jupiter makes me very sleepy', the word 'narrow' being used for 'thin' and the word 'tired' being used for 'sleepy'. The other words in the message can be extrapolated from existing codes.

Option A, 'planet', is not needed because 'Jupiter' could be extrapolated from Z ▲ 'similar Mars'.

Option C, 'chilly', is not needed because 'cold' could be extrapolated from T W, 'opposite hot'.

Option E, 'atmosphere', is not needed because 'air' could be extrapolated from Z ◆, 'similar oxygen'.

Question 21

Answer and rationale
X V(903, 904), ♦ , 506, V(♦ ✳), 502, ▢

The code combines the words 'enlarge unite aggression tense', 'me', 'aliens', 'unite me others', 'damage', 'home'.

Option C, 'It makes me very hostile when aliens attack our planet', is the correct answer as it uses all the codes, with 'enlarge unite aggression tense' being used as 'very hostile', 'me' being used as 'I', 'unite me others' being used as 'our', 'damage' being used as 'attack' and 'home' being used as 'planet'.

Option A has failed to use 'unite aggression tense' as 'hostile'.

Option B has not used the code 'aliens'.

Option D has not used the code 'me' as 'I' or the code 'unite me others' as 'our'.

Option E has failed to use 'unite aggression tense' as 'hostile' and has omitted the code 'unite me others' as 'our'.

Question 22

Answer and rationale
Option E would be the best way to encode the message 'The fire damage to the warp drive is a very tense situation for us'.

♦ V✳, ♥, 502, 904X, 501

This option has the correct codes by using ♦ V✳ 'me unite others' as 'us', and 904X 'tense enlarge' as 'very tense', and 501 'warp' as 'warp drive'.

Option A has used the code for 'aliens' instead of the code for 'warp'.

Option B is the same as Option A but ordered differently.

Option C has not 'enlarged' tense to 'very tense'.

Option D has missed the code V 'unite' between 'me others' to form 'us'.

Question 23

Answer and rationale
→, X♥, XT902, 506, V(♦ ✳)

The code combines the words 'ship', 'enlarge fire', 'enlarge opposite sociable', 'aliens', 'unite me others'.

Option A, 'The aliens were very unfriendly and fired at our ship', is the correct answer as it uses all the codes, with 'enlarge fire' being used as 'fired', 'enlarge opposite sociable' being used as 'very unfriendly' and 'unite me others' being used as 'our'.

Option B has failed to interpret 'enlarge fire' as 'fired' and has omitted the code 'enlarge opposite sociable' as 'very unfriendly'.

Option C has not 'enlarged' unfriendly to 'very unfriendly' and has used 'unite me others' as 'we'.

Option D has not used the code 'unite me others' as 'our'.

Option E has not used the code 'aliens' and has failed to interpret 'enlarge opposite sociable' as 'very unfriendly'.

Question 24

Answer and rationale
Option D would be the best way to encode the message 'Martians have the capacity to be both friendly and aggressive just like us.'

503, ▲506, V(902 903), V(♦ ✷), Z

This option has the correct codes by using ▲506 'Mars aliens' as 'Martians', V(902 903) 'unite sociable aggression' as 'both friendly and aggressive', V(♦ ✷) 'unite me others' as 'us' and Z 'similar' as 'just like'.

Option A has omitted the V to 'unite sociable aggression'.

Option B has failed to combine 'Mars' and 'aliens' as 'Martians' and has omitted to combine 'me' with 'others' to form 'us'.

Option C has omitted the code 'capacity'.

Option E has replaced the code 'capacity' with the code 'prefer'.

Question 25

Answer and rationale
V(Z♣◆), ✷, →, ■X, 501

The code combines the words 'unite similar hydrogen oxygen', 'others', 'ship', 'heavy enlarge' and 'warp'.

Option B, 'Some gases are heavier than others and affect the ship's speed', is the correct answer as it uses all the codes, with 'unite similar hydrogen oxygen' being used as 'some gases', 'heavy enlarge' being used as 'heavier' and 'warp' being used as speed.

Option A has failed to interpret 'unite similar hydrogen oxygen' as 'some gases' and has not used 'warp' as 'speed'.

Option C has repeated the code 'warp' by using it as both 'warp' and 'speed'.

Option D has used the code 'unite similar hydrogen oxygen' as both 'gases' and 'like oxygen and hydrogen'.

Option E has failed to use the codes 'others' and 'heavy enlarge'.

Question 26

Answer and rationale

Options C and E, 'bounces' and 'colours', would be the **two** most useful additions to the codes when attempting to convey the message 'The red and orange glow from Mars reflects off our ship'. The word 'bounces' could be used for 'reflects off' and the word 'colours' could stand for 'red and yellow'. The other words in the message can be extrapolated from existing codes or are irrelevant.

Option A 'mirror' could be used for 'reflects' but it would not convey 'reflects off' as well as 'bounces'.

Option B, 'ember', could be used for 'glow' but we could already extrapolate 'glow' from 'hot'.

Option D, 'shine', could be used for 'reflects' but it would not convey 'reflects off' as well as 'bounces'.

Question 27

Answer and rationale

Option A would be the best way to encode the message 'Earthlings and Martians may be dissimilar but their spacecrafts use the same fuel'.

♥, Z, ❑X, ZT, ▲X, ▲◖✳→

This option has the correct codes by using ♥ 'fire' as 'fuel', Z 'similar' as 'same', ❑X 'home enlarge' as 'Earthlings', ZT 'similar opposite' as 'dissimilar', ▲X 'Mars enlarge' as 'Martians' and ▲◖✳→ 'Mars Moon Sun ship' as 'spacecrafts'.

Option B has not used the code 'enlarge' with 'home' to make 'Earthlings'.

Option C has used the code ◆ 'oxygen' instead of ♥ 'fire' as 'fuel' and has not used the code 'enlarge' with 'Mars' to make 'Martians'.

Option D has used the code ◆ 'oxygen' instead of ♥ 'fire' as 'fuel'.

Option E has not used the code → 'ship' with ▲◖✳ 'Mars Moon Sun' to make 'spacecrafts'.

Question 28

Answer and rationale

502, V ✦ ✳506, ✳ ♥, WTX

The code combines the words 'damage', 'unite me others aliens', 'Sun fire', 'hot opposite enlarge'.

Option D, 'Sunburn and frostbite afflict all of us', is the correct answer as it uses all the codes, with 'damage' being used as 'afflicts', 'unite me others aliens' being used as 'all of us', 'Sun fire' being used as 'sunburn' and 'hot opposite enlarge' being used as 'frostbite'.

Option A has failed to use the codes 'me' and 'others'.

Option B has failed to use the code 'damage' and has misinterpreted the codes 'Sun fire' and 'hot opposite enlarge'.

Option C has failed to use the code 'unite me others aliens' and has misinterpreted the codes 'Sun fire' and 'hot opposite enlarge'.

Option E has failed to use the code 'unite me others aliens' and has separated them into 'some' and 'others'.

Chapter 5
The Situational Judgement Test

This chapter will help you to:

- understand the purpose and the format of the Situational Judgement Test (SJT);
- prepare for the SJT using general SJT questions;
- test your knowledge and understanding of SJT-type questions;
- identify those situational judgement skills where development is required.

Introduction

Pearson VUE describes the purpose of the SJT as follows:

> The test measures your capacity to understand real world situations and to identify critical factors and appropriate behaviour in dealing with them.

What are Situational Judgement Tests?

Since the late 1990s Situational Judgement Tests (SJTs) have been widely used by employers when they are recruiting staff, particularly at graduate level. Organisations currently using SJTs include PricewaterhouseCoopers, John Lewis, Sony, Wal-Mart, Deloitte and the NHS. In the NHS they are used in medical selection, including the selection of Foundation Doctors, General Practitioners and other medical specialties.

SJTs are basically a measure of an individual's behaviour and attitudes to work-related or life scenarios. Essentially, for the purposes of the UKCAT, the questions do not require any medical or procedural knowledge, although some of the questions may be based around hypothetical medical scenarios.

The test assesses integrity, perspective taking and team involvement, and it should be reasonably obvious from a scenario and associated questions which of these three areas is being tested. Obviously, there may be a scenario or questions where more than one area is involved.

'Integrity' is generally an assessment of a person's honesty. A scenario might relate to a person receiving a 'thank you' gift in the workplace that might be construed as bribery. Another scenario might relate to an ethical issue such as breaching a confidence or failing to act when witnessing the unethical behaviour of others in the workplace.

'Perspective taking' can best be described as assessing an individual's point of view in dealing with the differing scenarios. Probably a pragmatic approach to this type of 'problem solving' would be favoured where any issues involved can be dealt with at an appropriate level.

In the practice questions produced by the UKCAT themselves there does appear to be a bias towards resolving issues at a local level where this is appropriate.

'Team involvement' is essentially concerned with the dynamics of working within a team. In the medical profession, teamwork has a significant role to play in dealing with patients, often in life-threatening scenarios, in an effective and efficient way. The test is used to assess your understanding of how teams work and how you would react within a team in certain scenarios.

SJTs are considered to provide a predictable measure to identify candidates with the right attributes and behaviours required by an organisation. They are seen as being particularly effective for organisations screening large volumes of applicants for regularly recruited roles (in this instance, students). SJTs can provide a highly effective sift to identify candidates with the best fit in order to focus time and resources.

The Situational Judgement Test

As with the other tests, before attempting the SJT practice test it would be beneficial to work through the following scenarios, response formats and example questions that have been formatted in the style used in the UKCAT.

Scenarios, response formats and example questions

Most of the scenarios in the test will be reasonably short and specific and, as mentioned previously, they will not expect any prior medical or procedural knowledge. However, it might be useful, if you have not already done so, to look at a copy of the General Medical Council's 'Good medical practice'. This document sets out the responsibilities of all doctors towards society, their patients and their colleagues, and can be found on the www.gmc-uk.org website. Although a large part of the document is concerned with issues that would not be tested in the SJT, there are certain areas such as confidentiality and unethical behaviour that might be included in the test.

The questions are divided into two sets. In the first set you will be asked to rate the **appropriateness** of a series of options in response to the scenario. When considering how to respond to the scenario, the options are:

A   **A very appropriate thing to do** if it will address at least one aspect (not necessarily all aspects) of the situation.

B   **Appropriate, but not ideal** if it could be done, but is not necessarily a very good thing to do.

C   **Inappropriate, but not awful** if it should not really be done, but would not be terrible.

D   **A very inappropriate thing to do** if it should definitely not be done and would make the situation worse.

For the second set of questions you will be asked to rate the **importance** of a series of options in response to the scenario. When considering how to respond to the scenario, the options are:

A **Very important** if this is something that is vital to take into account.

B **Important** if this is something that is important but not vital to take into account.

C **Minor importance** if this is something that could be taken into account, but it does not matter if it is considered or not.

D **Not important** if this is something that should definitely not be taken into account.

In relation to either set of questions, a response should not be judged as if it is the only thing that is done. Response options should be treated independently. You should make a judgement as to the appropriateness or importance of a response option independent from the other. Within a scenario, each rating can be used **more than once or not at all – for example**, all response options can be given the same rating, such as very appropriate or very important. The response options provided are not intended to represent all of the possible options and it may be that the response you consider most appropriate or important is not present. In selecting a response option you must consider what an individual should actually do, rather that what they may be likely to do.

Some options may be appropriate or important in the *short term* (i.e. immediately addressing a wrongdoing) and some are appropriate or important in the *long term* (discussing the implications of the wrongdoing after the event). Consider response options irrelevant of the time frame.

For a test in the SJT format it is usual that full marks are awarded for an item if your response matches the 'ideal' answer as decided by the examiners. You will also be awarded marks dependent on how much your own answer deviates from the 'ideal' answer.

The UKCAT consortium makes the point that because the SJT is a measure of non-cognitive attributes, it will be considered by universities in a different manner to the cognitive subtests. This means that universities will differ in their interpretation of the test scores in determining their importance in the overall recruitment procedure.

Situational Judgement practice test: example questions

The following provides examples of the two sets of questions used in the SJT, i.e. those requiring 'appropriate' responses and those requiring 'important' responses.

Example item 1 (appropriate response)

George is shadowing a GP as part of his work-experience placement. On one occasion George is present when the GP sees Caroline, a young patient who is suffering from anxiety and panic attacks. After the observation the GP asks George to go to the adjoining pharmacy to collect some medical items. At the pharmacy George again sees Caroline who is waiting for her prescription. They speak to each other for a few minutes before Caroline leaves with the prescription. Two days later George receives a 'friend' request from Caroline on his social media site.

How appropriate is each of the following responses by George to this situation?

Question 1

George decides to ignore the 'friend' request from Caroline.

A A very appropriate thing to do.

B Appropriate, but not ideal.

C Inappropriate, but not awful.

D A very inappropriate thing to do.

Answer and rationale

Option D, 'A very inappropriate thing to do', is correct. This is a very inappropriate thing to do as it does not provide George with an opportunity to offer an explanation to Caroline as to why he is declining the request. Forming friendships with patients is not acceptable for doctors and although George is not even a medical student, it would be expected that he should act accordingly where he has observed a doctor–patient examination.

Question 2

George accepts the request as he is only a medical student and will not be returning to the GP practice again.

A A very appropriate thing to do.

B Appropriate, but not ideal.

C Inappropriate, but not awful.

D A very inappropriate thing to do.

Answer and rationale

Option D, 'A very inappropriate thing to do' is correct. In this event George has been present during a medical examination and it could be reasonably argued that even when only on work experience George would be subject to doctor–patient confidentiality. Caroline would probably not be aware of George's status and may have assumed he was a medical student or junior doctor. In fact, George could be seen as part of the medical team in Caroline's examination and therefore it would be very inappropriate for him to accept the 'friend' request.

Question 3

George informs the GP of Caroline's 'friend' request on social media.

A   A very appropriate thing to do.

B   Appropriate, but not ideal.

C   Inappropriate, but not awful.

D   A very inappropriate thing to do.

Answer and rationale

Option A, 'A very appropriate thing to do', is correct. George would not be expected to be conversant with the guidelines applying to social media requests and it would be very appropriate for him to inform the GP of the 'friend' request. This would allow the GP to provide advice to George and it would not preclude him contacting Caroline at a later time to explain his situation in refusing the request.

Question 4

George declines the request, informing Caroline that by accepting it he may be in breach of medical guidelines.

A   A very appropriate thing to do.

B   Appropriate, but not ideal.

C   Inappropriate, but not awful.

D   A very inappropriate thing to do.

Answer and rationale

Option A, 'A very appropriate thing to do' is correct. George has quite rightly responded to Caroline's request and although not accepting it, has provided good reason for his refusal. This course of action has shown integrity and sensitivity and is a very appropriate thing to do.

Example item 2 (important response)

Sanita, a Sixth Form student, joins the student branch of one of the main political parties. Within six months she is appointed as vice-chair of the party's regional 'Equality for Women' committee. One evening, prior to a meeting of the committee, she is approached by Ghania, a Muslim student who wears a burqa. She is shaking and visibly upset. Ghania tells Sanita that she has just been confronted by Clara, a white female member of the committee, who made disparaging comments about her wearing a burqa and that she was not doing herself or the committee any favours by wearing it.

How important is it to take into account the following considerations for Sanita when deciding how to respond to the situation?

Question 1

Sanita tells Ghania to ignore Clara's comments.

A Very important.

B Important.

C Minor importance.

D Not important.

Answer and rationale

Option D, 'Not important', is correct. This would really be an easy way out for Sanita but, as stated in the scenario, Ghania 'is shaking and visibly upset'. Telling Ghania to ignore Clara's comments does not address the issue or provide an acceptable solution. The response is therefore not important at all.

Question 2

Sanita asks Ghania to provide full details of Clara's actions and what was said and any relevant previous history between the two. Sanita then confronts Clara about the allegation.

A Very important.

B Important.

C Minor importance.

D Not important.

Answer and rationale

Option A, 'Very important', is correct. In Sanita's position as vice-chair, it is obviously very important to obtain an accurate record of what actually occurred and any history that there might be between Ghania and Clara. It is also very important that Sanita then speaks to Clara in an effort to resolve the situation.

Question 3

Sanita immediately contacts the chair of the Equality for Women committee and informs her what has occurred.

A Very important.

B Important.

C Minor importance.

D Not important.

Answer and rationale

Option C, 'Minor importance', is correct. Protocol would really determine that the chair of the Equality for Women should be informed of what had occurred. However, informing the chair could be something that would wait, while resolving the matter at the earliest opportunity at a local level would be more appropriate. Immediately informing the chair would therefore be of minor importance and can be dealt with later.

Question 4

Sanita reports the incident to the police.

A Very important.

B Important.

C Minor importance.

D Not important.

Answer and rationale

Option D, 'Not important' is correct. This is almost certainly an inappropriate course of action. It is not made clear in the scenario exactly what was said apart from the fact that Clara obviously objected to Ghania wearing a burqa. This alone would not support any police involvement and therefore the option is not important.

The Situational Judgement practice test: scenarios and questions

As with the other test, the SJT is an on-screen test that consists of 20 scenarios and 67 associated items. The 67 items have between two and six response options, and you are only allowed to select what you consider the 'one-best' option. A period of 27 minutes is allowed for the test, with 1 minute for instruction and the remaining 26 minutes for items.

If you want to simulate 'test conditions' you are advised to use rough paper to mark down your choice for each of the questions (i.e. A, B, C or D).

The correct answer and rationale for each of the questions are produced in the section following the practice test.

Question set 1

After his lunch break, Isaac, a dental student, enters the surgery where he is undertaking a short placement. In the surgery car park he sees one of the senior dentists, who is working that day, sitting in his stationary car drinking from a bottle of vodka. He has heard staff at the surgery gossiping about this dentist having an alcohol problem. Isaac sees the dentist back in the surgery a short time later and he does not appear to be drunk.

How appropriate are each of the following responses by Isaac in this situation?

Question 1

As the dentist did not appear to be drunk, Isaac should keep his own counsel and not mention it to anyone else.

A   A very appropriate thing to do.

B   Appropriate, but not ideal. *

C   Inappropriate, but not awful.

D   A very inappropriate thing to do.

Question 2

Isaac has witnessed the dentist drinking alcohol immediately before returning to work and should report the matter to a senior manager at the surgery.

A   A very appropriate thing to do. *

B   Appropriate, but not ideal.

C   Inappropriate, but not awful.

D   A very inappropriate thing to do.

Question set 2

A group of four dental students are in the local café having their lunch break during a training day. They are discussing their course and the tutors for the day. Gustav raises the sexual persuasion of one of the tutors and makes several homophobic comments directly about this tutor. Anna and Amelia immediately leave the café in disgust leaving Gustav with Harry.

How appropriate is each of the following responses by Harry in this situation?

Question 3

Harry should immediately challenge Gustav about his homophobic comments.

A   A very appropriate thing to do. *

B   Appropriate, but not ideal.

C   Inappropriate, but not awful.

D   A very inappropriate thing to do.

Question 4

Harry should first speak to Anna and Amelia and seek their views on what Gustav had said.

A A very appropriate thing to do.

B Appropriate, but not ideal.

C Inappropriate, but not awful.

D A very inappropriate thing to do.

Question 5

Harry should speak later with Gustav about his comments and the impact they obviously had on Anna and Amelia who immediately left the café.

A A very appropriate thing to do.

B Appropriate, but not ideal.

C Inappropriate, but not awful.

D A very inappropriate thing to do.

Question 6

Harry reports Gustav's homophobic comments as soon as possible to a senior member of the college staff.

A A very appropriate thing to do.

B Appropriate, but not ideal.

C Inappropriate, but not awful.

D A very inappropriate thing to do.

Question set 3

Irena, a medical student, and five other students are working as a team to produce a joint assignment that will impact on their final marks. The marking of the assignment not only includes the structure and content but also the way in which the group was able to work together throughout. Irena is concerned about one of the group members, Lydia, who doesn't appear to be pulling her weight. Although she does what she has to, Lydia is very quiet, does not contribute in their discussions about the project and never challenges any decisions that are made, always acquiescing to other group members. Irena knows Lydia better than anyone else in the group and Lydia has confided in her about her current domestic situation that is causing her considerable issues and affecting her work. Other members of the group are getting fed up with Lydia's failure to contribute to their work.

How appropriate is each of the following responses by Irena in this situation?

Question 7

Irena should seek advice from the course tutor or other staff member as to the best course of action.

A   A very appropriate thing to do.

B   Appropriate, but not ideal.

C   Inappropriate, but not awful.

D   A very inappropriate thing to do.

Question 8

During a group session Irena raises the issue of every member having a responsibility to contribute to the group's work, providing an opportunity to deal with any issues.

A   A very appropriate thing to do.

B   Appropriate, but not ideal.

C   Inappropriate, but not awful.

D   A very inappropriate thing to do.

Question 9

Lydia does what she has to in the group and in view of her current domestic problems it is probably best that Irena does nothing.

A   A very appropriate thing to do.

B   Appropriate, but not ideal.

C   Inappropriate, but not awful.

D   A very inappropriate thing to do.

Question 10

Irena should ask the other group members their views on Lydia's performance and how any issues might be resolved.

A   A very appropriate thing to do.

B   Appropriate, but not ideal.

C   Inappropriate, but not awful.

D   A very inappropriate thing to do.

Question set 4

Francesca is a junior doctor undertaking work experience at a GP's surgery. One morning she is in the reception area waiting to accompany one of the GPs on her external visits to patients. She overhears Alice, who has only been a receptionist for a short while, talking to a patient about the results of some tests. The receptionist informs the patient that his doctor has quite a backlog of test results to deal with which she can't understand because all the other doctors are up to date. She says that everyone speaks very highly of the doctor but he is a bit lazy in dealing with test results.

How appropriate is each of the following responses by Francesca in this situation?

Question 11

As soon as the patient has gone Francesca speaks to the receptionist in private and asks her to explain her comments.

A   A very appropriate thing to do.

B   Appropriate, but not ideal.

C   Inappropriate, but not awful.

D   A very inappropriate thing to do.

Question 12

Francesca interrupts the conversation between Alice and the patient, and tells Alice in the patient's hearing that her comment about the doctor being a bit lazy is inappropriate.

A   A very appropriate thing to do.

B   Appropriate, but not ideal.

C   Inappropriate, but not awful.

D   A very inappropriate thing to do.

Question 13

Francesca waits until the doctor she accompanies on her visits arrives and informs her what has happened.

A   A very appropriate thing to do.

B   Appropriate, but not ideal.

C   Inappropriate, but not awful.

D   A very inappropriate thing to do.

Question 14

Francesca should immediately go to the practice manager and inform them about what she witnessed.

A   A very appropriate thing to do. •

B   Appropriate, but not ideal.

C   Inappropriate, but not awful.

D   A very inappropriate thing to do.

Question set 5

Nicola is a medical student and in one of the classes she attends the lecturer, Dr Samuels, is renowned for his fiery temperament and his apparent delight at putting down students. Over the past few weeks he has been constantly picking on Ineke, one of Nicola's fellow students and friends, both in and outside the classroom environment. His remarks to Ineke have become increasingly personal, inferring she is dim-witted, obviously incapable of rational thought and highly unlikely to make the grade. These remarks are often said in a very threatening manner and Ineke is becoming increasingly upset. Nicola herself has had no issues with Dr Samuels.

How appropriate are each of the following responses by Nicola in this situation?

Question 15

Nicola tells Ineke to record each occasion on which Dr Samuels makes 'inappropriate' comments and note details of any other person who was present at the time.

A   A very appropriate thing to do. •

B   Appropriate, but not ideal.

C   Inappropriate, but not awful.

D   A very inappropriate thing to do.

Question 16

Nicola advises Ineke to speak to her course tutor at the college about Dr Samuels' behaviour.

A   A very appropriate thing to do. •

B   Appropriate, but not ideal.

C   Inappropriate, but not awful.

D   A very inappropriate thing to do.

Question 17

Nicola decides to speak to Dr Samuels herself about his behaviour towards Ineke and how it is affecting her.

A   A very appropriate thing to do.

B   Appropriate, but not ideal.

C   Inappropriate, but not awful.

D   A very inappropriate thing to do.

Question set 6

Simon, a medical student, is working on a placement in his local hospital. He is familiarising himself with work on one of the surgical wards which he visits daily. While talking to one of the patients, whom he has grown fond of, it is obvious she would like to be more than friends and offers her telephone number so they can meet up when she is discharged.

How appropriate is each of the following responses by Simon in this situation?

Question 18

Simon accepts the patient's telephone number.

A   A very appropriate thing to do.

B   Appropriate, but not ideal.

C   Inappropriate, but not awful.

D   A very inappropriate thing to do.

Question 19

Simon refuses the patient's telephone number.

A   A very appropriate thing to do.

B   Appropriate, but not ideal.

C   Inappropriate, but not awful.

D   A very inappropriate thing to do.

Question 20

Simon reports the behaviour of the patient to his manager.

A   A very appropriate thing to do.

B   Appropriate, but not ideal.

C   Inappropriate, but not awful.

D   A very inappropriate thing to do.

Question 21

Simon informs the patient that he is not allowed to befriend her as her approach is unethical.

A   A very appropriate thing to do.

B   Appropriate, but not ideal.

C   Inappropriate, but not awful.

D   A very inappropriate thing to do.

Question set 7

Siobhan is with a group of seven medical students undertaking a placement at the Royal Infirmary. Towards the end of the first week Siobhan is approached by one of the ward sisters who asks her if someone could speak to Kevin, one of the medical students. The sister has received several complaints from both nurses and patients about Kevin's dishevelled appearance and the fact that he smells of stale tobacco and body odour.

How appropriate is each of the following responses by Siobhan in this situation?

Question 22

Siobhan should speak to the other medical students to canvass their views on how to resolve the situation.

A   A very appropriate thing to do.

B   Appropriate, but not ideal.

C   Inappropriate, but not awful.

D   A very inappropriate thing to do.

Question 23

Siobhan should tell the ward sister at the time that this is an issue for her, the matron or consultant to deal with.

A A very appropriate thing to do.

B Appropriate, but not ideal.

C Inappropriate, but not awful.

D A very inappropriate thing to do.

Question 24

Siobhan should confront Kevin with what the ward sister has said to her.

A A very appropriate thing to do.

B Appropriate, but not ideal.

C Inappropriate, but not awful.

D A very inappropriate thing to do.

Question 25

Siobhan decides to send Kevin an anonymous letter signed 'a well-meaning friend'.

A A very appropriate thing to do.

B Appropriate, but not ideal.

C Inappropriate, but not awful.

D A very inappropriate thing to do.

Question set 8

Dr Patel has been treating Stephan during his four days stay on the cardiac ward. As he is being discharged, Stephan gives Dr Patel an envelope containing £250 in cash saying it's a thank you for the excellent treatment he has received.

How appropriate is each of the following responses by Dr Patel in this situation?

Question 26

Dr Patel refuses to accept the money telling Stephan it would be unethical.

A A very appropriate thing to do.

B Appropriate, but not ideal.

C Inappropriate, but not awful.

D A very inappropriate thing to do.

Question 27

Dr Patel accepts the £250, telling Stephan that it will be shared among the staff on the ward.

A A very appropriate thing to do.

B Appropriate, but not ideal.

C Inappropriate, but not awful.

D A very inappropriate thing to do.

Question 28

Dr Patel accepts the gift and asks Stephan not to mention it to anyone else.

A A very appropriate thing to do.

B Appropriate, but not ideal.

C Inappropriate, but not awful.

D A very inappropriate thing to do.

Question 29

Dr Patel accepts the £250 and tells Stephan he will pay the money to the nurses' benevolent fund and send him a receipt, which he does.

A A very appropriate thing to do.

B Appropriate, but not ideal.

C Inappropriate, but not awful.

D A very inappropriate thing to do.

Question set 9

Lucian is a junior doctor working in the oncology unit at the general hospital. One night after work he sees that one of his colleagues from oncology, Rowena, has posted a message on her social media site. The message says she'd had a bad day at work. She thought that they were having a television personality (naming the personality) admitted to the ward but it turned out that it was a patient with the same name as a television personality. Lucian has to decide whether he should report the matter to a senior manager.

How appropriate is each of the following responses by Lucian in this situation?

Question 30

Lucian decides to warn Rowena that she may have breached patient confidentiality and she should be more careful in future as to what she puts on social media.

A   A very appropriate thing to do.

B   Appropriate, but not ideal.

C   Inappropriate, but not awful.

D   A very inappropriate thing to do.

Question 31

The following day Lucian reports what Rowena has done to a senior manager.

A   A very appropriate thing to do.

B   Appropriate, but not ideal.

C   Inappropriate, but not awful.

D   A very inappropriate thing to do.

Question 32

Lucian telephones Rowena and tells her she must speak to the patient she has identified and apologise for what she's done or otherwise he will report the matter.

A   A very appropriate thing to do.

B   Appropriate, but not ideal.

C   Inappropriate, but not awful.

D   A very inappropriate thing to do.

Question set 10

Jordan, a dental student, is late for work but stops at his local convenience store to buy some food, parking his car in the store's car park. After visiting the store he returns to his car. He then reverses out of the parking place and accidentally collides with a van parked in an opposite bay. Jordan gets out of his car and on examining the unattended van he has just hit sees there is minor damage to the front wing.

How appropriate is each of the following responses by Jordan in this situation?

Question 33

Because he's late for work Jordan writes his name and phone number on a piece of paper and places it on the windscreen of the damaged car, apologising for the damage.

A   A very appropriate thing to do.

B   Appropriate, but not ideal.

C   Inappropriate, but not awful.

D   A very inappropriate thing to do.

Question 34

As the driver of the other vehicle is not present, Jordan calls 999 to report the accident to the police.

A   A very appropriate thing to do.

B   Appropriate, but not ideal.

C   Inappropriate, but not awful.

D   A very inappropriate thing to do.

Question set 11

While continuing her studies as a dental student, Rhianna has had a part-time job in a town centre pub where she is a bar sub-manager. One busy Friday evening Ayana, a recent member of the bar team, asks to speak to Rhianna away from the bar. She appears very upset and complains that a customer has just sworn at her and made racist comments.

How important is it for Rhianna to take into account the following considerations when deciding how to respond to the situation?

Question 35

Rhianna tells Ayana that it is just part of the job and to take no notice of the customer's behaviour.

A   Very important.

B   Important.

C   Minor importance.

D   Not important.

Question 36

Rhianna asks Ayana for all the circumstances surrounding the customer's actions and as to what was actually said. Rhianna then speaks to the customer in question about their inappropriate behaviour.

A Very important.

B Important.

C Minor importance.

D Not important.

Question set 12

Ranjit, a medical student, is currently on a placement at his local hospital clinic. One night his sister returns home and tells Ranjit that one of her friends, Julia, who works as a part-time receptionist at the hospital clinic, told her that one of their mutual friends Anna had been to the clinic with a lump in her breast and was being referred urgently to the Royal Infirmary for further tests. Ranjit's sister says that Julia told her this in confidence and she said she wouldn't say anything.

How important is it for Ranjit to take into account the following considerations when deciding how to respond to the situation?

Question 37

Ranjit should confront Julia the next time she is working at the clinic.

A Very important.

B Important.

C Minor importance.

D Not important.

Question 38

Ranjit should inform the manager at the clinic of the conversation between Julia and his sister.

A Very important.

B Important.

C Minor importance.

D Not important.

Question 39

Ranjit should inform Anna about what has occurred.

A   Very important.

B   Important.

C   Minor importance.

D   Not important.

Question 40

Ranjit should not identify his sister as the source of the information as it was said to her in confidence.

A   Very important.

B   Important.

C   Minor importance.

D   Not important.

Question set 13

Giles is a medical student and has recently undertaken work experience at his local GP practice. One Friday evening he is socialising with friends. One of his friends has brought along Sara who has recently moved to the area. During the evening Sara tells him she is going to sign up for the GP practice where you have been on work experience. She asks him which one of the five doctors at the practice it is best to sign up with. She has heard some criticisms about a couple of the doctors and is keen to sign up with the best one. Giles is aware that two of the GPs haven't got a very good reputation and has heard rumours that they are being investigated for malpractice.

How important is it for Giles to take into account the following considerations when deciding how to respond to the situation?

Question 41

Giles tells Sara that as far as he is concerned there are no issues with any of the doctors at the practice.

A   Very important.

B   Important.

C   Minor importance.

D   Not important.

Question 42

Giles tells Sara that he had heard rumours, but that's all they are, and if she wants to believe them she should sign on with another practice.

A Very important.

B Important.

C Minor importance.

D Not important.

Question set 14

Raja is a junior doctor in the Emergency Assessment Unit (EAU) and on doing her rounds a patient tells her that a £10 note has been taken from her purse. She knows this because she only had a £20 note, a £10 note and some loose change in her purse.

How important it is for Raja to take into account the following considerations when deciding how to respond to the situation?

Question 43

Raja decides to call the police.

A Very important.

B Important.

C Minor importance.

D Not important.

Question 44

Raja attempts to reassure the patient by taking full details of what has occurred and that the matter will be brought to the attention of senior staff and all those working in EAU.

A Very important.

B Important.

C Minor importance.

D Not important.

Question 45

At the following morning meeting Raja requests that all the nursing staff be made aware of the theft and asks them to tell their patients to safeguard their belongings and to be especially careful with their cash.

A Very important.

B Important.

C Minor importance.

D Not important.

Question 46

At the morning meeting, in addition to informing staff of the theft, Raja also asks that the culprit should replace the money stolen from the patient.

A Very important.

B Important.

C Minor importance.

D Not important.

Question set 15

Ludmila is a dental student undertaking a placement in a dental unit within a large hospital. On one day she is working with three of the dental technicians, Mahesh, Rose and Ellen, who are employed at the dental unit. At the coffee break Ludmila and the three technicians sit together at a table in the hospital restaurant. Members of the public and staff from other departments are present. Ludmila is talking to Mahesh when she overhears Rose and Ellen talking about the recruitment of a new assistant. During the conversation she hears Rose say 'I can't believe they've employed someone who's morbidly obese. She's gross. I can't imagine what the patients will think.' By their reaction you realise that some of the other people present have overheard this conversation.

How important is it for Ludmila to take into account the following considerations when deciding how to respond to the situation?

Question 47

Before Rose can say anything further, Ludmila confronts her about the inappropriate remarks.

A Very important.

B Important.

C Minor importance.

D Not important.

Question 48

After the coffee break Ludmila finds an opportunity to be alone with Rose and to confront her about the inappropriate remarks.

A Very important.

B Important.

C Minor importance.

D Not important.

Question 49

After the coffee break Ludmila talks separately to Mahesh and Ellen and asks them to join her in confronting Rose about her inappropriate remarks.

A Very important.

B Important.

C Minor importance.

D Not important.

Question 50

Speak to Rose's line manager about the incident.

A Very important.

B Important.

C Minor importance.

D Not important.

Question 51

Ludmila finds out the name of the person who has been recruited as an assistant technician and intends to speak to them about Rose's remarks when they start work.

A Very important.

B Important.

C   Minor importance.

D   Not important.

Question set 16

Dr Phillips is a junior doctor who has just started working at a new hospital. Later one evening, on going into the doctors' lounge, he finds one of his colleagues watching adult pornography on a hospital computer.

How important is it for Dr Phillips to take into account the following considerations when deciding how to respond to the situation?

Question 52

Dr Phillips should tell the police at the earliest opportunity.

A   Very important.

B   Important.

C   Minor importance.

D   Not important.

Question 53

Dr Phillips should confront his colleague about the inappropriateness of watching adult pornographic images at work and using hospital property.

A   Very important.

B   Important.

C   Minor importance.

D   Not important.

Question 54

Dr Phillips should report the matter to medical personnel as the colleague is misusing hospital property.

A   Very important.

B   Important.

C   Minor importance.

D   Not important.

Question 55

Dr Phillips should report the matter to a senior colleague.

A Very important.

B Important.

C Minor importance.

D Not important.

Question set 17

Dr Mwanga, a junior doctor, is treating Kristina who has been admitted to A&E with a suspected fractured jaw and severe bruising to her left arm and upper body. While no other members of staff are present, Kristina tells Dr Mwanga that her husband had found out that she had been having an affair and had beaten her up. She tells the doctor that she has told her this in confidence and insists that she must not tell anyone else because she passionately wants to save her marriage for the sake of her two small children.

How important is it for Dr Mwanga to take into account the following considerations when deciding how to respond to the situation?

Question 56

Dr Mwanga must involve the police and social services as soon as possible.

A Very important.

B Important.

C Minor importance.

D Not important.

Question 57

Dr Mwanga informs Kristina that she must document their conversation, including her husband's liability but would not allow the police access to her notes unless Kristina agrees to it.

A Very important.

B Important.

C Minor importance.

D Not important.

Question 58

Dr Mwanga informs Kristina that she has a duty of care towards her and will inform her senior colleague of their conversation.

A   Very important.

B   Important.

C   Minor importance.

D   Not important.

Question set 18

Dr Singh is a junior doctor working in a very busy A&E unit. One Saturday morning a colleague, Dr Peterson, calls the ward from home, saying that she will not be coming in because she is feeling unwell. Subsequently, Dr Singh finds out that his colleague has, in fact, spent the weekend in the country with her boyfriend and that she had not suffered any illness. Dr Singh is not aware that his colleague has previously taken 'sick' leave without good cause.

How important is it for Dr Singh to take into account the following considerations when deciding how to respond to the situation?

Question 59

Dr Singh informs his consultant of the circumstances as soon as reasonably practicable.

A   Very important.

B   Important.

C   Minor importance

D   Not important.

Question 60

Dr Singh speaks to Dr Peterson on her return to work and warns her that if there is any repetition he will report the matter.

A   Very important.

B   Important.

C   Minor importance.

D   Not important.

Question set 19

Aaron is undertaking work experience with his local GP practice and observes a consultation with a patient who has been suffering from depression for several months and who has self-harmed during that time. After a short time Aaron realises that the patient is one of his sister's best friends, although he has rarely spoken to her and he now lives away from the family home.

How important is it for Aaron to take into account the following considerations when deciding how to respond to the situation?

Question 61

As soon as Aaron realises the patient's relationship with his sister, he excuses himself and leaves the consulting room.

A Very important.

B Important.

C Minor importance.

D Not important.

Question 62

Aaron speaks to the GP immediately after the consultation has finished.

A Very important.

B Important.

C Minor importance.

D Not important.

Question 63

Aaron speaks to the patient as soon as possible after the event to reassure her.

A Very important.

B Important.

C Minor importance.

D Not important.

Question set 20

Omar and Alex are both medical students, having started their training together and often socialise with each other. One night after several drinks Alex asks Omar to lend him some money. He eventually confides in Omar that he has been using cocaine for some time and needs the money to buy some drugs. He says he will pay the money back at the end of the month. He asks Omar not to tell anyone about his addiction and that he needs his support.

How important is it for Omar to take into account the following considerations when deciding how to respond to the situation?

Question 64

Omar agrees not to tell anyone about Alex's cocaine addiction.

A Very important.

B Important.

C Minor importance.

D Not important.

Question 65

Omar tells Alex that he needs to tell his manager himself about his addiction. If Alex doesn't, even though he will support him, Omar will have no option but to report him.

A Very important.

B Important.

C Minor importance.

D Not important.

Question 66

Omar decides to observe how Alex performs and if he sees any problems would then report these to a senior manager or consultant.

A Very important.

B Important.

C Minor importance.

D Not important.

Question 67

Omar reports Alex's addiction to a senior manager.

A Very important.

B Important.

C Minor importance.

D Not important.

Situational Judgement practice test: answers

Question number	Correct response	Question number	Correct response
1	D	35	D
2	A	36	A
3	B	37	B
4	C	38	A
5	A	39	B
6	C	40	D
7	B	41	A
8	A	42	C
9	D	43	D
10	A	44	A
11	A	45	C
12	D	46	D
13	C	47	B
14	B	48	A
15	B	49	C
16	B	50	A
17	A	51	D
18	C	52	D
19	A	53	A
20	A	54	C
21	D	55	B
22	C	56	B
23	B	57	A
24	A	58	A
25	D	59	C
26	A	60	A
27	B	61	C
28	D	62	B
29	B	63	D
30	D	64	D
31	A	65	B
32	D	66	D
33	B	67	A
34	C		

Situational Judgement practice test: explanation of answers

Question set 1

Question 1

Answer and rationale

Answer D, 'A very inappropriate thing to do', is correct. The major issue with this scenario is patient safety and it would be inappropriate for Isaac to ignore what he had witnessed. Diplomacy of any description is not an option as a practitioner's fitness to practise is paramount. At the very least it is likely that patients (and staff) will smell alcohol on the dentist's breath that is unprofessional.

Question 2

Answer and rationale

Answer A, 'A very appropriate thing to do', is correct. By informing a senior manager at the surgery of what Isaac has witnessed, action can be taken to ensure that patient safety is not compromised. Obviously, it is for the senior manager to determine what action is taken but Isaac has fulfilled his responsibility in this situation.

Question set 2

Question 3

Answer and rationale

Answer B, 'Appropriate, but not ideal', is correct. To immediately challenge Gustav about his homophobic comments would be appropriate, but not ideal. There is a possibility that Gustav may become defensive about his remarks said in what he considered to be a 'safe' environment, i.e. among friends. It may also be that Anna and Amelia would not support this course of action as they may themselves have wanted to confront Gustav's behaviour but did not feel it appropriate at this time.

Question 4

Answer and rationale

Answer C, 'Inappropriate, but not awful', is correct. Having heard Gustav's comments, Harry should take responsibility and not wait to be supported by the views of Anna and Amelia. He should take whatever course of action is appropriate. However, although failing to take action himself would be inappropriate, it would not be awful if he decided to discuss the matter further with Anna and Amelia before doing so.

Question 5

Answer and rationale

Answer A, 'A very appropriate thing to do', is correct. Allowing time after the event provides both Harry and Gustav the opportunity to reflect on what was said and the repercussions, as opposed to a knee-jerk reaction immediately after the event. It is likely that Gustav would be less defensive about his comments rather than being confronted immediately after they were made. It also recognises that there is a problem that requires some form of resolution.

Question 6

Answer and rationale

Answer C, 'Inappropriate, but not awful', is correct. Although Gustav's comments are not acceptable, they were said in a situation where he felt 'safe' to express his views. Such situations, where possible, should be resolved locally, in this case among the group of students involved. However, the reaction to Gustav's comments might be such that reporting the matter to a senior member of the college staff seems justifiable. Although it would be better for the matter to be dealt with at a local level, such an action, though inappropriate, would not be awful.

Question set 3

Question 7

Answer and rationale

Answer B, 'Appropriate, but not ideal', is correct. In the first instance, the best resolution should be a matter for the group itself, and asking the tutor or other staff member is appropriate, but not ideal. Opening up the disaffection within the group, albeit only applying to one member, may have other unforeseen ramifications, including the tutors' or staff members' subsequent assessment of how the group was able to deal with its own problems.

Question 8

Answer and rationale

Answer A, 'A very appropriate thing to do', is correct. Purposefully raising the issue within the group would provide an opportunity to seek a local resolution. It is a very appropriate thing to do and can only be healthy for the working of the group to get things out in the open.

Question 9

Answer and rationale

Answer D, 'A very inappropriate thing to do', is correct. When working in groups, especially where there is some form of academic, skills and behavioural assessment, group members are entitled to expect that all their members take an effective part. It is not appropriate for one member to have limited contributions, as appears to be the case with Lydia. It might be argued that Lydia should share with the group that she is having external problems that are affecting her performance or determine that she should leave the group.

Question 10

Answer and rationale

Answer A, 'A very appropriate thing to do', is correct. This approach again provides for a local resolution of the issues surrounding Lydia's performance. It provides an opportunity for everyone in the group to express their views and be part of the resolution.

Question set 4

Question 11

Answer and rationale

Answer A, 'A very appropriate thing to do', is correct. Francesca has witnessed the conversation and is in the best position to confront Alice about her inappropriate comments. This also gives Alice the opportunity to explain why she said what she said and Francesca the opportunity to identify the need for sensitivity when dealing with patients and expressing opinions about doctors' abilities.

Question 12

Answer and rationale

Answer D, 'A very inappropriate thing to do', is correct. It would be inappropriate for Francesca to make comments to the receptionist in front of the patient. What has been said cannot be undone and can be dealt with more appropriately without both the receptionist and patient being present. There is no need for an immediate intervention.

Question 13

Answer and rationale

Answer C, 'Inappropriate, but not awful', is correct. The situation has now moved on and a solution that addresses the incident itself would be preferable. In this instance the doctor may only really give Francesca advice on addressing the matter and not its resolution. However, in view of the transitory nature of Francesca's presence at the practice, it would probably be remiss of her not to inform the doctor of what she witnessed.

Question 14

Answer and rationale
Answer B, 'Appropriate, but not ideal', is correct. Talking to the practice manager, who will undoubtedly have responsibility for the staff and their training and development, would be appropriate in that what Francesca witnessed does identify development needs for Alice in her receptionist role, even though this may be an isolated incident. However, the most appropriate thing to do would be for Francesca to confront Alice about her actions immediately after the event.

Question set 5

Question 15

Answer and rationale
Answer B, 'Appropriate, but not ideal', is correct. Where Nicola or Ineke feel that they cannot deal with Dr Samuels informally, recording details of 'inappropriate' incidents, together with names of witnesses, is an acceptable strategy. This would probably result in the matter being dealt with more formally at a later date.

Question 16

Answer and rationale
Answer B, 'Appropriate, but not ideal', is correct. This course of action would still allow the matter to be resolved at a local level, although it is not as preferable as Nicola or Ineke confronting Dr Samuels. Telling the course tutor would allow them to speak with Dr Samuels about his 'inappropriate' behaviour without the situation becoming more formal should it be successful.

Question 17

Answer and rationale
Answer A, 'A very appropriate thing to do', is correct. Nicola appears to have a good relationship with Dr Samuels and is not daunted by his manner towards others. This option would resolve the matter at a local level without involving other senior staff. This could also have an immediate impact, whereas reporting the matter to more senior staff would prolong the process.

Question set 6

Question 18

Answer and rationale
Answer C, 'Inappropriate, but not awful', is correct. There may be occasions where it is acceptable for a doctor to befriend a patient no longer under their care. However, the GMC

may see such befriending as a breach of the patient's trust or their vulnerability, and a doctor may be found to be in breach of duty. In this instance, Simon is a medical student and not a qualified doctor, but adherence to the profession's code of conduct might still be expected. Although taking the patient's number is not unethical, it may give the wrong impression. However, where the patient might get upset at a refusal to take the number, it could be taken so long as there was no further contact of a befriending nature. So, although basically it would be inappropriate to take the number, in certain circumstances it would not be awful.

Question 19

Answer and rationale
Answer A, 'A very appropriate thing to do', is correct. As discussed in the answer above, refusing the patient's telephone number would be the most appropriate thing to do, thereby avoiding any conflict with the profession's code of conduct.

Question 20

Answer and rationale
Answer A, 'A very appropriate thing to do', is correct. It is particularly important that Simon reports the matter to his manager (or consultant) in the event of the patient making any future allegations about his conduct that could be made following the refusal to accede to her 'befriending' request.

Question 21

Answer and rationale
Answer D, 'A very inappropriate thing to do', is correct. Irrespective of the fact that Simon is a medical student, the approach by the patient is not unethical as she is not bound by any code of ethics. It is the acceptance of a future friendship that would be unethical.

Question set 7

Question 22

Answer and rationale
Answer C, 'Inappropriate, but not awful', is correct. It could be argued that there is absolutely no need to canvass the views of the other medical students as the fact is that Kevin's appearance is dishevelled and he smells of stale tobacco and body odour. However, it would not be awful to consult fellow students in finding the best way to approach what is to an extent a sensitive matter.

Question 23

Answer and rationale

Answer B, 'Appropriate, but not ideal', is correct. It would be appropriate for Kevin to be confronted directly about the issues surrounding his personal hygiene. Whether this is done by the ward sister, matron or consultant is really immaterial. However, because of the sensitivity of the situation, the preferred resolution would be for Siobhan, a colleague, to make the approach to Kevin.

Question 24

Answer and rationale

Answer A, 'A very appropriate thing to do', is correct. This is a very appropriate thing to do as it allows the matter to be dealt with sensitively by a colleague, Siobhan, causing the minimum of embarrassment for Kevin.

Question 25

Answer and rationale

Answer D, 'A very inappropriate thing to do', is correct. This course of action is simply an avoidance strategy that is both unprofessional and insensitive.

Question set 8

Question 26

Answer and rationale

Answer A, 'A very appropriate thing to do', is correct. Gifts from patients must always be dealt with sensitively as they may impact on the doctor–patient relationship. However, it must be ensured that any such gifts cannot be construed as bribery. In this situation it would be very appropriate for Dr Patel to refuse the gift.

Question 27

Answer and rationale

Answer B, 'Appropriate, but not ideal', is correct. The care of Stephan has been the responsibility of all those concerned with his care and to share the gift with the rest of the ward team would be more appropriate. It demonstrates that any allegations of bribery against Dr Patel would be significantly mitigated by his selfless act of sharing the gift.

Question 28

Answer and rationale

Answer D, 'A very inappropriate thing to do', is correct. To accept the £250 is unethical and in telling Stephan not to mention it to anyone else clearly shows a level of dishonesty on the part of Dr Patel.

Question 29

Answer and rationale

Answer B, 'Appropriate, but not ideal', is correct. The most appropriate thing to do would be to refuse the gift. However, accepting the money and paying it into the nurses' benevolent fund would still be appropriate but not achieve the ideal of refusal. There would be no detriment in Dr Patel's actions, especially in view of the fact that he has receipted the payment to the fund and it would be doubtful that there would be any adverse impact on the doctor–patient relationship.

Question set 9

Question 30

Answer and rationale

Answer D, 'A very inappropriate thing to do', is correct. It is clear from the scenario that the name of the patient has been disclosed. Also, the ward and hospital will be known to some, if not all, of Rowena's social media friends. This is a clear breach of patient confidentiality and it would not be appropriate for it to be resolved at a local level. Lucian has little option other than to report the matter to a senior manager.

Question 31

Answer and rationale

Answer A, 'A very appropriate thing to do', is correct. It is paramount that patient confidentiality is maintained, and in this case patient information has been shared with countless others across social media. Albeit that only the patient's name has been disclosed to those accessing Rowena's social media site, there will be a number of her friends (both personal and social media) who are aware of where she works and in which department. Reporting the matter to a senior manager is a very appropriate thing to do.

Question 32

Answer and rationale

Answer D, 'A very inappropriate thing to do', is correct. Although an apology directly to the patient may appear to be the right thing to do, it does not address the issue of Rowena breaching patient confidentiality, which should be reported. Lucian's actions are unacceptable both in not directly reporting the matter and demanding the apology under threat of disclosure. This would make him a party to the breach of patient confidentiality and culpable for his actions.

Question set 10

Question 33

Answer and rationale

Answer B, 'Appropriate, but not ideal', is correct. The ideal would have been for Jordan to attempt to trace the driver. There is a strong possibility that the driver may have been in the convenience store. Being a few more minutes late for work would not make that much difference. However, the fact that he has left his personal details accepting responsibility for the damage is an appropriate thing to do, but not the ideal. The medical profession is seeking individuals who display honesty and probity, and who can admit when they have made mistakes. Jordan has displayed these attributes in his actions.

Question 34

Answer and rationale

Answer C, 'Inappropriate, but not awful', is correct. The 999 system is for emergency calls only and in this scenario the accident is certainly not an emergency. No persons were injured as a result of the accident and it took place on a convenience store car park, so there was little danger to other road users. It was therefore an inappropriate thing to do, but not awful.

Question set 11

Question 35

Answer and rationale

Answer D, 'Not important', is the correct answer. This might appear to be a reasonable course of action given the circumstances of a busy pub on a Friday night with customers who may have consumed too much alcohol. However, this does not address what has taken place and the upset it has caused Ayana, and therefore the response is 'not important'.

Question 36

Answer and rationale

Answer A, 'Very important', is correct. Before deciding on a course of action, it is essential that Rhianna is fully conversant with what actually took place. If another member of the bar team or other customers overheard the conversation between Ayana and the customer it might be useful for Rhianna to confirm what had taken place. Rhianna should then speak to the customer who made the offending comments. The response is therefore 'very important'.

Question set 12

Question 37

Answer and rationale

Answer B, 'Important', is correct. There is little doubt that Julia has breached patient confidentiality in telling Ranjit's sister about Anna's medical condition. However, although it is important that Julia is confronted about this as a matter of some urgency, it would be preferable for any confrontation or action to be undertaken by a manager at the clinic and not Ranjit as a medical student, who is also related to the 'informant'.

Question 38

Answer and rationale

Answer A, 'Very important', is correct. It is very important that Ranjit informs the manager at the clinic in order that the necessary action in relation to a breach of patient confidentiality can be taken. Obviously, there are rules and procedures in place within the clinic to deal with this type if situation.

Question 39

Answer and rationale

Answer B, 'Important', is correct. Although it would be important for Anna to be informed about what has occurred, Ranjit would probably not be the best person to undertake this task in view of his sister's involvement and the clinic manager would be best placed to ensure this was done in accordance with any rules and procedures.

Question 40

Answer and rationale

Answer D, 'Not important', is correct. Obviously, the seriousness of breaching patient confidentiality is paramount, so the issue of Ranjit's sister is of no consequence. In fact, by the act of informing Ranjit, the sister has breached Julia's confidence probably because of the seriousness of the matter.

Question set 13

Question 41

Answer and rationale

Answer A, 'Very important', is correct. That two of the GPs do not have a very good reputation is based on rumour only. Giles has no evidence to support negatively commenting on the ability of any of the doctors. Even where Giles might feel the rumours have some foundation after seeing the GPs at first hand, it is very important that he does not disclose these rumours to Sara.

Question 42

Answer and rationale
Answer C, 'Minor importance', is correct. Giles has been honest with Sara that there are rumours, but has not been specific about these or named any of the related GPs. He is rightly passing the responsibility back to Sara to make her own decision. It is therefore of minor importance in the fact of confirming there are rumours but nothing beyond that.

Question set 14

Question 43

Answer and rationale
Answer D, 'Not important', is correct. In this case there is only a small amount of money involved and the possible culprit could be a whole host of people, including all the medical staff with access to the wards, domestic staff, visitors, etc. It is highly unlikely that the police would be able to do a great deal in these circumstances. If there were a sequence of such thefts over a period of time, or a substantial sum of money stolen, then the police may well be involved in tracing the offender. Summoning the police in such cases would normally require the consent of a senior manager.

Question 44

Answer and rationale
Answer A, 'Very important', is correct. It is very important that Raja should attempt to reassure the patient by taking an interest in and showing concern for what has occurred, and that the theft will be brought to the attention of staff within the EAU.

Question 45

Answer and rationale
Answer C, 'Minor importance', is correct. Although this seems to be common sense, it should already be a matter that has been raised. Patients should know they have a responsibility for their possessions and in particular their money. There is no harm in reminding them of this, but in this situation the most important thing is to reassure the patient from whom money has been stolen.

Question 46

Answer and rationale
Answer D, 'Not important', is correct. It is highly unlikely that the strategy of asking the culprit to replace the money will work, even though the suggestion is probably done with the best intentions. Although not stated directly, it appears that this strategy is assuming that the culprit is part of the medical team and it is highly likely this will have a negative effect on the team. In effect, this strategy is not important at all in resolving the theft.

Question set 15

Question 47

Answer and rationale

Answer B, 'Important', is correct. Although it is important to stop the conversation to ensure that Rose makes no further inappropriate comments that can be overheard, this may well embarrass her. A better strategy might be to change the subject of the conversation and then speak to Rose later.

Question 48

Answer and rationale

Answer A, 'Very important', is correct. It is very important that Ludmila confronts Rose about her inappropriate comments and this would be best done in private away from the café. It is assumed that Ludmila would then determine any further action dependent on Rose's response, although the seriousness of such comments should involve further steps.

Question 49

Answer and rationale

Answer C, 'Minor importance', is correct. Ludmila actually witnessed the inappropriate remarks so would be in the best position to confront Rose. Although also witnessed by Mahesh and Ellen, there is really no need for them to be present at the confrontation as it may appear heavy-handed. However, their presence would support Ludmila's actions, so it can't be described as having no importance.

Question 50

Answer and rationale

Answer A, 'Very important', is correct. It is very important that Ludmila raises the matter with Rose's line manager. The incident was witnessed by a number of people in the café and the line manager must make sure there is no reoccurrence of this type of behaviour, whatever course of action may be taken.

Question 51

Answer and rationale

Answer D, 'Not important', is correct. There is absolutely no need for Ludmila to speak to the recruited assistant about this matter. It will have been dealt with by the hospital management, and to speak to the assistant may well have serious negative consequences. The remarks were not made about the individual as a person and informing her of the remarks could be very upsetting.

Question set 16

Question 52

Answer and rationale

Answer D, 'Not important', is correct. Viewing adult pornography is not a criminal offence and therefore informing the police would not be appropriate in these circumstances.

Question 53

Answer and rationale

Answer A, 'Very important', is correct. Although not a criminal offence, it must still be considered inappropriate both to view adult pornographic images while at work and make use of hospital property for these purposes. It is very important that Dr Phillips confront his colleague about this and the course of action that would hopefully stop any future occurrence. This would ensure that the matter is resolved at a local level. Should Dr Phillips be aware of any future similar behaviour by his colleague, then reporting this to the hospital authorities might be a necessary step.

Question 54

Answer and rationale

Answer C, 'Minor importance', is correct. At this stage, it would be important for Dr Phillips to nip the problem in the bud by confronting the colleague. Reporting the matter to medical personnel at this time would not be appropriate, but should the problem reoccur, reporting the matter might then seem to be the proper course of action.

Question 55

Answer and rationale

Answer B, 'Important', is correct. It would not be appropriate for Dr Phillips to inform a senior colleague about his colleague's misuse of hospital property and viewing adult pornography while on duty. The preferred action is for Dr Phillips to confront the colleague but, dependent on his response or any concern about a repetition, informing a colleague is quite acceptable.

Question set 17

Question 56

Answer and rationale

Answer B, 'Important', is correct. In these circumstances, Kristina is a 'vulnerable adult' and Dr Mwanga has a duty of care towards her beyond her treatment at the hospital.

Dr Mwanga should inform Kristina that she is unable to agree to maintain confidence when Kristina is at serious risk of further harm. Also, the mention of young children in the family unit further exacerbates the risk. The normal procedure would be for Dr Mwanga to inform a senior colleague, when procedures for informing the police and social services would be put into operation.

Question 57

Answer and rationale

Answer A, 'Very important', is correct. It is very important that Dr Mwanga fully documents the conversation with Kristina, including the fact that her husband was responsible for causing her injuries. However, the doctor should reassure Kristina that these notes are confidential and that only her senior colleague will see them at the outset. Obviously, they may not be able to be held in confidence if it is considered that the risk of harm to Kristina or her family is such that it requires the intervention of other agencies. In the event of a criminal prosecution, the documented conversation would be admissible in any proceedings.

Question 58

Answer and rationale

Answer A, 'Very important', is correct. It is appropriate that Dr Mwanga talks to her senior colleague about Kristina's situation. The duty of care to her patient demands this, whether or not she is a junior doctor. Kristina is obviously in a 'high-risk' category of further abuse and there is also a possible risk relating to the two young children. In speaking with a senior colleague, it could be argued that she is not breaching her patient's confidence as it would be expected that a senior member of the team should be consulted in such circumstances.

Question set 18

Question 59

Answer and rationale

Answer C, 'Minor importance', is correct. This course of action would seem particularly hard, especially where the feigned sickness was probably a one-off affair. Although Dr Peterson's absence would have required covering in some way, reporting the matter to a senior manager would not allow her an opportunity to ensure there was no reoccurrence.

Question 60

Answer and rationale

Answer A, 'Very important', is correct. It is very important that Dr Peterson is confronted about her behaviour and given the chance to ensure that it is not repeated. The proviso of reporting any future similar misdemeanour is quite proper in these circumstances.

Question set 19

Question 61

Answer and rationale

Answer C, 'Minor importance', is correct. This course of action may appear to be acceptable where Aaron as a third party (not the GP) is hearing the medical history of a close friend of his sister. The reality of being a GP is that such 'conflicts' occur quite often where the GP is dealing with a patient within their social circle. However, the confidentiality that exists between a GP and their patients is accepted as sacrosanct. Therefore, Aaron's actions in leaving the room are of minor importance.

Question 62

Answer and rationale

Answer B, 'Important', is correct. Aaron would not be expected to know if there are any guidelines in relation to this type of situation, but seeking help and guidance as soon as possible is important in that the doctor would clarify the situation with regard to patient confidentiality.

Question 63

Answer and rationale

Answer D, 'Not important', is correct. It would not be important to speak to the patient even if Aaron had remained in the consulting room for the duration of the examination. No doubt there would have been an acceptance by the patient that anything that occurred or was discussed would be confidential. The only purpose here would be to reassure the patient that Aaron would not disclose any information to a third party, in this instance probably his sister.

Question set 20

Question 64

Answer and rationale

Answer D, 'Not important', is correct. Omar cannot ignore such an important issue as Alex's cocaine addiction. It is highly likely that patient safety would be jeopardised because of this addiction.

Question 65

Answer and rationale

Answer B, 'Important', is correct. This is an important thing to do as it places the responsibility firmly with Alex. He needed to make this decision due to the impact the addiction may well have on his medical performance. However, Omar also has a responsibility to report this matter irrespective of what Alex decides.

Question 66

Answer and rationale

Answer D, 'Not important', is correct. Omar might find that there are no problems with Alex's performance at this time, but his continuing addiction might well cause problems in the future. Therefore, this is a very inappropriate thing to do in a situation with such serious possible outcomes.

Question 67

Answer and rationale

Answer A, 'Very important', is correct. It is very important that Omar reports Alex's cocaine addiction to senior management. There is every likelihood that the addiction would impact on Alex's ability to perform his duties to the required standards. Additionally, cocaine use is a criminal offence and it would be for senior managers to determine whether or not this should be reported to the police.

Part III
Practice tests, questions and answers for the UKCAT

This part of the book aims to support you to further develop your UKCAT skills and exam technique. Working through these questions should enable you to reach your potential through developing a better understanding of the areas being tested.

In total, this section provides over **300** questions across the four subtests.

Chapters 6 and 7 each contain full tests comprising Verbal Reasoning, Quantitative Reasoning, Abstract Reasoning and Decision Analysis. The answers and rationale for each question are included in Chapter 8.

It is anticipated that you may wish to sit the tests simulating examination conditions, and instructions in relation to timing have been provided before each subtest. You will need a paper and pencil in order to write down the answers to the questions and for the Quantitative Reasoning subtest to undertake mathematical calculations.

Chapter 6
Practice test 1

1. Verbal Reasoning practice subtest 1

Answers on page 292.

The Verbal Reasoning subtest is an on-screen test that consists of 44 items associated with 11 reading passages. For each reading passage there are four questions in the form of statements. Three answer options are provided for each statement: True; False; Can't Tell. Only one of these options is correct. A period of 22 minutes is allowed for the subtest, with 1 minute for instruction and the remaining 21 minutes for items.

The answers and rationale for this subtest can be found on page 292.

Passage 1: discrimination and mental health

Social stigma and prejudice are examples of discrimination, and mental health service users can often find that society and the community are unwilling to engage with them. This can be expressed directly in the form of explicit rejection, ridicule or aggression, or indirectly in the form of dismissal or avoidance. This is largely based on fear and misunderstanding of what mental health means, and it is not uncommon for questions of capability and risk to be presented as reasons for exclusion. Indirect discrimination is often more complex to identify, as it results from a misunderstanding and adaptation rather than a direct and explicit rejection or exclusion. For those with mental health issues, it is based more on attitudes and social norms. Some types of stigma and stereotyping can be defined as indirect discrimination, for example presuming that an individual is unable to make decisions or unable to take part in a cognitive activity.

Passage 1: question 1
Discrimination affects the recipient's sense of self-worth and overall self-image.

A True

B False

C Can't Tell

Passage 1: question 2
A lack of awareness can lead to people with mental health issues being excluded from society.

A   True

B   False

C   Can't Tell

Passage I: question 3
Rarely questions of capability and risk are presented as reasons for excluding those with mental health problems.

A   True

B   False

C   Can't Tell

Passage I: question 4
Mental health creates a barrier to social interaction, services, employment and training.

A.   True

B.   False

C.   Can't Tell

Passage II: patient choice

If your GP refers you to a specialist, you can choose the hospital at which you want to be treated. You can choose any hospital in England that meets the NHS standards and this could include independent or private hospitals which are free as part of the Choice agenda. To support Choice, most GP practices use a national IT system called Choose and Book. You can choose the hospital with the best reputation, shortest waiting times, or simply the one that is most convenient. Choice of hospitals may not be appropriate for all services. Services where speedy access to diagnosis and treatment are particularly important are not required to offer a choice of hospital. This includes emergency attendances or admissions, patients attending a Rapid Access Chest Pain Clinic under the two-week maximum waiting time, and patients attending cancer services under the two-week maximum waiting time. Mental health and maternity services are also not included, although your GP may offer you a choice of providers if you are referred for these services.

Passage II: question 5
Because of the Choice agenda you will always be able to choose the hospital which you want to be treated at except for mental health and maternity services.

A   True

B   False

C   Can't Tell

Passage II: question 6

Patients suffering from cancer and chest pains do not have to be offered a choice of which hospital they can attend.

A True

B False

C Can't Tell

Passage II: question 7

GPs in Wales and Scotland do not have access to the Choose and Book IT system.

A True

B False

C Can't Tell

Passage II: question 8

Rapid Access Chest Pain Clinics and cancer services are not provided by independent and private hospitals.

A True

B False

C Can't Tell

Passage III: *diabetes and sleeping disorders*

According to the NHS, type 2 diabetes, which is often associated with obesity, affects about 2.3 million people in the UK, with at least 500,000 more who are not aware that they have the condition. Research has linked type 2 diabetes and sleeping disorders, suggesting there is a connection between diabetes and the way the body responds to the 24-hour cycle of light and dark. New genetic research points to a gene involved in detecting melatonin – a hormone that is part of the body's internal clock – and an increased risk of diabetes. The findings of the research will raise the possibility of genetic tests to identify people vulnerable to developing type 2 diabetes.

Passage III: question 9

People who are obese are more likely to suffer from sleeping disorders.

A True

B False

C Can't Tell

Passage III: question 10
Genetic tests are available to identify people with type 2 diabetes.

A True

B False

C Can't Tell

Passage III: question 11
There are about 2.8 million people in the UK affected by type 2 diabetes.

A True

B False

C Can't Tell

Passage III: question 12
People with type 2 diabetes are often awake during the night and sleep during the day.

A True

B False

C Can't Tell

Passage IV: cost of life-saving drugs reduced

A radical deal has been struck between drug companies and the Health Service for the cost of life-saving drugs to be significantly reduced. Currently, a number of effective drugs are not used because they are too expensive. Previously, drug companies would charge what they believed the market would bear, but under the new agreement companies will offer flexible prices. They will still be able to charge what they want, say, for new cancer or heart drugs, but companies will enter into negotiations with the Health Service for a realistic 'value' to be placed on the drug. The new scheme may see savings of about £200m, in the first year, rising to £300m in subsequent years.

Passage IV: question 13
In offering more flexible prices for their products the profits made by drug companies will decline.

A True

B False

C Can't Tell

Passage IV: question 14

People are dying because the Health Service cannot afford to buy drugs that would keep them alive.

A   True

B   False

C   Can't Tell

Passage IV: question 15

The fact that drug companies are willing to enter into negotiations with the Health Service about drug pricing shows they are more concerned with people living and dying rather than profiting from the misfortune of others.

A   True

B   False

C   Can't Tell

Passage IV: question 16

When the Health Service can afford to buy more effective drugs the death rate in relation to people suffering heart disease and cancer will be significantly reduced.

A   True

B   False

C   Can't Tell

Passage V: cross-curriculum themed classes

In an overhaul of education for 5–11-year-olds it is proposed that history, geography and science will be removed from the curriculum and their content taught through cross-curriculum themed classes. It is considered that the teaching of rigid subject areas in primary schools was making children's knowledge and understanding shallow. In addition to the curriculum changes, there is a proposal that teachers should encourage children's social and emotional well-being in an explicit recognition that schools must help to cure some of the 'social ills' facing society.

Passage V: question 17

History, geography and science will no longer be taught in primary schools.

A   True

B   False

C   Can't Tell

Passage V: question 18

Teachers have a responsibility for the social fabric of society.

A   True

B   False

C   Can't Tell

Passage V: question 19

Children under 11 have only a superficial understanding of history, geography and science.

A   True

B   False

C   Can't Tell

Passage V: question 20

Cross-curriculum themed classes will result in primary school children having a better understanding of history, geography and science.

A   True

B   False

C   Can't Tell

Passage VI: educational success and communication skills

A think tank has reported that children growing up in the most deprived homes need to be taught to speak and have lessons in empathy and self-control. Some children from the most deprived homes have only been 'grunted' at by their parents, and empathy and self-control will not have been learnt at home. Communication skills are seen as the road to educational success, but in poorer homes children only hear 500 different words a day compared to 1,500 in a better-off household. From this it is estimated that about one in ten children start school unable to talk in sentences or understand simple instructions. In some parts of the country this can rise to 50% of four- and five-year-olds. It is believed that parents in deprived areas often feel alienated from a child they did not want, may be depressed by their circumstances or not be functioning socially and emotionally because of drugs or alcohol.

Passage VI: question 21

Children from deprived homes will not attain the same educational standards as children from middle-class homes.

A True

B False

C Can't Tell

Passage VI: question 22
In poorer homes less articulate conversations take place between carers and children.

A True

B False

C Can't Tell

Passage VI: question 23
Parents who are drug addicts or alcoholics are more likely to have children who have difficulty communicating when they first attend school.

A True

B False

C Can't Tell

Passage VI: question 24
In better-off households children are likely to hear five times as many different words spoken in the home each day as children from deprived homes.

A True

B False

C Can't Tell

Passage VII: patterns of communicable disease

The patterns of communicable disease are the result of the interactions between the infectious agent, the host and the environment. The source of infection may be human, there may be animal reservoirs such as brucellosis in cattle or leptospirosis in rats, or reservoirs may exist in the environment in the water or soil. There are a number of modes of transmission between the source and the host through direct or indirect transmission (by vectors or vehicles). Vehicles such as water or food carry the infective agent while vectors such as mosquitoes for malaria are part of the life cycle. The transmission of infection may be by inhalation, ingestion, direct skin or mucosal contact, sexual contact, injection, or cross-placental routes. The susceptibility of the host is influenced by age, natural immunity, artificial immunity (active or passive), nutritional status and immune suppression.

Passage VII: question 25
Immunisation can protect people from contacting certain communicable diseases.

A True

B False

C Can't Tell

Passage VII: question 26
Communicable diseases are continually changing and new communicable diseases emerging.

A True

B False

C Can't Tell

Passage VII: question 27
A person's age, diet and lifestyle choices have little impact on their susceptibility to disease.

A True

B False

C Can't Tell

Passage VII: question 28
The atmosphere is a vehicle that can carry an infective agent.

A True

B False

C Can't Tell

Passage VIII: the meaning of 'normal'

Different people use the word 'normal' in different ways. A philosopher views the normal as the most usual. Psychologists and statisticians refer to normal as the middle range of a distribution of values (i.e. statistically normal). A sociologist defines 'normal' as that which is in line with a rule for a particular social or cultural group in society. The *Oxford English Dictionary* defines 'normal' as 'conforming to a standard'. In medicine 'normal' is often used to mean an absence of physiological pathology. In common speech, 'normal' may simply mean 'not abnormal, not strange'.

Passage VIII: question 29

'Normal' can refer to the lack of a significant deviation from the average.

A True

B False

C Can't Tell

Passage VIII: question 30

Violating social norms or standards may be normal dependent on the social and cultural group to which a person belongs.

A True

B False

C Can't Tell

Passage VIII: question 31

People are often referred to as 'strange' if they are seen not to agree with the views and principles of the majority.

A True

B False

C Can't Tell

Passage VIII: question 32

In medicine, everyone who has a disease is considered to be 'abnormal'.

A True

B False

C Can't Tell

Passage IX: Internet restrictions

A survey of managers aged 35 and under found that two-thirds of employers monitor staff use of the Internet during working hours and block access to sites deemed irrelevant to the job. This has been branded as 'old-fashioned', with senior executives not encouraging the benefits of exploiting new technology. Some 16% of managers described their senior executives as dinosaurs. Senior executives were pessimistic that staff wanted access to the Internet for research, professional development and other aspects of getting the job done. A total of 65% of organisations monitored Internet usage, and this rose to 88% in the police. Also, 65% blocked access to 'inappropriate' sites, with this rising to 89% in local government and 90% in the utilities.

Passage IX: question 33

There is a 'generation gap' in views about the use of Internet technology at work.

A   True

B   False

C   Can't Tell

Passage IX: question 34

Senior executives consider Internet usage as a waste of time.

A   True

B   False

C   Can't Tell

Passage IX: question 35

Monitoring Internet usage is higher in the police because of their accountability.

A   True

B   False

C   Can't Tell

Passage IX: question 36

Around 35% of organisations do not block access to 'inappropriate' Internet sites.

A   True

B   False

C   Can't Tell

Passage X: Europe sets working week limit

The European Parliament has scrapped the special treatment granted to some sovereign states to allow people to work in excess of the 48 hours a week limit set by the European Union. However, the UK government intends to carry on the battle to retain the right to longer working hours, believing it gives a choice to UK workers to work in excess of 48 hours if they so wish. The trade unions are in favour of the European maximum 48-hour limit that is averaged out over a one-year period. The government believe the working hours limit would cost the UK economy tens of billions of pounds over the next ten years. In addition to the 48-hour working week, the European Parliament has also decided that 'inactive' on-call time for employees, such as doctors, should be counted as working hours, a position the government considers will hamper the National Health Service.

Passage X: question 37

If the European Parliament decision is accepted by the UK, no one will work more than 48 hours a week.

A True

B False

C Can't Tell

Passage X: question 38

Because 'inactive' on-call time for doctors will be counted as working hours, the National Health Service will need to recruit more doctors.

A True

B False

C Can't Tell

Passage X: question 39

Trade unions are not in favour of their members working overtime.

A True

B False

C Can't Tell

Passage X: question 40

People working in excess of the 48-hour working time limit make a significant contribution to the UK economy.

A True

B False

C Can't Tell

Passage XI: new technology helps the disabled

Access to education for people with disabilities and learning difficulties is now being helped by new technology. Sophisticated software turns speech into written form for the hearing impaired, while printed words are transformed into sounds at the click of a button for the blind. Those suffering from dyslexia can alter the size or colour on a printed document to make it easier to read. The ability to make effective use of this new technology can depend on a student's age and IT literacy. This is particularly true of mature disabled students who did not grow up with new technology. However, the difficulties in accessing learning tend to lie not in the student's disability or learning problem, but in the task they are expected to perform where time may be a crucial factor. What can take an able-bodied person a few minutes can mean hours of work for someone with a disability. Overall, disabled students have generally become agile users of new technologies, developing personal strategies depending on their needs and making full use of whatever technical support is on offer.

Passage XI: question 41

Technology is more of a benefit than a barrier to learning.

A   True

B   False

C   Can't Tell

Passage XI: question 42

Technology will help all people with disabilities and learning difficulties obtain academic qualifications.

A   True

B   False

C   Can't Tell

Passage XI: question 43

Universities have to offer all students equal learning opportunities.

A   True

B   False

C   Can't Tell

Passage XI: question 44

New technology allows students to study in previously unimagined ways.

A   True

B   False

C   Can't Tell

2. Quantitative Reasoning practice subtest 1

Answers on page 300.

The Quantitative Reasoning subtest consists of 36 items associated with tables, charts and/or graphs. A period of 25 minutes is allowed for the test, with one minute for instruction and 24 minutes for items.

Remember that each of the questions is always accompanied by five possible answers, A, B, C, D and E, and that only ONE answer is correct. Also remember to read through all five competing answers before selecting what you consider to be the correct answer. By reading the four 'incorrect' answers you should confirm that your choice is in fact correct.

The answers and rationale for this subtest can be found on page 300.

Questions I to 4 relate to the table below. This provides the 'scores' of a sample of men and women who have sat the on-screen hazard simulation test as part of the driving licence test requirement. The test has a maximum possible score of 70 and the pass mark is a minimum of 37 correct responses.

Respondent	Score	Respondent	Score
1 (Female)	38	11 (Male)	40
2 (Male)	29	12 (Female)	57
3 (Female)	47	13 (Female)	39
4 (Female)	39	14 (Female)	35
5 (Male)	44	15 (Female)	46
6 (Male)	23	16 (Male)	33
7 (Male)	37	17 (Female)	31
8 (Male)	43	18 (Male)	37
9 (Female)	54	19 (Female)	45
10 (Male)	36	20 (Female)	41

1. What is the percentage of the sample who successfully passed the on-screen hazard simulation test?

   A 50%

   B 55%

   C 60%

   D 65%

   E 70%

2. What is the mode of the females' scores who sat the on-screen hazard simulation test?

   A 31

   B 39

   C 41

   D 46

   E 57

3. What is the range of the males' scores who sat the on-screen hazard simulation test?

   A 21

   B 23

   C 33

   D 39

   E 44

4. In relation to the scores for the on-screen hazard simulation test, which one of the following statements is correct?

   A More than half of the respondents scored above the mean.

   B The ratio of males that passed the test compared to the number of successful females was 1:3.

   C Less than half of the respondents scored above the mean.

   D More than half of the male respondents attained a score above the mean.

   E Less than half of the female respondents attained a score above the mean.

Questions 5 to 8 relate to a medium-sized enterprise whose products are mainly for markets outside the European Union (EU). The table below provides a list of the current postal charges to non-EU countries.

	SURFACE MAIL				AIRMAIL		
Weight	**Letters**	**Packets**		**Weight**	**Letters**	**Packets**
Not over	**Price**	**Price**		**Not over**	**Price**	**Price**
				10g	£6.60	£7.45
20g	58p	99p		20g	£6.60	£7.45
60g	£1.00	99p		60g	£7.25	£7.45
100g	£1.41	99p		100g	£7.86	£7.45
150g	£1.99	£1.32		140g	£8.51	£7.76
500g	£5.86	£3.65		180g	£9.16	£8.10
750g	£8.62	£5.32		220g	£9.74	£8.42
1,000g	£11.36	£6.98		240g	£10.04	£8.57
1,500g	£16.87	£10.31		280g	£10.61	£8.89
2,000g	£21.64	£13.22		300g	£10.91	£9.06

Surface mail: Letters over 2,000g cannot be sent by surface mail; packets over 2,000g, for each 50g thereafter add 28p.

Airmail: Letters/packets over 300g, for every 20g up to 500g add 16p; every 20g up to 1kg add 20p; every 200g above 1kg add 18p.

5. The company has four letters each weighing 150g and five packets, three of which weigh 200g and the remainder each weighing 300g. As a percentage, how much cheaper would surface mail be compared to airmail?

   A 30.6%

   B 32.5%

   C 57.8%

   D 67.5%

   E 74.2%

6. Unlike surface mail, airmail rates are currently subject to VAT at 20%. If VAT were not charged on airmail rates, what would be the cost of sending 25 letters each weighing 100g?

   A £158.20

   B £164.10

   C £170.20

   D £180.80

   E £191.48

7. Which one of the following statements is correct?

   A Airmail letters weighing 1 kilogram cost an extra £6.60 in addition to the price of a 300g letter.

   B Compared to airmail it is cheaper to send a packet weighing 2.5kg by surface mail.

   C It is always cheaper to send packets by airmail compared to letters by airmail.

   D Sending a 100g letter by surface mail is about $\frac{1}{10}$ of the price of sending a 100g letter by airmail.

   E The cost of sending a 4 kilogram packet by surface mail would be £32.84.

8. The company secretary has 27 letters to post with each letter being of the same weight. The total weight of the letters is 4.5 kilograms. What would be the cost of surface mail for 27 letters?

   A £53.73

   B £79.60

   C £117.20

   D £146.50

   E £158.22

Questions 9 to 12 are about a town bookshop, and shown in the table below are some of the broad classifications used by the bookshop in cataloguing their books and the number of books in stock per classification.

Book Classifications	Current Stock Level
Paperback Fiction	12,750
Biography	3,800
History	5,700
Science	3,450
Geography	2,275
Medical	3,500
Nature	4,125
Education	7,600
Reference	10,300
Ancient World	1,900

9. To the nearest whole number, what percentage of stock in the bookshop is classified as 'history'?

   A 3%

   B 5%

   C 7%

   D 10%

   E 12%

10. The total selling price of the paperback fiction books currently in stock is £101,362.50. How much is the actual selling price, per paperback fiction book, where there is a promotion of 4 for the price of 3 on all paperback fiction books?

   A £4.46

   B £5.16

   C £5.96

   D £6.17

   E £6.45

11. The total selling price of the medical books currently in stock is £31,324.00. If the bookshop buys the medical books for $\frac{2}{3}$ of the selling price how much profit would it make if $\frac{2}{8}$ of the current stock were sold (to 2 decimal places)?

A £1,305.17

B £1,976.43

C £2,610.34

D £3,915.50

E £10,441.33

12. What is the range of the number of books currently in stock in the bookshop by classification?

A 2,450

B 5,150

C 7,050

D 9,250

E 10,850

Questions 13 to 16 relate to the information contained in the pie chart below. This information shows the average number of text messages per person per month, for last year, across ten countries. The percentage change over the past five years for each country is shown in parentheses.

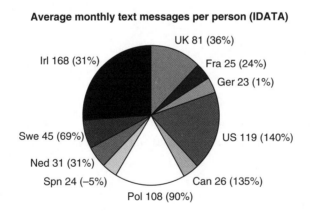

Average monthly text messages per person (IDATA)

UK 81 (36%)

Irl 168 (31%)

Fra 25 (24%)

Ger 23 (1%)

Swe 45 (69%)

US 119 (140%)

Ned 31 (31%)

Spn 24 (–5%)

Can 26 (135%)

Pol 108 (90%)

13. From the information contained in the pie chart, which one of the following statements is correct?

A The number of countries in which people average more than 80 text messages a month exceeds those with less than this number.

B Countries whose average number of text messages per person per month is less than 25 account for one-tenth of those included in the survey.

C The average number of texts per person for Ireland (Irl) is 2,016 per annum, up from 128 per month five years ago.

D The average percentage change over the past five years for the top five countries where people send the most text messages per month is less than 70%.

E Spain (Spn) has the lowest average number of text messages per person per month.

14. What percentage of countries has an average number of text messages in excess of 32 per person per month?

A 25%

B 30%

C 40%

D 50%

E 60%

15. What is the ratio of the number of messages per person per month in the UK and US combined, compared to the total number of messages per person per month living in the other countries within the survey?

A 1:3

B 1:6

C 2:7

D 3:8

E 4:9

16. The average cost of a text message for all countries is £0.05p. How much would the annual average number of text messages per individual cost in Ireland (€1 = £0.80p) and the US ($1 = £0.68p)?

A €10.50 and $88.00

B €76.80 and $57.40

C €100.80 and $71.40

D €126.00 and $105.00

E €226.80 and $177.40

Questions 17 to 20 relate to the figure which shows the birth rates in Scotland over a four-year period according to the age range of the women who gave birth, shown as a percentage of the total births.

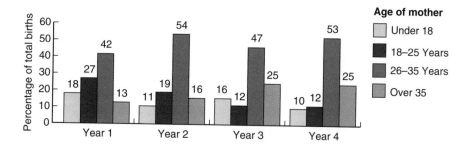

17. Which one of the following statements is supported by the information in the figure above?

    A Between Year 1 and Year 4 the birth rate for women over 35 was about a third more than for women under 18.

    B Between Year 1 and Year 4 the birth rate for women aged 26–35 remained within a margin of 12%.

    C Between Year 1 and Year 4 the birth rate for women under 18 decreased by nearly three-quarters.

    D Between Year 1 and Year 4 the average percentage birth rate for women aged 18–25 years was over 20%.

    E Between Year 1 and Year 4 the percentage of births for women aged over 35 increased by less than half.

18. If 750 women aged 26–35 gave birth to one child each in Year 2, how many women aged 18–25, to the nearest 50, gave birth in the same year, assuming that they each had one child?

    A 350

    B 300

    C 250

    D 200

    E 150

19. Which one of the following statements is supported by the information in the figure above?

    A Over the four years the percentage birth rate for women aged 26–35 was consistently three times greater than for the other age ranges of women added together.

    B The least significant rise or fall in birth rates over four years was in relation to women aged 26–35 years.

  C The lowest percentage swing in birth rates over the four years was in relation to women aged over 35.

  D The single highest fall in birth rates during the four years was in relation to women aged 18–25.

  E Between Year 3 and Year 4, women aged over 35 were twice as likely to give birth than women under the age of 18.

20. What is the average percentage of total births to women aged over 35, between Year 1 and Year 4?

  Closest to:

  A 25%

  B 20%

  C 15%

  D 12%

  E 10%

Questions 21 to 24 are about the table below. This shows the results of a survey about the weights of 120 people, 24 to 32 years of age, selected at random to participate in a study on obesity.

Weight in kilograms (kg)	<50	51–60	61–70	71–80	81–90	>90
Number of people	10	20	21	29	26	14

21. How many people weigh less than 71 kilograms?

  A 10

  B 20

  C 41

  D 51

  E 81

22. What can you say categorically about the weight of 25% of the people surveyed?

  A They are less than 70 kilograms.

  B They are more than 70 kilograms and less than 90 kilograms.

  C They are at most 60 kilograms.

  D They are less than 80 kilograms.

  E They are at least 71 kilograms.

23. What fraction of the people surveyed weigh in excess of 80 kilograms?

    A $\frac{3}{8}$

    B $\frac{1}{3}$

    C $\frac{1}{4}$

    D $\frac{1}{2}$

    E $\frac{3}{4}$

24. What is the ratio of the number of people who weigh less than 61 kilograms compared to the number who weigh 61 kilograms and above?

    A 1:3

    B 1:4

    C 2:3

    D 3:4

    E 3:5

Questions 25 to 28 are about a college and the student population. The college currently has 19,876 students registered and 8,241 of these are studying a science subject. Also, 6,037 of the students are part-time. It is not possible to study a science subject part-time.

25. Approximately, what is the percentage of students who are part-time?

    A 7%

    B 15%

    C 20%

    D 25%

    E 30%

26. What is the approximate ratio of students studying science compared to the rest of students at the college?

    A 2:3

    B 2:5

    C 3:2

    D 3:4

    E 3:5

27. Student loans are not available to part-time students, and those studying science subjects obtain grants and do not need to obtain a student loan. If all of those students entitled to a student loan actually obtain a loan, how much is the total cost, to the nearest £m, of providing the loans if each student is in receipt of £2,300?

    A £13m

    B £14m

    C £19m

    D £32m

    E £46m

28. The student accommodation for the college is divided into blocks: 21 blocks can hold 48 students in each, while 38 blocks can hold 93 students in each. What is the best approximation for the maximum capacity of students in the college accommodation blocks?

    A 1,000

    B 2,000

    C 3,500

    D 4,600

    E 6,000

Questions 29 to 32 relate to a floor layer who is tiling the floor of five bathrooms in a small hotel before the bathroom furniture is installed. Four of the five bathrooms are of the same dimensions, as shown in the figure below. The fifth bathroom is, in area, $\frac{3}{4}$ the size of one of the other bathrooms.

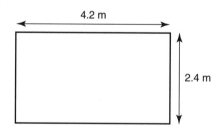

4.2 m

2.4 m

29. What is the total area of flooring that requires tiling to the nearest whole metre?

    A 40m²

    B 44m²

    C 48m²

    D 52m²

    E 56m²

30. The tiles that are being used measure 30cm². How many tiles, to the nearest whole tile, would be required for one of the larger bathrooms?

   A 82

   B 88

   C 92

   D 96

   E 112

Before laying the tiles, the hotel owner decides to fit showers in the four larger bathrooms, as shown in the diagram below. The floor area to be tiled has been reduced by the size of the shower. Note the measurements are now in millimetres.

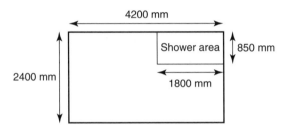

31. In order to find the new floor area of the bathroom that requires tiling, which one of the following is correct?

   A (4200 × 2400) − (1800 × 850)

   B (2400 − 850) + (4200 − 1800)

   C (4200 × 1800) − (2400 − 850)

   D ((2400 − 850) + (4200 − 1800)

   E (850 + 2400) − (4200 × 2400)

32. The floor layer has estimated that he will need about 500 tiles to complete the job. At the builders' merchants the tiles cost £2.75 each but there is a discount of 12% per hundred. Also, there is a buy-back policy of £1.25 per tile. If the builder uses 430 tiles, how much will he have paid if he returns the unused tiles?

   A £1,035.50

   B £1,080.00

   C £1,122.50

   D £1,210.00

   E £1,375.00

Questions 33 to 36 relate to the table below that provides information on strikes and stoppages in the United Kingdom over a 12-month period.

Strikes and stoppages in the UK: 12-month period

Number of disputes	Reasons for disputes	Working days lost
52	Pay	48,300
12	Pattern of hours	6,580
24	Redundancy	26,125
5	Union matters	2,460
11	Working conditions	4,900
25	Manning/work allocation	18,260
25	Dismissal/discipline	8,700

33. What is the mean of the number of disputes over the 12-month period?

    A 12

    B 22

    C 24

    D 25

    E 27

34. What is the mode of the number of disputes over the 12-month period?

    A 17

    B 21

    C 25

    D 28

    E 32

35. What is the range of the total working days lost over the 12-month period?

    A 8,700

    B 16,475

    C 25,425

    D 36,690

    E 45,840

36. In relation to the table, which one of the following statements is correct?

   A On average, redundancy had more days lost than any other reason for disputes.

   B The average number of working days lost in relation to disputes over pay is less than those in relation to union matters.

   C The lowest number of disputes accounted for the least number of working days lost.

   D Manning/work allocation and dismissal/discipline disputes together accounted for over half of the total number of working days lost.

   E Compared to pay, the number of pattern of hours disputes were about 10% less.

3. Abstract Reasoning practice subtest 1

Answers on page 308.

The Abstract Reasoning subtest is an on-screen test that consists of 55 items associated with 11 pairs of Set A and Set B shapes. Five test shapes are presented with each pair of Set A and Set B shapes, and there are three answer options for each test shape: Set A, Set B or Neither Set. Only ONE of the three answer options is correct. Each test shape is presented with the pair of Set A and Set B shapes on a separate screen with the three answer options below. A period of 14 minutes is allowed for the test, with one minute for instruction and the remaining 13 minutes for items.

N.B. An additional 20 questions have been included at the end of this section to offer you extra practice.

The answers and rationale for this subtest can be found on page 308.

Questions 1 to 5

Set A

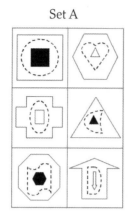

Set B

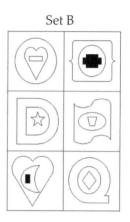

Test shapes

| Question 1 | Question 2 | Question 3 | Question 4 | Question 5 |

Questions 6 to 10

Set A

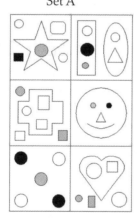

Set B

Test shapes

| Question 6 | Question 7 | Question 8 | Question 9 | Question 10 |

Questions 11 to 15

Set A

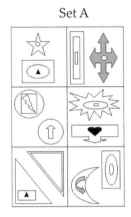

Set B

Test shapes

Question 11

Question 12

Question 13

Question 14

Question 15

Questions 16 to 20

Set A

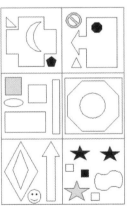

Set B

Test shapes

Question 16

Question 17

Question 18

Question 19

Question 20

Questions 21 to 25

Set A

Set B

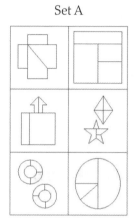

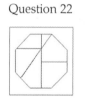

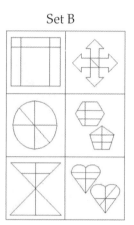

Test shapes

Question 21	Question 22	Question 23	Question 24	Question 25

Questions 26 to 30

Set A

Set B

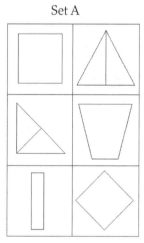

Test shapes

Question 26	Question 27	Question 28	Question 29	Question 30

Questions 31 to 35

Set A

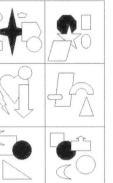

Set B

Test shapes

Question 31	Question 32	Question 33	Question 34	Question 35

Questions 36 to 40

Set A

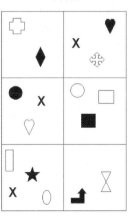

Set B

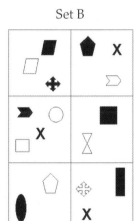

Test shapes

Question 36	Question 37	Question 38	Question 39	Question 40

Questions 41 to 45

Set A

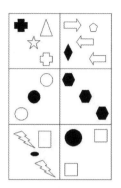

Set B

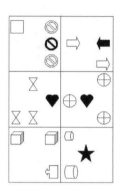

Test shapes

Question 41	Question 42	Question 43	Question 44	Question 45

Questions 46 to 50

Set A

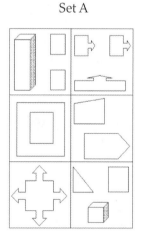

Set B

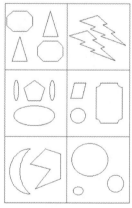

Test shapes

Question 46	Question 47	Question 48	Question 49	Question 50

Questions 51 to 55

Set A

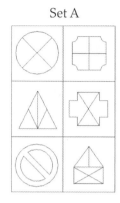

Set B

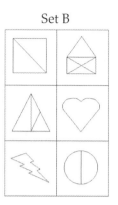

Test shapes

| Question 51 | Question 52 | Question 53 | Question 54 | Question 55 |

Questions 56 to 60

Set A

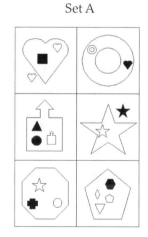

Set B

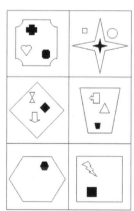

Test shapes

Question 56   Question 57   Question 58   Question 59   Question 60

Questions 61 to 65

Set A Set B

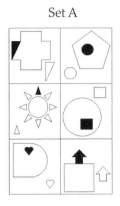

Test shapes

Question 61 Question 62 Question 63 Question 64 Question 65

Questions 66 to 70

Set A Set B

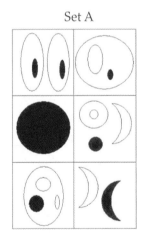

Test shapes

Question 66 Question 67 Question 68 Question 69 Question 70

Questions 71 to 75

Set A

Set B

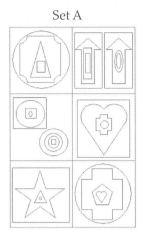

Test shapes

Question 71   Question 72   Question 73   Question 74   Question 75

 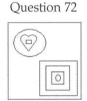 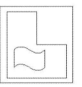

4. Decision Analysis practice subtest 1

Answers on page 315.

The Decision Analysis subtest is an on-screen test that consists of one scenario and 28 associated items. The scenario may contain text, tables and other types of information.

The 28 items have four or five response options, and for some items more than one of the options may be correct. Where more than one of the response options is correct, this is clearly identified within the item. A period of 32 minutes is allowed for the test, with one minute for instruction and the remaining 31 minutes for items.

The answers and rationale for this subtest can be found on page 315.

The Buzzards and the Kites

The Buzzards and the Kites are a group of ten children who regularly play together. They communicate with each other by using codes so that other children or adults cannot spoil their fun and games (of course, their parents have access to the codes). The Buzzards and the Kites would like to increase their group to twelve and they are going to select the two children who can interpret their codes in the quickest time by decoding 26 messages. To pass this test you will be required to interpret the coded questions and select the best option or options from those listed. The information from the codes may not always be complete and may be in any order, but you are asked to make your 'best judgement' based on this information and not on what you might consider to be reasonable.

Table: the Buzzards and the Kites codes

Action codes	People codes	Toy codes	Time codes	Like codes
A = run	☺ = me	☙ = bike	🍽 = dinner	11 = happy
B = walk	ᵐ = them	⚓ = boat	☽ = night	22 = sad
C = jump	♀ = mother	🚗 = car	⅄ = lunch	33 = cry
D = fly	⅄ = father	📄 = book	bb = breakfast	44 = laugh
E = fall	Ⓟ = police	✎ = crayon	ww = weekend	55 = jealous
F = ride	♥ = enemies	▥ = bucket	hh = holiday	66 = greedy
G = fight	101 = us	◗ = Frisbee	nn = now	77 = tall
H = climb	202 = we	&= scooter	tt = tomorrow	88 = small
I = opposite	303 = you	? = skipping rope	yy = yesterday	99 = smile
J = negative	404 = brother		cc = year	00 = angry
K = increase	505 = sister	# = paint	am = morning	
L = play	606 = cousin	^ = kite	pm = afternoon	
M = combine	707 = neighbour	} = skateboard		
⚓ = swim	808 = doctor	▶▶= spade		
⛵ = sail		◎ = ball		
🗨 = talk				
💤 = sleep				

Question 1

What is the best interpretation of the following coded message?

⛵ K, 📄K, 404, (11 99), ☺

A Sailing makes my brother happy.

B Books on sailing please my brother.

C My brother is pleased when I give him a book.

D Books on sailing make my brother smile.

E My brother gave me a book on sailing.

Question 2

What is the best interpretation of the following coded message?

(404 606), 404, 606, G, FK, &K, ☺

A My brother and cousin fight over scooters.

B Scooters are the cause of arguments in our family.

C My brother and cousin argue when riding their scooters.

D My cousin and brother ride their scooters together.

E My family argue over who will ride the scooter.

Question 3

What is the best interpretation of the following coded message?

(505 }), ☺, A, (Ⓟ 🚗)

A My sister skateboarded into the police car.

B The police car is faster than my sister's skateboard.

C The police told my sister not to skateboard near cars.

D The police car ran over my sister's skateboard.

E My sister left her skateboard and ran to the police car.

Question 4

What is the best interpretation of the following coded message?

(am pm), L, ☺👪, (J bb 🍸 🍽)

A We play all day and forget to eat.

B We play after breakfast, lunch and dinner.

C Eating gets in the way of play.

D When we play in the morning we forget breakfast.

E We are always ready for our meals when we play all day.

Question 5

What is the best interpretation of the following coded message?

⚬ K, 101, &K, 101, AK? (NB: **Two** options are correct.)

A   Their bikes are faster than our scooters.

B   Our bikes are faster than our scooters.

C   Our scooters aren't as fast as our bikes.

D   Our scooters aren't as fast as their bikes.

E   Our bikes and scooters are both fast.

Question 6

What is the best interpretation of the following coded message?

⚬ K, hh, ⚬ K, 11, ☺, M 505 ♦ ⅄ 404

A   My family swim and cycle on holiday.

B   Swimming and cycling are enjoyed by all of us.

C   Family holidays involve swimming and cycling.

D   Holidays are more enjoyable if you swim and cycle.

E   My family enjoy swimming and cycling on holiday.

Question 7

What is the best interpretation of the following coded message?

707, ♦ , ❧ , 808

A   Our neighbour telephoned mum about the doctor.

B   Mum telephoned the doctor for the lady next door.

C   Mum said the neighbour called the doctor.

D   The doctor is mum's neighbour.

E   The lady next door to mum is a doctor.

Question 8

What is the best interpretation of the following coded message?

●I, 202, ♦, 11, 101, Υ, M{202●I}

A Mum is not happy if we have lunch with our enemies.

B We are happy that mum lets us have lunch together.

C Our friends are happy when mum lets us have lunch together.

D Our friends like it when we ask them to lunch.

E Our enemies are not happy when we have lunch with mum.

Question 9

What is the best interpretation of the following coded message?

}, 202, ⋔, 707, 00

A We were angry and took the neighbour's skateboard.

B Our neighbour was angry and took their skateboard.

C Their neighbour was angry and took their skateboard.

D We were angry that the neighbour took our skateboard.

E Our neighbour does not like us skateboarding.

Question 10

What is the best interpretation of the following coded message?

33 K, 77 I, 505, E, &, ☺

A My big sister fell off her scooter and cried.

B I cried when my sister fell off her scooter.

C My small sister is always falling off her scooter.

D My sister and me often fall off the scooter.

E My small sister fell off her scooter and cried.

Question 11

What is the best interpretation of the following coded message?

🚗K, 202, J↩, ☽

A   We had to sleep in the car last night.

B   The cars did not keep us awake last night.

C   The cars kept us awake.

D   We had no sleep last night due to traffic.

E   Traffic is noisy at night outside our bedroom.

Question 12

What is the best interpretation of the following coded message?

⌂, 202, 101, 🗑K, hh, ▶▶K

A   We swim and play with our buckets and spades on holiday.

B   We take our buckets and spades on holiday.

C   We play with our buckets in the water on holiday.

D   Our holidays are spent on the beach with buckets and spades.

E   We either swim or play with our buckets and spades.

Question 13

What is the best interpretation of the following coded message?

Ⓟ, 🚲, C K, ⍵ , F

A   After lunch the policeman went for a bike ride.

B   The policeman skipped lunch and rode off on his bike.

C   The policeman jumped on to the bike and rode off for lunch.

D   Police cyclists take their lunch with them.

E   The policeman said he would jump on his bike and come over.

Question 14

What is the best interpretation of the following coded message?

M(404 505), ✝, ☺, ☺, M(K 22 33 00), G (NB: Two options are correct.)

A   Mum gets very emotional when my siblings and I argue.

B   Mum cries and gets angry when I fight with my brother.

C   Mother is angry when I make my brother and sister cry.

D   My siblings make me angry when they upset mum.

E   When I fall out with my siblings mother gets really upset.

Question 15

Which **two** of the following would be the most useful additions to the codes when attempting to convey the following message?

My family are flying off for a holiday in the sun later this year.

A   plane

B   hot

C   cold

D   time

E   airport

Question 16

What is the best interpretation of the following coded message?

L, tt, 202, 👥, 🗣, ☺, M(🚲 🛹 🚗 ⚽}◎)

A   I spoke to my friends to see whether we are playing tomorrow.

B   I chat with my friends about which toys we will play with tomorrow.

C   Tomorrow we are going bike riding, skateboarding and playing ball.

D   It is up to my friends which toys we will play with tomorrow.

E   My friends and I will discuss what we are playing tomorrow.

Question 17

What would be the best way to encode the following message?

My family smile and laugh a lot because we are very happy.

A ☺, M(404 ⚲ 505 ϒ), 202, 99, 44, K 11

B K(99 44), 202, K 11, ☺, M(404 ⚲ 505 ϒ)

C ☺, M(404 ⚲ 505 ⚲), K(99 33), 101, K 11

D K(99 44), 202, 11, ☺, (404 ⚲ 505 ϒ)

E 202, ☺, K(99 44), M(404 ⚲ 505 ϒ)

Question 18

What is the best interpretation of the following coded message?

⚲ , ϒ, 707, 🍴, I 66, ✊

A Mum and dad say the neighbour gives generous dinner portions.

B Mum and dad have invited the greedy neighbour to dinner.

C The neighbour says that mum and dad are greedy.

D Mum and dad asked the neighbour to dinner.

E The neighbour generously asked mum and dad to dinner.

Question 19

What is the best interpretation of the following coded message?

E, 88 ?, 101, I 🪑, ⚓

A We sailed the boat tied to the rope.

B The skipping rope made our boat sink.

C The rope fell off and our boat sank.

D The boat sank so we played with the skipping rope.

E Our boat sailed with the small rope attached.

Question 20

What is the best interpretation of the following coded message?

K D, ^, L, 202, nn ww, I, M(☺ 👫)

A This weekend we are having a kite-flying game against each other.

B We are going to play kite flying this weekend.

C I will not oppose my friends in the weekend kite-flying contest.

D This weekend's kite flying is for my friends and me only.

E I will fly my kite opposite my friends this weekend.

Question 21

Which **two** of the following would be the most useful additions to the codes when attempting to convey the following message?

The police said that the paint poured on our car was criminal damage.

A break

B throw

C drop

D harass

E crook

Question 22

What is the best interpretation of the following coded message?

M(bb ϒ 🍽️), 202, hh, M(👤 ϒ☺ 404 505)

A We eat our meals with mum and dad when on holiday.

B I have breakfast, lunch and dinner with my family.

C We have breakfast, lunch and dinner together on holiday.

D We have all our meals together when on holiday.

E We just have our main meal together when on holiday.

Question 23

What is the best interpretation of the following coded message?

#, E, 88 📖, 88 707

A The child from next door fell over the tin of paint.

B The neighbour's tin of paint fell over.

C The bucket of paint fell on the neighbour.

D The tin of paint fell on the child.0

E The neighbour fell on the bucket of paint.

Question 24

What is the best interpretation of the following coded message?

K M(A C H B⚓), 202, L, M(♦ Υ☺ 404 505 606)

A Our family swim, walk, run and climb together.

B We all play together.

C Our family have very active hobbies.

D Mother and father like us all to be very active.

E Very active play is good for us all.

Question 25

What would be the best way to encode the following message?

The doctor had to fight to stop my sister from drowning.

A J⚓, H, 808, ☺, 505, I B

B G, 808, ☺, 505, I B, J⚓

C 808, ☺, 505, I B, J⚓, D

D ⚓, H, 808, ☺, 505, I B

E G, 808, ☺, 404, I B, J⚓

Question 26

What is the best interpretation of the following coded message?

✏, Υ, #, nn, 🚗, 55

A The neighbour is jealous of dad's new car.

B The paint colour of dad's new car is green.

C   Father had to have the car painted.

D   Dad was jealous and wanted a new car.

E   Now dad has changed the car for a green one.

Question 27

What would be the best way to encode the following message?

My brother and I are cycling uphill to our cousins this weekend.

A   606, ☺404, 🚲K, H, nn ww, ☺404

B   ☺404, ww, H, ☺, 🚲, 606

C   606, ☺404, 🚲K, ☺, H, nn ww, ☺404

D   404, 606, ☺, 🚲K, H, nn, ☺404

E   nn ww, 606, ☺, ☺, H, 🚗K

Question 28

Which **two** of the following would be the most useful additions to the codes when attempting to convey the following message?

My parents are cross with next door's dog and cat because they dig in our garden.

A   cat

B   dog

C   pet

D   parents

E   outside

Chapter 7
Practice test 2

5. Verbal Reasoning practice subtest 2

Answers on page 322.

The Verbal Reasoning subtest is an on-screen test that consists of 44 items associated with 11 reading passages. For each reading passage there are four questions in the form of statements. Three answer options are provided for each statement: True, False or Can't Tell. Only one of these options is correct. A period of 22 minutes is allowed for the subtest, with one minute for instruction and the remaining 21 minutes for items.

The answers and rationale for this subtest can be found on page 322.

Passage 1: MRSA and *Clostridium difficile*

After a surprise inspection by the Healthcare Commission revealed dirty bedpans and concerns about the adequacy of training for staff, a big London hospital has been warned that it must raise hygiene standards. The hospital has a good record on MRSA and *Clostridium difficile*, the two most rampant hospital superbugs, but the Commission says its systems are not sound enough to prevent a potentially serious hygiene lapse. Inspectors found bedpans and commodes that had been cleaned but were visibly dirty and marked as being ready for use. In the endoscopy suite it was not clear whether flexible tubes that are inserted into the body for diagnosis and treatment were ready for sterilisation or had already been decontaminated, even though this had previously been brought to the hospital's attention. An audit by the hospital's own trust also found that only six out of ten staff were washing their hands properly, but the trust's board was not informed. The board had also been informed that attendance for mandatory infection-control training by staff was acceptable, but in fact it was low. Only three out of nine hygiene audits planned for the previous 12 months had been carried out. These breaches of the government's hygiene code gave the Commission cause for concern, in spite of the low incidence of infections. The hospital reported 22 cases in *C. difficile* between April and June.

Passage 1: question 1
The Healthcare Commission is responsible for hygiene inspections of National Health Service and trust hospitals.

A   True

B   False

C   Can't Tell

Passage I: question 2

One of the major issues at the hospital inspected appears to be a lack of communication between the staff and the trust board.

A True

B False

C Can't Tell

Passage I: question 3

Twenty-two cases of *Clostridium difficile* at the hospital in a three-month period is considered particularly high.

A True

B False

C Can't Tell

Passage I: question 4

This is not the first inspection of the hospital by inspectors from the Healthcare Commission.

A True

B False

C Can't Tell

Passage II: cultural identity

We all have a cultural identity and shared outlook which provide us with a sense of 'belonging'. This belonging may be to a small group, such as a university sports team, or a large group, such as a nation or religion. Within those groups we have shared prejudices about other teams, other nations and other religions. A confrontation or even an interaction with another group, or culture, can be threatening because it implies a difference of opinion with different answers to fundamental questions of why we live the way we do. Culture shock is a phrase used to describe our reaction when we encounter behaviour that we would not necessarily consider appropriate even if it is the norm in another culture. A common reaction to different cultures is fear, which can lead to distrust and hostility.

Passage II: question 5

It is often a natural reaction for a person to be prejudiced when encountering other cultures.

A True

B False

C Can't Tell

Passage II: question 6

All wars can be traced back to fundamental cultural differences.

A True

B False

C Can't Tell

Passage II: question 7

In a multicultural society such as Britain there is a greater acceptance and tolerance of differing religious beliefs than is the case in other countries.

A True

B False

C Can't Tell

Passage II: question 8

The membership of both small and large social groups encourages a competitive and even prejudicial outlook in relation to other such social groups.

A True

B False

C Can't Tell

Passage III: jet aircraft biofuels

Air travel generates 3% of global carbon dioxide emissions. It is one of the fastest rising contributors to climate change, but the search for a greener alternative to kerosene jet fuel has been problematic. Airlines cannot use standard first-generation biofuels such as ethanol because these would freeze at high altitude. In addition, environmentalists argue that manufacturing biofuels can produce more emissions than they absorb when growing, and can also displace agricultural crops and push up the price of food. However, the search for an environmentally friendly fuel for aeroplanes is moving forward. The world's first flight powered by a second-generation biofuel, derived from plants that do not compete with food crops, has recently taken place in New Zealand. An Air New Zealand jumbo jet with a 50–50 mix of jet fuel and oil from jatropha trees in one of its four engines successfully undertook a two-hour test flight, without the need for any modification of the engines. The biofuel was made from jatropha nuts, which are up to 40% oil, harvested from trees grown on marginal land in India, Mozambique, Malawi and Tanzania. An American airline is shortly to run a test flight that will use a mixture of jatropha-derived biofuel and fuel made from algae in one of its engines. Again, algae are not a food source and can be grown in arid regions and virtually anywhere. However, Greenpeace has warned against over-interpreting the results from the test flights. They believe it will not mean an end to the use of kerosene jet engines, as the amount of jatropha that would be needed to power the entire aviation section can never be produced in a sustainable way.

Passage III: question 9
The oils from jatropha nuts and algae are the preferred oils for use with kerosene jet fuel.

A True

B False

C Can't Tell

Passage III: question 10
It is likely that eventually the use of kerosene jet engines will be a thing of the past.

A True

B False

C Can't Tell

Passage III: question 11
Algae and the jatropha trees can be grown in the arid regions of the world and virtually anywhere.

A True

B False

C Can't Tell

Passage III: question 12
The use of biofuels is of particular concern to environmentalists because of the increase in emissions caused by growing crops specifically for biofuel use.

A True

B False

C Can't Tell

Passage IV: universities defy government cap

Universities have accepted 35,000 more students than in the previous year despite a government cap of 13,000. This capping followed the finding that there was a £200 million black hole in their university financing. The government are intending to fine universities for every student admitted over the official limit, which could cost universities millions of pounds.

There were an additional 60,000 applications for places in the current year, comprising a 10% increase in students overall but a 19.5% rise among students over 25 years of age. The universities themselves believe that to some extent the anxieties in the media about the government capping could have exacerbated the natural urge for students to sort out their applications. University applications for the following year are already up 14% on the previous year with the number of applications standing at 150,000. There are also record numbers of non-EU students opting to study in the UK, the number of overseas students doubling in the past 10 years. Fees for non-EU students are not regulated and they are now the biggest source of income for universities after the government.

Passage IV: question 13
A large number of suitably qualified students were not prevented from starting a degree due to universities defying an order to restrict the number of places.

A True

B False

C Can't Tell

Passage IV: question 14
The number of over-25s successfully applying for university places now exceeds the number of under-25s.

A True

B False

C Can't Tell

Passage IV: question 15
The rise in the number of mature students enrolling at universities has been prompted by the over-25s being made, or being at risk of being made redundant and job insecurity.

A True

B False

C Can't Tell

Passage IV: question 16
Universities welcome non-EU students to apply for places in order to provide much needed income.

A True

B False

C Can't Tell

Passage V: speed limiters

A transport advisory body has recommended that speed limiters should be fitted to cars and lorries to reduce carbon emissions and cut accidents. The Commission for Integrated Transport and the Motorists' Forum claim that accidents involving injuries could be cut by 12 per cent if the system were adopted universally – with a manual override system – and by more if the speed limiter was mandatory and always on. Speed limiters would use satellite navigation technology to read the road's speed limit and adjust the vehicle's accelerator. Using the system on urban roads with a 30mph limit could increase fuel consumption and emissions, because cars operate more efficiently above that speed. However, there should be significant reductions on roads where the limit is 70mph. It is recommended that in the first instance speed limiters should be fitted to vehicles for newly qualified drivers and those convicted of dangerous driving. However, some people believe that the use of speed limiters could have dangerous consequences and could make road safety worse. For example, drivers may not be able to accelerate out of dangerous situations. Also there is an understandable deep-rooted concern about Big Brother!

Passage V: question 17
Cars and lorries operate more efficiently between 30 and 70mph.

A True

B False

C Can't Tell

Passage V: question 18
The introduction of speed limiters might lead to a greater infringement of civil liberties.

A True

B False

C Can't Tell

Passage V: question 19
The impact in relation to lorries would be minimal as engines on lorries are already fitted with speed limiters.

A True

B False

C Can't Tell

Passage V: question 20
Fitting speed limiters to the vehicles of newly qualified drivers would not see a reduction in the number of accidents involving injuries.

A   True

B   False

C   Can't Tell

Passage VI: excessive alcohol

Research has shown that high alcohol intake can affect mental abilities and damage someone's ability to pay attention, remember things and make good judgements. Heavy drinkers are already known to be at increased risk of having an accident, being involved in violence and engaging in unprotected sex, but research identifying permanent brain damage is a new phenomenon. The research indicated that in the UK 23% of men and 15% of women drink more than twice the government's recommended daily limit. It also showed that people who have a few heavy drinking sessions undergo subtle brain changes, making it harder to learn from mistakes and new ways of tackling problems because their brain function has been impaired. Alcohol-related brain damage is an increasing burden on the NHS, and patients who do not die early with the condition need long-term care costing £1,000 a week for the rest of their lives.

Passage VI: question 21

Research shows that 23% of men and 15% of women are running the risk of suffering permanent brain damage from excessive alcohol consumption.

A   True

B   False

C   Can't Tell

Passage VI: question 22

People who have unprotected sex are more likely to drink excessive amounts of alcohol.

A   True

B   False

C   Can't Tell

Passage VI: question 23

The majority of people with alcohol-related brain damage have a shorter life expectancy.

A   True

B   False

C   Can't Tell

Passage VI: question 24

Men are twice as likely as women to be heavy drinkers.

A True

B False

C Can't Tell

Passage VII: influences on health

The normal internal environment (body status) is called homeostasis. The homeostatic reserve of the very young and very old is less than that of those in early and middle adult life; for example, there are more frequent occurrences of delirium with infection at the extremes of the age spectrum. Early upbringing will also influence health in later life. There are the possible positive and negative effects of childhood diet and exercise, parental smoking and alcohol use, and good and bad parenting. Many elderly people with multiple pathologies still consider themselves to be normal and healthy by virtue of the fact they can go about their day-to-day lives. Generally, older people see their health as functioning even in the presence of chronic disease while young people see health more as fitness.

Passage VII: question 25

People who have had bad parents are more at risk of chronic disease later in their lives.

A True

B False

C Can't Tell

Passage VII: question 26

Those in middle adult life are less likely to suffer delirium with infection than old people.

A True

B False

C Can't Tell

Passage VII: question 27

Parental smoking or alcohol abuse has no adverse effect on the health of their children's health in later life.

A True

B False

C Can't Tell

Passage VII: question 28

Generally, older people are less concerned about their levels of fitness than simply being able to function in their daily lives.

A True

B False

C Can't Tell

Passage VIII: community service

People who have been convicted of a criminal offence in England and Wales and sentenced to community service are now required to wear bright orange bibs when undertaking their community work. These controversial bibs are designed as public reminders that offenders cleaning graffiti or laying pavements are being punished and not paid. Some people have suggested that the scheme is medieval and not dissimilar to putting offenders in stocks; that it is about shaming people. However, the government consider that any shame felt by offenders is the shame and humiliation of having committed an offence and the resulting criminal record. They believe the public want to see that justice is being done, that community punishments are seen as effective and tough, and that such sentences may result in fewer people being sent to prison. However, the Probation Service has highlighted the fact that there have been a number of attacks on offenders undertaking community service and that the use of bright orange bibs is almost certain to increase the risk.

Passage VIII: question 29

The orange bib scheme will mean that fewer offenders will be sentenced to terms of imprisonment.

A True

B False

C Can't Tell

Passage VIII: question 30

Those offenders who are sentenced to community service are ashamed at having committed and been convicted of a criminal offence.

A True

B False

C Can't Tell

Passage VIII: question 31

Offenders who don't wear orange bibs when undertaking community service are less likely to be attacked than those wearing orange bibs.

A True

B False

C Can't Tell

Passage VIII: question 32

People were put in stocks in medieval times to be shamed for their wrongdoing.

A True

B False

C Can't Tell

Passage IX: cow tax

Green Party activists are pressuring the government to introduce a 'cow tax' to penalise farmers for owning belching and flatulent cattle and pigs. They consider this an environmental issue and say that farmers should be charged for rising levels of methane and other polluting nitrous gases emitted by farm animals. It is calculated that a farm with 30 dairy cows, 40 beef cattle or 200 pigs emits more than 100 tons of carbon equivalent each year. The 'cow tax' would demand a fee of about £100 for each cow and £20 for each pig. The farming lobby is up in arms about such a tax and believes even moderate size farms could see tax bills in thousands of pounds. This could put many farmers out of business, with a knock-on effect of wide-scale closures of food outlets across the country.

Passage IX: question 33

If the 'cow tax' were introduced farms with 200 pigs would see a reduction in the current 100 tons of carbon equivalent produced each year.

A True

B False

C Can't Tell

Passage IX: question 34

If farms closed as a result of the 'cow tax' there would be a shortage in the supply of cattle and pig products.

A True

B False

C Can't Tell

Passage IX: question 35

The emission of methane and other nitrous gases from cattle and pigs is considered a real environmental issue.

A True

B False

C Can't Tell

Passage IX: question 36

Farm animals' belching and flatulence have a significant carbon footprint.

A True

B False

C Can't Tell

Passage X: offenders' benefit claims

Two years after being released from prison, 47% of offenders were on out-of-work benefits. During the two-year period overall, 75% of offenders made a new claim to an out-of-work benefit at some point. On average, offenders leaving prison spent 48% of the next two years on out-of-work benefits. After being released from prison, 11% of offenders are back in prison two years later. During the two-year period overall nearly half (46%) of offenders started another prison sentence at some point. Offenders discharged from custody who claimed Job Seeker's Allowance (JSA) within 13 weeks of release spent 57% of the next three years on out-of-work benefits, compared with 42% for the average JSA claimant.

Passage X: question 37

Within two years of being released from custody, 46% of offenders started another prison sentence.

A True

B False

C Can't Tell

Passage X: question 38

Non-offenders in receipt of Job Seeker's Allowance accounted for 42% of all claimants.

A True

B False

C Can't Tell

Passage X: question 39

Within two years of their release from prison, 89% of offenders commit no further offences.

A True

B False

C Can't Tell

Passage X: question 40

Offenders leaving prison spent on average 47% of the next two years on out-of-work benefits.

A True

B False

C Can't Tell

Passage XI: fuel poverty

Data from a recent survey indicates that 4 million households in England were classified as being in fuel poverty (18% of all households). This is three times the number of households that were in fuel poverty six years ago. As might be expected, the vast majority of people who have both low incomes and live in very energy-inefficient housing are in fuel poverty. Less obviously, two of the low-income groups with high rates of fuel poverty are single-person households of working age and those who live in rural areas. This is notable because these two groups have not been the focus of the last government's more general anti-poverty strategy. Households are considered by the government to be in 'fuel poverty' if they would have to spend more than 10% of their household income on fuel to keep their home in a 'satisfactory' condition. It is thus a measure which compares income with what the fuel costs 'should be' rather than what they actually are. Whether a household is in fuel poverty or not is determined by the interaction of a number of factors, but the three obvious ones are: the cost of energy, the energy efficiency of the property and household income. The focus of government's more general anti-poverty strategy has tended to focus on children, older people and deprived urban areas.

Passage XI: question 41

Loft insulation and double-glazing have a considerable impact on the energy efficiency of a house.

A True

B False

C Can't Tell

Passage XI: question 42

'Fuel poverty' is a measure that compares household income with the actual costs of fuel.

A True

B False

C Can't Tell

Passage XI: question 43

People who live in rural communities are more likely to be classified as being in fuel poverty compared to people living in urban areas.

A True

B False

C Can't Tell

Passage XI: question 44

'Fuel poverty' disproportionately affects single-person households of working age who are on low incomes.

A True

B False

C Can't Tell

6. Quantitative Reasoning practice subtest 2

Answers on page 331.

The Quantitative Reasoning subtest consists of 36 items associated with tables, charts and/or graphs. A period of 25 minutes is allowed for the test, with 1 minute for instruction and the remaining 24 minutes for items.

Remember that each of the questions is always accompanied by five possible answers, A, B, C, D and E, and that only ONE answer is correct. Also remember to read through all five competing answers before selecting what you consider to be the correct answer. By reading the four 'incorrect' answers you should confirm that your choice is in fact correct.

The answers and rationale for this subtest can be found on page 331.

Questions 1 to 4 are about a registered charity that offers services and activities to adults with learning disabilities. The table below shows the activities on offer, the session length, the individual's cost per session and the actual cost to the charity.

Activity	Time	User cost	Charity cost
Theatre company	6 hours	£37.50	£25.75
Art and crafts	4 hours	£15.00	£9.75
Wednesday life-links	6 hours	£12.00	£8.40
Friday life-links	6 hours	£12.00	£8.40
Shop training	6 hours	£32.50	£23.25
Rural crafts	3 hours	£7.75	£4.00
Weaving to work	2 hours	£2.50	£1.75
Yoga	1 hour	£4.00	£2.85
Football	2 hours	£2.00	£1.45
Badminton	1 hour	£2.50	£1.65
Sewing	2 hours	£2.50	£1.65
Discotheque	3 hours	£3.00	£2.00

1. The charity is offering a reduction of 15% for service users who book a block of twelve sessions with the theatre company. What would be the total cost to the user for these twelve sessions?

   A £318.75

   B £351.05

   C £382.50

   D £405.00

   E £450.00

2. What is the range of user costs for all activities?

   A £6.88

   B £8.40

   C £11.10

   D £24.00

   E £35.50

3. The charity cost relates to the cost of running the activity. The 'profit' made between the user cost and charity cost covers central overhead costs. In relation to shop training, what percentage of the user cost covers the central overheads?

A 18%

B 21%

C 25%

D 28%

E 32%

4. One of the service users has a personal budget of £78.20 per week. Their preferences are to attend the theatre company for one day, two sessions of rural craft, one session of badminton and one session of yoga. How much more money would they need if they also wanted to do one-day shop training?

A £9.45

B £13.80

C £18.70

D £21.55

E £25.10

Questions 5 to 8 relate to the table below that shows the top ten results of a half marathon (13 miles) for the categories of men and women. The time is shown in hours and minutes.

MEN	Time	WOMEN	Time
A Taylor	2.35	C Akabusi	2.49
F Simkins	2.36	A Bakewell	2.51
L Glossop	2.40	Y Jeavons	2.52
B Smith	2.41	P Karlson	2.58
M Khan	2.42	T Zukova	3.01
C Denston	2.46	S Pearson	3.02
K Verma	2.48	D Pearson	3.02
J Yani	2.48	B Collins	3.07
T Price	2.50	P Johnson	3.09
K Benson	2.52	D Fellows	3.10

5. What is the mean running time, in minutes, for the top ten women runners in the half marathon?

   A 86.10 minutes

   B 128.40 minutes

   C 180.10 minutes

   D 188.40 minutes

   E 240.10 minutes

6. What is the difference in minutes between the mode running times for the men's and women's half marathon?

   A 14 minutes

   B 17 minutes

   C 21 minutes

   D 28 minutes

   E 35 minutes

7. What is the median running time, in hours and minutes, for the top ten men runners in the half marathon?

   A 2 hours 42 minutes

   B 2 hours 44 minutes

   C 2 hours 45 minutes

   D 2 hours 46 minutes

   E 2 hours 48 minutes

8. The half-marathon event was recognised by the Amateur Athletics Association as a qualifying event for the forthcoming regional championships. The time required to qualify for the championships was under 2 hours 46 minutes for men and under 3 hours 5 minutes for women. What percentage of the men and women runners in the top ten obtained the qualifying time?

   A 35%

   B 40%

   C 45%

   D 50%

   E 55%

Questions 9 to 12 refer to the pie chart below which groups the level of turnover of a number of professional rugby league clubs included in a 'UK Sport for All' survey. The number of rugby league clubs per group is shown in parentheses.

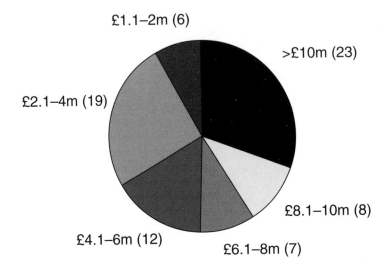

£1.1–2m (6)

>£10m (23)

£2.1–4m (19)

£8.1–10m (8)

£4.1–6m (12)

£6.1–8m (7)

9. What percentage, rounded to the nearest whole number, of rugby league clubs has a turnover in excess of £8m?

A 30%

B 37%

C 41%

D 45%

E 50%

10. 'UK Sport for All' wish to publish the results of the survey in Australia because of their close ties with rugby league and want the figures shown in Australian dollars. If £1 = A$2.10, what would be the minimum turnover in Australian dollars for those organisations with a turnover of £4.1–6m, to the nearest A$500,000?

A A$8,000,000

B A$8,500,000

C A$9,000,000

D A$9,500,000

E A$13,000,000

11. The rugby league clubs comprising this survey employ a total of 900 people, of whom 60% are employed by those clubs with a turnover in excess of £8m. The remaining employees are spread pro rata across the other clubs. How many employees, to the nearest round number, work for each rugby league club with a turnover of £2.1m to £4m?

   A 8

   B 10

   C 12

   D 15

   E 21

12. What is the ratio of the number of rugby league clubs with a turnover of £6.1m to £10m compared to the rest of the rugby league clubs?

   A 1:2

   B 1:3

   C 2:3

   D 1:4

   E 1:5

Questions 13 to 16 are about the job of a painter and decorator who has been given the job of redecorating a lounge. The lounge is 7.5 metres long, 3.5 metres wide and 2.75 metres high and is shown in the diagram below.

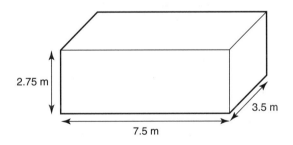

13. The owner of the property where the lounge is being redecorated wants the two long walls and one side wall painted in arctic white emulsion. A 5-litre tin of arctic white emulsion costs £9.75 and will apply one coat to an area of 12 square metres. What is the total cost of paint required to apply two coats of paint, taking into account any excess paint?

   A £29.25

   B £36.55

C £48.75

D £87.75

E £107.25

14. The side wall that is not painted needs to be wallpapered using woodchip paper. One roll of wallpaper is 55 centimetres wide and 5 metres long. How many rolls of wallpaper will the decorator need, rounded up to the nearest whole number?

A 3

B 4

C 5

D 6

E 7

15. Before the decorator starts wallpapering, the owner decides he wants to fit a door in the side wall to lead out into a conservatory he is having built and also wallpaper the other side wall which has just been painted. The dimensions of the door are detailed in the drawing below.

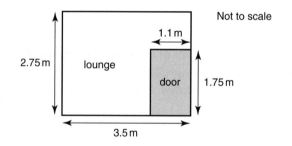

Assuming the wallpaper is 55cm wide, what is the total length of wallpaper in metres the decorator needs to wallpaper the two side walls?

A 12m

B 15m

C 19m

D 27m

E 35m

16. Before painting and papering the lounge, the decorator has estimated the cost of the job including his hourly rate. He has calculated that he will need about seven 5-litre tins of emulsion paint and no more than eight rolls of woodchip wallpaper. The paint normally costs £9.75 per tin but he gets it at trade with a 15% discount

per tin. The woodchip wallpaper is £2.65 a roll with the same discount as the paint. He believes the job will take him 20 hours to complete and his labour charges are £18.50 an hour plus VAT at 20%. What is the total estimated cost for this job to the nearest £10.00?

A £600.00

B £575.00

C £550.00

D £520.00

E £510.00

Questions 17 to 20 relate to an extract from an article on how crimes are being dealt with.

'More than 207,500 spot fines for disorder were issued last year, alongside 104,000 cannabis warnings and 362,900 police cautions. The increase means that for only the second time more crime was dealt with through summary justice than through the courts. The figures show that only 49% of 1.37m crimes detected last year resulted in a charge or court summons.'

17. Last year, how many more people were dealt with by spot fines for disorder, cannabis warnings or police cautions than were dealt with by a charge or court summons?

A 24,300

B 14,900

C 7,450

D 3,100

E 2,800

18. In relation to all crime detected last year, what percentage of crime (to two decimal places) was dealt with by spot fines for disorder?

A 7.59%

B 15.15%

C 20.28%

D 26.50%

E 30.34%

19. What was the approximate ratio of cannabis warnings compared to police cautions?

A 1:5

B 2:3

C 2:7

D 2:9

E 3:5

20. In ten years from these figures being published, detected crimes are forecast to increase by 18% when, if current trends continue, only 40% of these detected crimes will result in a charge or court summons. If this were the case, what would be the number of police cautions in ten years' time, assuming they rise proportionately to spot fines and warnings, to the nearest whole number?

A 503,797

B 593,870

C 674,400

D 737,200

E 969,960

Questions 21 to 24 are about 'stopovers' and associated flying times (in hours) when travelling by air from the UK to Australia and New Zealand. These are presented in the table below.

Country	Local time	UK to stopover	Stopover to Australia	Stopover to New Zealand
Bali	GMT +8	16 hours 9,700 miles	$5\frac{1}{2}$ hours 2,800 miles	8 hours 4,125 miles
Dubai	GMT +4	$7\frac{1}{2}$ hours 3,750 miles	14 hours 7,300 miles	$18\frac{1}{2}$ hours 11,300 miles
Hawaii	GMT −10	17 hours 10,500 miles	10 hours 5,300 miles	$9\frac{1}{4}$ hours 4,900 miles
Fiji	GMT +12	23 hours 12,800 miles	$4\frac{1}{2}$ hours 2,300 miles	3 hours 1,500 miles
China	GMT +8	$11\frac{1}{4}$ hours 6,250 miles	$10\frac{3}{4}$ hours 5,650 miles	16 hours 9,750 miles

21. From the UK, how much longer in hours does it take to get to New Zealand if you include a stopover in China of 4 days, than it does to get to Australia including a stopover in Dubai of 3½ days?

A $17\frac{3}{4}$ hours

B $18\frac{1}{4}$ hours

C $20\frac{3}{4}$ hours

D $24\frac{1}{4}$ hours

E $25\frac{3}{4}$ hours

22. The cost of a single business class fare from the UK to China has been calculated at £0.15 per mile, with the mileage from China to New Zealand calculated at an additional £0.05 per mile. The cost of a return fare is 15 per cent less than the total cost of a two-way individual single fare. From UK to China is 6,250 miles, and from China to New Zealand is 9,750 miles. What is the cost of the return fare to New Zealand via China?

A £2,310.00

B £3,176.25

C £4,052.50

D £4,908.75

E £5,775.00

23. Two flights leave the UK on Monday at 10.00 hours, one bound for Dubai and one for Hawaii. The Dubai flight is adversely affected by inclement weather conditions and arrives at its destination 1 hour and 12 minutes behind schedule. The flight to Hawaii develops technical problems and is forced to land at New York JFK. It is grounded for 5 hours and 20 minutes before continuing on to Hawaii without any further disruption. What is the difference in local time between the two planes landing at their destination?

A 2 minutes

B 2 hours 58 minutes

C 4 hours 2 minutes

D 8 hours 58 minutes

E 12 hours 2 minutes

24. The airlines using the routes to Australia and New Zealand mainly use the Boeing 757 aircraft that has an average cruising speed of 550mph. The airlines are now looking at taking into service a new aeroplane, the Boeing 787, that has an average cruising speed of 570mph. When the 787 is taken into service, what will be the

flight duration for an aircraft travelling to Australia with a stopover at Fiji to the nearest $\frac{1}{2}$ hour?

A   25 hours

B $25\frac{1}{2}$ hours

C   26 hours

D $26\frac{1}{2}$ hours

E   27 hours

Questions 25 to 28 relate to the population figures of the United Kingdom for the twentieth century as shown in table below.

UK population (thousands) 1901 to 2001

	United Kingdom	England & Wales	Scotland	Northern Ireland
1901	38,328	32,612	4,479	1,237
1911	42,138	36,136	4,751	1,251
1921	44,072	37,932	4,882	1,258
1931	46,074	39,988	4,843	1,243
1941	48,216	41,748	5,160	1,308
1951	50,290	43,815	5,102	1,373
1961	52,807	46,196	5,184	1,427
1971	55,928	49,152	5,236	1,540
1981	56,352	49,634	5,180	1,538
1991	57,808	51,099	5,107	1,601
2001	59,009	52,211	5,123	1,675

25. If the population of the United Kingdom continues to grow at the rate it did between 1981 and 2001, what would be the projected population (thousands) in 2021?

A   60,984

B   61,782

C   62,237

D   62,808

E   63,115

26. Which one of the following statements is correct?

    A Between 1901 and 1911 the growth rate of the UK population averaged 5% per annum.

    B The twentieth century saw the population of Northern Ireland increase by over half a million.

    C The populations of England and Wales, Scotland and Northern Ireland have all grown at a similar rate.

    D In the twentieth century the percentage growth rate in Northern Ireland exceeded that in Scotland.

    E The population in England and Wales increased by almost 50% over the twentieth century.

27. Expressed as a fraction, approximately what was the population of Scotland compared to that of England and Wales in 1941?

    A $\dfrac{1}{2}$

    B $\dfrac{1}{3}$

    C $\dfrac{1}{4}$

    D $\dfrac{1}{6}$

    E $\dfrac{1}{8}$

28. The UK population is growing older. In 1951 the proportion of the population over 50 was about 25% and by 1991 it was about 31%. Assuming a similar increase to the 1951 and 1991 figures, how many people (thousands) would be over 50 by 2001?

    A 18,708

    B 18,992

    C 19,178

    D 19,709

    E 21,833

Questions 29 to 32 are about Reginald Smythe who has entered the biannual Laconda Touring Rally driving his vintage Laconda motor vehicle from London to Le Mans in France.

29. The first stage of the rally is from London to Dover, a distance of 70 miles. Smythe drives the first 20 miles at an average speed of 30mph, the next 40 miles at an

average of 60mph and the last 10 miles at an average of 30mph. How long did it take Smythe to drive from London to Dover?

A 1 hour 35 minutes

B 1 hour 40 minutes

C 1 hour 45 minutes

D 1 hour 50 minutes

E 1 hour 55 minutes

30. Shortly after leaving the ferry in Calais, Smythe joins the E1 motorway in the direction of Paris. After three hours he pulls into a service area. For the first quarter of this journey he travels at a steady 90 kilometres per hour (kph) and for the remainder of the journey he travels at 120 kph. How far has Smythe travelled in miles (to two decimal places) between Calais and the service area (1 mile = 1.6 kilometres)?

A 170.67 miles

B 192.35 miles

C 210.94 miles

D 277.27 miles

E 337.50 miles

31. Before leaving Calais, Smythe filled his car with 75 litres of petrol as the petrol gauge was on empty. By the time he reached Le Mans Smythe estimated that the car had a third of a tank of petrol remaining even though he stopped to fill it up with another 75 litres at Rouen. Smythe estimates his car does 5.75 kilometres per litre of petrol. How many kilometres has Smythe travelled between Calais and Le Mans?

A 575 kilometres

B 628.75 kilometres

C 668.25 kilometres

D 718.75 kilometres

E 862.50 kilometres

32. Smythe is allowed to drive his Lagonda round the Le Mans racing circuit, which measures 5 miles for one lap. In driving round the circuit Smythe drives at 80mph for 3 minutes, 110mph for 12 minutes and 140mph for 15 minutes. How many full laps of the Le Mans circuit does Smythe complete?

A 6 laps

B 8 laps

C   10 laps

D   12 laps

E   14 laps

Questions 33 to 36 relate to the figure below which shows the number of deaths in a county over four five-year periods according to the age range of the people who have died, shown as a percentage of the total deaths.

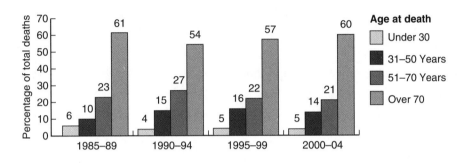

33. 575 women aged over 70 died between 1995 and 1999, accounting for $\frac{1}{3}$ of all deaths of people over 70. How many men aged over 70 died in the same period?

A   385

B   775

C   950

D   1,050

E   1,150

34. Which one of the following statements is supported by the information in the figure above?

A   Between 1985 and 2004 the average death rate for people over 70 exceeded the average death rate for people aged 31–50 by over 44%.

B   Between 1985 and 2004 the death rate for people aged 51–70 remained within a margin of 5%.

C   Between 1985 and 2004 the average percentage death rate for people 31–50 was in excess of 15%.

D   Between 1985 and 2004 the death rate for people under 30 remained constantly under 5% of the total number of deaths.

E   Between 1990 and 2004 the death rate for people aged 51–70 decreased by over three quarters.

35. Between 2000 and 2004 what is the approximate ratio of deaths of the over-70s compared to the 31–50-year-olds?

  A 2:5

  B 1:3

  C 3:1

  D 4:1

  E 5:2

36. Which one of the following statements is supported by the information in the figure above?

  A The percentage death rate for people aged 51–70 increased over the last two five-year periods.

  B The largest percentage change in the death rate has occurred in people aged over 70.

  C The largest percentage change in the death rate for people aged 51–70 exceeded that of people aged 31–50.

  D The largest percentage change in the death rate has occurred in people aged 51–70.

  E The percentage change in the death rate for people aged under 30 remained constant.

7. Abstract Reasoning practice subtest 2

Answers on page 340.

The Abstract Reasoning subtest is an on-screen test that consists of 55 items associated with 11 pairs of Set A and Set B shapes. Five test shapes are presented with each pair of Set A and Set B shapes, and there are three answer options for each test shape: Set A, Set B or Neither Set. Only ONE of the three answer options is correct. Each test shape is presented with the pair of Set A and Set B shapes on a separate screen with the three answer options below.

A period of 14 minutes is allowed for the test, with one minute for instruction and the remaining 13 minutes for items.

N.B. An additional 20 questions have been included at the end of this section to offer you extra practice.

The answers and rationale for this subtest can be found on page 340.

Questions 1 to 5

Set A

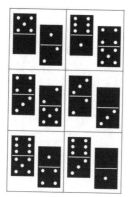

Set B

Test shapes

Question 1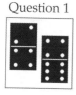

Question 2

Question 3

Question 4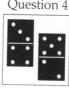

Question 5

Set A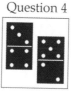

Questions 6 to 10

Set A

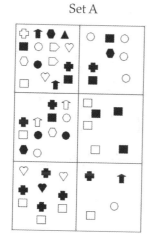

Set B

Test shapes

Question 6

Question 7

Question 8

Question 9

Question 10

Questions 11 to 15

Set A

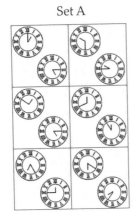

Set B

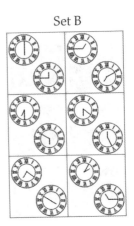

Test shapes

Question 11	Question 12	Question 13	Question 14	Question 15

Questions 16 to 20

Set A

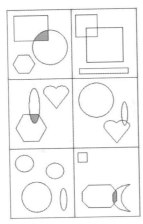

Set B

Test shapes

Question 16	Question 17	Question 18	Question 19	Question 20

Questions 21 to 25

Set A
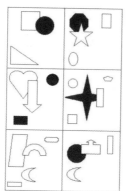

Set B
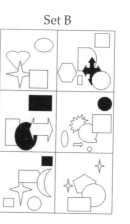

Test shapes

Question 21	Question 22	Question 23	Question 24	Question 25
	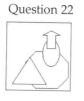	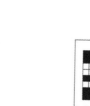		

Questions 26 to 30

Set A
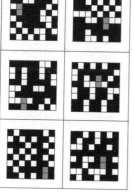

Set B
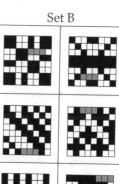

Test shapes

Question 26	Question 27	Question 28	Question 29	Question 30

Questions 31 to 35

Set A

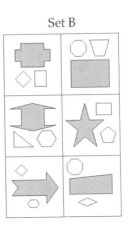

Set B

Test shapes

Question 31

Question 32

Question 33

Question 34

Question 35

Questions 36 to 40

Set A

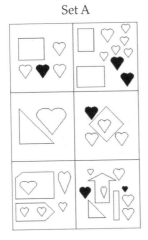

Set B

Test shapes

Question 36

Question 37

Question 38

Question 39

Question 40

Questions 41 to 45

Set A

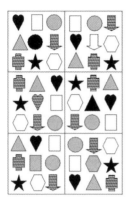

Set B

Set B content shown in grid

Test shapes

Question 41	Question 42	Question 43	Question 44	Question 45

Questions 46 to 50

Set A

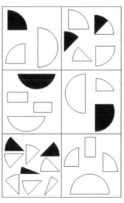

Set B

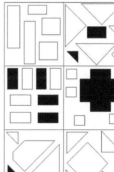

Test shapes

Question 46	Question 47	Question 48	Question 49	Question 50

Questions 51 to 55

Set A

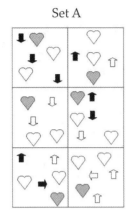

Set B

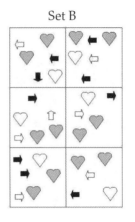

Test shapes

Question 51

Question 52

Question 53

Question 54

Question 55

Questions 56 to 60

Set A

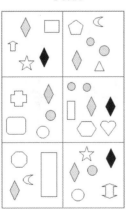

Set B

(Set B diagram)

Test shapes

Question 56

Question 57

Question 58

Question 59

Question 60

Questions 61 to 65

Set A   Set B

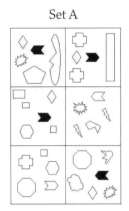

Test shapes

Question 61   Question 62   Question 63   Question 64   Question 65

Questions 66 to 70

Set A   Set B

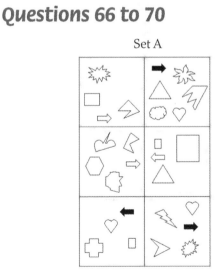

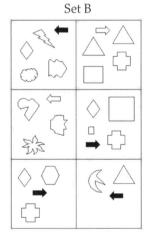

Test shapes

Question 66   Question 67   Question 68   Question 69   Question 70

Questions 71 to 75

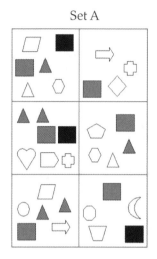

Set A

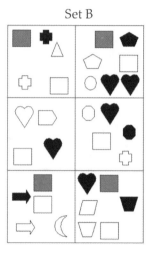

Set B

Test shapes

Question 71

Question 72

Question 73

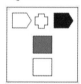

Question 74

Question 75

8. Decision Analysis practice subtest 2

Answers on page 348.

The Decision Analysis subtest is an on-screen test that consists of one scenario and 28 associated items. The scenario may contain text, tables and other types of information.

The 28 items have four or five response options and for some items more than one of the options may be correct. Where more than one of the response options is correct, this is clearly identified within the item. A period of 32 minutes is allowed for the test, with one minute for instruction and the remaining 31 minutes for items.

The answers and rationale for this subtest can be found on page 348.

The Mesopotamian codes

In the early part of the nineteenth century a cache of codes was discovered that had been used across the Mesopotamian empire towards the end of the sixth century when other countries were emerging in the Middle East. These codes substantially consisted of letters and numbers of Greek and Cyrillic origin. Together with the cache of codes, there was also a number of actual coded messages and from these the code's structure was determined. The codes were used for political and military purposes and also social insurrection. The information from the codes may not always be complete, but you are asked to make your 'best judgement' based on this information and not on what you might consider to be reasonable.

Table: The Mesopotamian codes

Political codes	Military codes	Social codes	Other codes
Σ = government	123 = Mongolia	Я = peace	β = unlawful
T = police	213 = Greece	Γ = terrorists	γ = comparison
U = budget	231 = Mesopotamia	Ъ = conscription	δ = converse
φ = opposition	312 = Persia	Љ = rich	¥ = combine
λ = transport	Э = allies	999 = weak	ə = opposite
ψ = meeting	κ = gunpowder	666 = public	η = less
χ = health	λλ = secret	333 = inside	œ = greater
010 = policy	Ю = war	Z = people	+ = negative
101 = housing	Ж = insurgents	E = include	= = achieve
110 = employment	Ф = attack	π = female	~ = day
	Ω = army		

Question 1

What is the best interpretation of the following coded message?

312, 213 Z, œ, U, 123, Ω

A The Greek army budget is greater than that of Persia or Mongolia.

B Persia and Mongolia have smaller armies than Greece.

C The Greek army budget is greater than that of Persia but is smaller than that of Mongolia.

D Greece is greater than Persia or Mongolia due to its army.

E The Greek army budget is less than that of Persia or Mongolia.

Question 2

What is the best interpretation of the following coded message?

Ω, + 110, ə π, 231, Ђ

A Conscription is compulsory for men in Mesopotamia.

B Unemployed men are forced to join the Mesopotamian army.

C Women are employed in the Mesopotamian army.

D Mesopotamia uses conscription to battle unemployment.

E Unemployed women do not have to join the Mesopotamian army.

Question 3

What is the best interpretation of the following coded message?

Σ, ¥ (Φ œ), 101 η, Ж, Γ η Z

A Insurgents attacked the terrorist group at government house.

B Government insurgents attacked the terrorist group.

C Government house was invaded by terrorists and insurgents.

D Terrorist groups took over government house during the attack.

E Terrorist groups and insurgents attacked government house.

Question 4

What is the best interpretation of the following coded message?

η, Ω, Γ, β, Τ, 999 œ

A   The army and the police were no match for the terrorists.

B   Unlawful attacks were made on the police and the army.

C   Terrorists broke the law and the police were powerless without the army.

D   Terrorists have illegally joined the army and the police.

E   Unlawful terrorists attacked the army and the police.

Question 5

What is the best interpretation of the following coded message?

231, Z, χ +, œ + Љ

A   The population of Mesopotamia are healthy and rich.

B   Mesopotamia is a poor and unhealthy country.

C   The population of Mesopotamia suffer from absolute poverty.

D   Suffering and poverty are widespread in Mesopotamia.

E   The people of Mesopotamia are healthy but very poor.

Question 6

What is the best interpretation of the following coded message?

U, η, Σ, κ, 010 œ, 101, 110, (123 312 213 231)

A   The governments of all countries are cutting housing budgets during this volatile time.

B   The governments of Persia, Mongolia and Greece are cutting housing budgets.

C   Jobs will be lost in all countries and building will cease due to a loss of budget.

D   Politically explosive policies on housing and jobs will cut budgets in all countries.

E   Governments of all countries will face political and economic challenges.

Question 7

What is the best interpretation of the following coded message?

Ω, Ω, 333, Җ œ, δ, λλ, ψ

A The army are having a meeting behind closed doors to discuss insurgency within the ranks.

B Insurgents have secretly attended army meetings and this has conversely affected security.

C Insurgents are to be found within all ranks of the armed forces, therefore meetings are held in secret.

D The army is going to hold a secret meeting with the insurgents to discuss a way forward.

E High-ranking members of the army are holding a secret meeting with the insurgents.

Question 8

What is the best interpretation of the following coded message?

¥ (Я Z), ψ, ¥(ə 666), λλ, T

A The secret police prevent people demonstrating for peace.

B The public protest against the war and the secret police.

C The secret police permit people to hold public meetings.

D People want peace and hold secret meetings with the police.

E Pacifists meet in private to avoid the secret police.

Question 9

Which **two** of the following would be the most useful additions to the codes when attempting to convey the following message?

Mesopotamia signed a peace treaty with Persia agreeing to release all enemy prisoners.

A confine

B capture

C concur

D write

E detainees

Question 10

What is the best interpretation of the following coded message?

Σ, η, U, Z, χ, γ, Ω

A   Government spending on health compares with that of the army.

B   The money raised from the people provides a strong army.

C   Government spending on the army exceeds that spent on citizens' health.

D   The health of the population is important to the government.

E   The government has both a health and military budget.

Question 11

What is the best interpretation of the following coded message?

Ω, Σ, 010, 123, ¥(œ Φ), ¥(γ Γ)

A   The Mongolian government's policy is to execute all terrorists.

B   The Mongolian government and army undertake concerted attacks on terrorists.

C   A military junta is in charge in Mongolia and deals brutally with acts of disaffection.

D   The army and government of Mongolia deal savagely with insurgents.

E   The Mongolian military junta trains its own terrorists in the art of war.

Question 12

What would be the best way to encode the following message?

Persia won the war with Mongolia and they are now our strong allies.

A   312, œ, Ю, 123, Э, ¥ (η Ω)

B   312, =, Ю, 123, ¥(γ ~), ¥(ə, 999), Э

C   312, =, δ, ψ, 123, ~, ¥(γ η), Ω

D   312, œ, ə, 123, ¥(ə 999)

E   312, =, Ю, 123, ¥(γ ~), ¥(γ η), Э

Question 13

What is the best interpretation of the following coded message?

213, ¥(γ δ),Ю, 231

A   The Mesopotamian army attacks the Greek army.

B   The Greek army is under attack from the Mesopotamian army.

C   Mesopotamia at war with Greece.

D   Greece declares war on Mesopotamia.

E   Mesopotamia is under attack from the Greek army.

Question 14

What is the best interpretation of the following coded message?

213, 010, ¥(η β), β, 101, κ, ¥(ə E), Ω, Z

A   Greece requires all stores of gunpowder to be surrendered by both the military and the population.

B   It is unlawful in Greece for any person, military or civilian, to store gunpowder.

C   Greece is clamping down on armed terrorists' use of explosives.

D   It is against Greek law to be in possession of gunpowder without authority.

E   Greece passed a law forbidding the storage of explosives except by military personnel.

Question 15

What is the best interpretation of the following coded message?

213, δ, ¥(ə ~), ¥(β Z ψ), 333, 213

A   Greece declares a night-time curfew across the country.

B   Greeks have declared that a curfew imposed by the government is unlawful.

C   Greece subjects all non-Greeks to a night-time curfew.

D   Greeks who have a criminal conviction are subject to a night-time curfew.

E   Greece's night-time curfew excludes the native Greek population.

Question 16

What is the best interpretation of the following coded message?

123, 213, 110, Г, ¥(ə 333 123 213), œ, ¥(123 213 Ω)

A Terrorists from Middle Eastern countries often infiltrate the enemy's armed forces.

B Mongolia and Greece make use of terrorists from other countries to increase the size of their armies.

C Terrorists from Mongolia and Greece are trained to fight by their respective armies.

D Mongolia and Greece have a pact that terrorists from their countries will not attack each other's army.

E Terrorists of Mongolian and Greek origin mainly commit acts of terrorism against the armed forces of their own country.

Question 17

What would be the best way to encode the following message?

Persia is demanding that some Greek soldiers face war crime charges.

A 312, ¥ (ə δ), 213, Ω, Z,Ж, ¥(Φ Ю β)

B 312, ¥(ə δ), 213, Ω, Z, Г, Φ, Ю, β

C 312, ¥(ə , 999, δ), 213, Ω, Z, ¥(Ю β Φ)

D 312, ¥(ə δ), 213, Ω, Z, Г, β, Φ

E 312, ¥(ə 999), δ, 213, Ω, Ж, ¥(Ю β Φ)

Question 18

What is the best interpretation of the following coded message?

Z, 312, Я, ψ, ¥(ə η), Φ, γ(Φ Т)

A The Persian people are a peace-loving nation, although they are subjected to marshal law.

B People in Persia are not used to peace, having problems with insurgents and a brutal police force.

C The Persian people are often harassed by the police without just cause.

D People in Persia holding peaceful demonstrations are often fired on by riot police.

E The Persian people are law abiding and know the police will crack down on any dissent.

Question 19

What is the best interpretation of the following coded message?

¥(η ~), Ж, κ, 213, Σ, 101, ¥(œ Z), ¥(œ Φ)

A Today in the Greek parliament there was an explosion, believed to be caused by terrorists, killing several people.

B Members of the Greek government exploded over the recent killing of some of its ministers.

C Insurgents are believed to be responsible for a bomb that killed a minister and several others in the Greek parliament building.

D Recently, a bomb was planted in the Greek parliament building that could have killed hundreds of people.

E Yesterday, insurgents blew up the Greek parliament building and a large number of people were killed.

Question 20

What is the best interpretation of the following coded message?

¥(+ 123 213 231 312), Φ, ¥(123 213 231 312), +, =

A People from outside Mongolia, Greece, Mesopotamia and Persia often fight as mercenaries for these countries.

B Mongolia, Greece, Mesopotamia and Persia are often at war with each other.

C Other countries sometimes fight alongside Mongolia, Greece, Mesopotamia or Persia to help them win.

D Mongolia, Greece, Mesopotamia and Persia have often defeated other countries.

E Other countries sometimes invade the Middle East but without success.

Question 21

What is the best interpretation of the following coded message?

γ(E Ю), ¥(œ Z Φ), 213, Ю, 231, π, δ(œ Z)

A In the war between Greece and Mesopotamia the most significant casualties were civilians.

B Like all wars women and children were used to fight in the war between Greece and Mesopotamia.

C Comparatively, the number of people killed in the war between Greece and Mesopotamia were mainly civilians.

D As with all wars, the main casualties when Greece fought Mesopotamia were women and children.

E In comparison to other wars, a large number of females were killed in the war between Greece and Mesopotamia.

Question 22

What is the best interpretation of the following coded message?

123, λλ, T, γ(Φ Z), ¥(+ Σ), ¥(+ =), Ω, Σ, ¥(γ Φ)

A The Mongolian secret police are rounding up dissidents to prevent the military government being overthrown.

B Mongolian police are devising secret plans to detain people known to oppose the government.

C The military police of Mongolia are helping in the overthrow of insurgents infiltrating the government.

D The Mongolian secret police have discovered a large-scale plan to destabilise the current government.

E Mongolian police have discovered an underground network of people determined to overthrow the government.

Question 23

Which **two** of the following would be the most useful additions to the codes when attempting to convey the following message?

To safeguard its borders Greece often came to Mesopotamia's assistance during its wars with Mongolia.

A help

B boundary

C frequent

D protect

E restore

Question 24

What is the best interpretation of the following coded message?

¥(Z 312 Σ), Э, γ(ΓZ), ¥(123 213 231)

A The people of Persia support their government in clamping down on terrorists from Mongolia, Greece and Mesopotamia.

B Members of the Persian government have close ties with different terrorist groups in other countries.

C The Persian population has its own terrorists just like those in Mongolia, Greece and Mesopotamia.

D The people who govern Persia are looking at different ways of dealing with terrorists from other countries.

E Persia is trying to ally itself with the terrorist groups operating in Mongolia, Greece and Mesopotamia.

Question 25

What are the **two** best interpretations of the following coded message?

231, Ω, œ, 123, Ω, γ, 312, Ω, +, œ, 213, Ω

A The Mesopotamian army is bigger than the Mongolian army, comparative to the Persian army, but not as big as the Greek army.

B The Mongolian army is bigger than the Persian army.

C The Persian army is smaller than both the Mongolian and the Mesopotamian armies.

D The Mongolian army is the second smallest army in the Middle East.

E Greece's army is bigger than those of Mesopotamia, Mongolia or Persia.

Question 26

What is the best interpretation of the following coded message?

¥ (γ Я), ¥(+ Ю), δ, œ, 213

A War and peace have been a part of Greece's legacy.

B Peace has been declared after a long war with Greece.

C Make love not war was a phrase used by the ancient Greeks.

D The Greeks have had enough of war and are suing for peace.

E The majority of Greeks want peace not war.

Question 27

What would be the best way to encode the following message?

The heads of Mongolia, Greece, Mesopotamia and Persia are holding a peace summit with a ceasefire.

A Я, ψ, Σ, 123, 213, 231, 312, ЮФ

B Ю, ψ, Σœ, 213, 231, 312, ЮФ+

C Я, ψ, 666, 123, 213, 231, 312, ЮФ

D Я, ψ, Σœ, 123, 213, 231, 312, ЮФ+

E Ю, ψ, Σœ, 123, 213, 231, 312, ЮФ+

Question 28

What is the best interpretation of the following coded message?

œ, γ, χ, 101, 110, Љ, Љә

A The difference in well being, property and occupations between the rich and the public cannot be compared.

B The difference in well being, property and occupations between the wealthy and the poor is significant.

C The difference in well being, property and occupations between the wealthy and the poor is marginal.

D The difference in health and occupations between the rich and the poor is significant.

E The wealthy and the poor have some differences in terms of health and housing.

Chapter 8
Answers and rationale

1. Verbal Reasoning practice subtest 1

Question number	Correct response	Question number	Correct response
1	C	23	A
2	A	24	B
3	B	25	A
4	C	26	C
5	B	27	B
6	A	28	A
7	C	29	A
8	C	30	C
9	C	31	A
10	B	32	B
11	A	33	A
12	C	34	B
13	C	35	C
14	A	36	A
15	B	37	B
16	C	38	C
17	B	39	C
18	B	40	A
19	A	41	A
20	C	42	C
21	C	43	C
22	A	44	A

Passage I: question 1

C. Can't Tell

Although one would assume that being subjected to 'rejection, ridicule or aggression' would affect the recipient's sense of self-worth and overall self-image, this is not actually stated in the passage.

Passage I: question 2

A. True

The 'lack of awareness' is clearly identified in the third sentence of the passage, i.e. 'largely based on fear and misunderstanding of what mental health means, and it is not uncommon for questions of capability and risk to be presented as reasons for exclusion. Indirect discrimination is often more complex to identify, as it results from a misunderstanding and adaptation rather than a direct and explicit rejection or exclusion.'

Passage I: question 3

B. False

This is the opposite of what the passage actually states, i.e. 'it is not uncommon for questions of capability and risk to be presented as reasons for exclusion'.

Passage I: question 4

C. Can't Tell

Although there is little doubt that in reality this statement is true, the passage only makes reference to 'social interaction'. More information would be needed to include 'services, employment and training'.

Passage II: question 5

B. False

The question does not take account of the restrictions relating to 'services where speedy access to diagnosis and treatment are particularly important' (e.g. emergency attendances or admissions).

Passage II: question 6

A. True

It is quite explicit in the passage that 'patients attending a Rapid Access Chest Pain Clinic under the two-week maximum waiting time, and patients attending cancer services under the two-week maximum waiting time' do not qualify for the Choice agenda.

Passage II: question 7

C. Can't Tell

Although the passage specifically relates to GPs in England, there may or may not be similar systems in Wales and/or Scotland. Further information would be required to determine this.

Passage II: question 8

C. Can't Tell

Although it might be assumed that Rapid Access Chest Pain Clinics and cancer services are provided by independent and private hospitals, this is not clear in the passage. The passage only states that patients using these services do not qualify for the Choice agenda.

Passage III: question 9

C. Can't Tell

Although the passage states that type 2 diabetes is often associated with obesity and type 2 diabetes is linked with sleeping disorders, further information would be required as the research is only 'suggesting' such a connection.

Passage III: question 10

B. False

The final sentence of the passage states: 'The findings of the research will raise the possibility of genetic tests to identify people vulnerable to developing type 2 diabetes.' Therefore, these tests are not yet available, and in any case would identify only a potential vulnerability to diabetes, rather than the disease itself.

Passage III: question 11

A. True

The passage states that type 2 diabetes affects 'about 2.3 million people in the UK, with at least 500,000 more who are not aware that they have the condition', and adding these together makes 2.8 million people.

Passage III: question 12

C. Can't Tell

Although the passage refers to how the body responds to the '24-hour cycle of light and dark' and 'a hormone that is part of the body's internal clock', there is no actual information about people being awake during the night and sleeping during the day, and further information would be required to authenticate this or otherwise.

Passage IV: question 13

C. Can't Tell

This is a very general statement. Although there may be a profit reduction in relation to some drugs purchased by the Health Service, the paragraph does state 'they will still be able to charge what they want', and therefore without additional information a 'true' or 'false' answer cannot be determined.

Passage IV: question 14

A. True

It is made quite clear in the passage that 'Currently, a number of effective drugs are not used because they are too expensive.' It can be inferred from the rest of the passage that this includes more effective treatments for heart disease and cancer.

Passage IV: question 15

B. False

Drug companies, as with all other private companies, operate in a world where profit ensures their existence and satisfies shareholders. The passage itself states that drug companies will enter negotiations for a 'realistic' value to be agreed but also goes on to say 'they will still be able to charge what they want'.

Passage IV: question 16

C. Can't Tell

Although it might be assumed that there would be a reduction in the death rate from heart disease and cancer, there is no indication of how 'significant' this may be and how this might be measured. Without further information, this question cannot be answered in the affirmative or negative.

Passage V: question 17

B. False

It is quite clear that under the new proposals history, geography and science will be 'taught through cross-curriculum themed classes'.

Passage V: question 18

B. False

Although the passage refers to teachers encouraging children's social and emotional well-being to cure some of the 'social ills' facing society, there is nothing that can be inferred from the passage about their responsibility for the social fabric of society.

Passage V: question 19

A. True

This is actually stated within the passage: 'It is considered that the teaching of rigid subject areas in primary schools was making children's knowledge and understanding shallow.'

Passage V: question 20

C. Can't Tell

Although this is undoubtedly the desired outcome from the recommended changes, further information will be required over time to assess and compare the children's performance in these subject areas.

Passage VI: question 21

C. Can't Tell

The passage essentially deals with younger children and, although it is suggested that a lack of communication skills will reduce children's chances of educational success, it does not comment on the attainment of educational standards. Further information would be required in relation to this area.

Passage VI: question 22

A. True

This is true as it actually states in the passage that 'in poorer homes children only hear 500 different words a day compared to 1,500 in a better-off household'.

Passage VI: question 23

A. True

This statement can be extrapolated from the passage where it states the following to support the general premise: 'It is believed parents in deprived areas often feel alienated from a child they did not want, may be depressed by their circumstances or not be functioning socially and emotionally because of drugs or alcohol.'

Passage VI: question 24

B. False

The passage states that 'in poorer homes children only hear 500 different words a day compared to 1,500 in a better-off household': 500 to 1,500 is a ratio of 1:3, therefore children in better-off households are likely to hear three times (not five times) as many different words spoken as those from deprived homes.

Passage VII: question 25

A. True

Although the passage does not directly use the term 'immunisation', this is referred to in the passage as 'artificial immunity (active or passive)'.

Passage VII: question 26

C. Can't Tell

The passage makes no mention of changes in communicable diseases or the emergence of new communicable diseases.

Passage VII: question 27

B. False

The passage states: 'The susceptibility of the host is influenced by age, natural immunity, artificial immunity (active or passive), nutritional status and immune suppression', so age, diet and lifestyle choice do have an impact on a person's susceptibility to disease.

Passage VII: question 28

A. True

Although the passage does not specifically state that 'the atmosphere is a vehicle that can carry an infective agent', it does state that 'transmission of infection may be by inhalation', which has the same meaning.

Passage VIII: question 29

A. True

The passage states: 'Psychologists and statisticians refer to normal as the middle range of a distribution of values.' The 'middle range' can also be referred to as the 'average', so a lack of significant deviation from the average is 'normal'.

Passage VIII: question 30

C. Can't Tell

The passage states: 'A sociologist defines "normal" as that which is in line with a rule for a particular social or cultural group in society.' The statement is suggesting that normality for a particular group may be the violation of norms and standards. The passage does not really provide a definitive answer to this, so more information would be required.

Passage VIII: question 31

A. True

The passage states: 'normal as the most usual' or 'as conforming to a standard' and 'In common speech, "normal" may simply mean "not abnormal, not strange."' Therefore, 'strange' is used as a synonym for 'abnormal', i.e. not normal.

Passage VIII: question 32

B. False

The passage states: 'In medicine "normal" is often used to mean an absence of physiological pathology.' The adverb 'often' is used, which means 'frequently' or 'many times'. The statement uses the word 'everyone' – hence the answer is 'false'.

Passage IX: question 33

A. True

This is apparent from the passage, which says that views on the use of Internet technology differ considerably between managers (and especially those under 35) and senior executives.

Passage IX: question 34

B. False

It does not state this in the passage. Internet access was allowed, albeit sometimes restricted. Senior executives were generally pessimistic about some of the benefits, but they still allow Internet access.

Passage IX: question 35

C. Can't Tell

Although it states in the passage that '65% of organisations monitored Internet usage, and this rose to 88% in the police', and it might be assumed that this would be the case because of their accountability, it is not actually stated in the passage and therefore further information would be required to authenticate this as a fact.

Passage IX: question 36

A. True

This item relates to the statement, 'Also, 65% blocked access to "inappropriate" sites, with this rising to 89% in local government and 90% in the utilities.' In relation to the '65%' figure, it could be said that 35% do not block access to 'inappropriate' Internet sites.

Passage X: question 37

B. False

Workers will be able to work in excess of 48 hours a week as the maximum working hours limit is averaged out over a one-year period.

Passage X: question 38

C. Can't Tell

This may well be the outcome but it cannot be stated without further information being provided.

Passage X: question 39

C. Can't Tell

The passage states: 'The trade unions are in favour of the European maximum 48-hour limit'; however, this does not necessarily relate to overtime. It would be possible for overtime to be worked up to the 48-hour limit. Further information would be required to assess the trade unions' position in relation to overtime.

Passage X: question 40

A. True

There is no doubt that this answer is true, as in the passage it states: 'The government believe the working hours' limit would cost the UK economy tens of billions of pounds over the next 10 years.'

Passage XI: question 41

A. True

The whole tenet of the passage is about the benefit of technology and not about it being a barrier to learning, and especially the benefit in relation to people with disabilities and learning difficulties.

Passage XI: question 42

C. Can't Tell

No information is given in the passage about academic qualifications, so the answer must be 'Can't Tell'.

Passage XI: question 43

C. Can't Tell

Although one might assume that a policy exists in universities for offering students equal learning opportunities, this is not stated in the passage and more information would be required.

Passage XI: question 44

A. True

The ways in which new technology helps students with disabilities and learning difficulties is amply qualified within the passage.

2. Quantitative Reasoning practice subtest 1

Question number	Correct response	Question number	Correct response
1	E	19	D
2	B	20	B
3	A	21	D
4	C	22	C
5	D	23	B
6	C	24	A
7	A	25	E
8	E	26	A
9	D	27	A
10	C	28	D
11	D	29	C
12	E	30	E
13	C	31	A
14	D	32	C
15	E	33	B
16	D	34	C
17	B	35	E
18	C	36	A

Question 1

Answer E is correct: 70%

The minimum score required on the on-screen hazard simulation test is 37, and there were 14 respondents who scored 37 or higher. Write this number as a fraction of the total and multiply by 100 to attain the percentage, i.e. $\frac{14}{20} \times 100 = 70\%$.

Question 2

Answer B is correct: 39.

The mode is the number in the distribution that has the highest frequency. In the information relating to females, the score of 39 appears twice and every other number only once.

Question 3

Answer A is correct: 21.

The range of a distribution is the difference between the highest and lowest values. The highest value is 44 and the lowest value is 23, therefore $44 - 23 = 21$.

Question 4

Answer C is correct: Less than half of the respondents scored above the mean.

To calculate the mean, sum the values of the distribution and divide by the number of values, i.e. $\frac{794}{20} = 39.70$. The number of scores above the mean is 9, therefore less than half of the respondents scored above the mean.

Question 5

Answer D is correct: 67.5%.

Surface mail would cost: 4 letters at £1.99 = £7.96; 5 × packets less than 500g at £3.65 = £18.25. Total cost £7.96 + £18.25 = £26.21.

Airmail would cost: 4 letters at £9.16 = £36.64; 3 × 200g packets at £8.42 = £25.26; 2 × 300g packets at £9.06 = £18.12 + 56p surcharge = £18.68. Total = £80.58.

Surface mail would be cheaper than airmail as a percentage: the difference between surface and airmail is £80.58 − £26.21 = £54.37, which as a percentage is $\frac{54.37}{80.58} \times 100 = 67.5\%$.

Question 6

Answer C is correct: £170.20.

The cost of sending 25 letters each weighing 100g would be 25 × £8.51 = £212.75.

20% of £212.75 is $\dfrac{212.75}{100} \times 20 = £42.55$

The cost of sending 25 letters each weighing 100g without VAT would be £212.75 − £42.55 = £170.20.

Question 7

Answer A is correct: Airmail letters weighing 1 kilogram cost an extra £6.60 in addition to the price of a 300g letter.

Airmail letters over 300g, for every 20g up to 500g add 16p, so 200g = 10 × 16p = £1.60; for every 20g up to 1kg add 20p, so 500g = 25 × 20p = £5.00. The extra cost of a 1 kilogram airmail letter is £1.60 + £5.00 = £6.60.

Question 8

Answer E is correct: £158.22

Each letter is of equal weight, so calculate the weight of each letter, 4.5 kilograms, or $\dfrac{4,500}{27} = 166.7\text{g}$.

The cost of one 166.7g surface mail letter is £5.86, so the cost of 27 letters is £5.86 × 27 = £158.22.

Question 9

Answer D is correct: 10%.

Calculate the total number of books, write the number of 'history' books as a fraction of the total and multiply by 100 to obtain the percentage, i.e. $\dfrac{5,700}{55,400} \times 100 = 10\%$.

Question 10

Answer C is correct: £5.96

The cost of a fiction paperback is the total stock selling price divided by the number of paperbacks, i.e. $\dfrac{101,362.50}{12,750} = £7.95$. The cost of 3 books is £7.95 × 3 = 23.85, therefore $\dfrac{23.85}{4} = £5.96$.

Question 11

Answer D is correct: £3,915.50.

The profit is $\dfrac{1}{3}$ of the selling price. For the total stock it would be $\dfrac{31,324}{3} = £10,441.33$. To obtain $\dfrac{3}{8}$ of the profit, first obtain $\dfrac{1}{8}$, i.e. $\dfrac{10,441}{8} = 1,305.17$, and then multiply this by 3, i.e. $1,305.17 \times 3 = £3,915.50$.

Question 12

Answer E is correct: 10,850.

The range of a distribution is the difference between the highest and lowest values. The highest value is 12,750 and the lowest value is 1,900, therefore the range is 12,750 – 1,900 = 10,850.

Question 13

Answer C is correct: The average number of texts per person for Ireland (Irl) is 2,016 per annum, up from 128 per month five years ago.

To obtain the average number of texts per person for Ireland per annum multiply 168 × 12 = 2,016. To obtain the average number of texts per month five years ago: $\dfrac{168}{131} \times 100 = 128$.

Question 14

Answer D is correct: 50%.

Five countries (UK, US, Can, Pol, Swe) have average monthly text messages in excess of 32 and there are 10 countries in total, so $\dfrac{5}{10} \times 100 = 50\%$.

Question 15

Answer E is correct: 4:9.

Any two numbers can be compared by writing them alongside each other separated by a ratio sign (:). There are 200 messages per person per month in the UK and US (81 + 119) and 450 in the other countries (25 + 23 + 26 + 108 + 24 + 31 + 45 + 168). Therefore, the ratio is 200:450, which can be simplified to 4:9 by dividing each value by 50.

Question 16

Answer D is correct: €126.00 and $105.00.

The annual average number of text messages in Ireland is 168 × 12 = 2016 × £0.05 = £100.80. The cost in euros is $\dfrac{100.80}{0.80} = €126.00$.

The annual average number of text messages in the US is 119 × 12 = 1428 × £0.05 = £71.40. The cost in dollars is $\dfrac{71.40}{0.68} = \$105.00$.

Question 17

Answer B is correct: Between Year 1 and Year 4 the birth rate for women aged 26–35 remained within a margin of 12%.

Between Year 1 and Year 4 the percentage of births for women aged 26–35 ranged from a low of 42% (Year 1) to a high of 54% (Year 2), therefore 54% − 42% = 12% which is within a margin of 12%.

Question 18

Answer C is correct: 250.

In Year 2 women aged 26–35 accounted for 54% of births. If this equated to 750 women giving birth, the number of women aged 18–25 giving birth would be $\frac{750}{54} \times 19 = 263.91$, which to the nearest 50 = 250.

Question 19

Answer D is correct: The single highest fall in birth rates during the four years was in relation to women aged 18–25.

The birth rate for women aged 18–25 had the highest fall between Year 1 (27%) and Year 2 (19%), an 8% drop.

Question 20

Answer B is correct: 20%.

Add together the percentages over the four years: 13% + 16% + 25% + 25% = 79%. Divide by the number of years to obtain the average percentage, $\frac{79}{4} = 19.75\%$, which is closest to 20%.

Question 21

Answer D is correct: 51.

Obtain the correct data from the table and add the figures together. The classifications less than 71 kilograms are <50, 51–60 and 61–70, so the number of people is 10 + 20 + 21 = 51.

Question 22

Answer C is correct: They are at most 60 kilograms.

Obtain 25% of the total sample of 120 people, i.e. $\frac{120}{100} \times 25 = 30$. Of the choices, the only option available to obtain 30 is by adding the first two columns together, i.e. <50kg (10) and 51–60kg (20), therefore 25% of the people surveyed 'are at most 60 kilograms'.

Question 23

Answer B is correct: $\dfrac{1}{3}$

A total of 120 people are surveyed and those who weigh in excess of 80 kilograms are:

26 (81–90kg) + 14 (>90kg) = 40 people. 40 as a fraction of 120 is $\dfrac{40}{120} = \dfrac{1}{3}$.

Question 24

Answer A is correct: 1:3.

The number of people weighing less than 61 kilograms is 30 and the number weighing 61 kilograms and above is 90. Therefore, the ratio is 30:90, which can be simplified to 1:3.

Question 25

Answer E is correct: 30%.

To obtain a percentage, divide the number of part-time students by the total number of students and then multiply this by 100, i.e. $\dfrac{6,037}{19,876} \times 100 = 30.37\%$. You are asked for an approximation, so 30% is correct.

Question 26

Answer A is correct: 2:3.

First obtain the number of students without the science students, 19,876 – 8,241 = 11,635. The ratio of science students compared to the rest of the students is 8,241:11,635. You are asked for an 'approximation', so round the numbers up or down to the nearest hundred, 8,200:11,600, which can be simplified to 41:58; round these numbers to 40:60, which can be simplified to 2:3. Alternatively, round the original numbers up or down to the nearest thousand, 8,000:12,000, which can be simplified to 2:3 by dividing both numbers by 4,000.

Question 27

Answer A is correct: £13m.

Obtain the number of students entitled to a loan, which is the total number of students minus the part-time students and science students, i.e. 19,876 – (6,037 + 8,241) = 19,876 – 14,278 = 5,598. The total cost of student loans is 5,598 × £2,300 = £12,875,400, which to the nearest £m is £13m.

Question 28

Answer D is correct: 4,600.

Find out the capacity of the two blocks, i.e. 21 × 48 = 1,008 and 38 × 93 = 3,534. Add the two figures together, 1,008 + 3,534 = 4,542, so the best approximation is 4,600.

Question 29

Answer C is correct: 48m².

The area of flooring for one bathroom is 4.2m × 2.4m = 10.08m², so for four bathrooms it is 10.08 × 4 = 40.32m².

One bathroom is $\frac{3}{4}$ of 10.08 = $\frac{10.08}{4} \times 3 = 7.56$m.

The total floor area is 40.32 + 7.56 = 47.88m², to the nearest whole metre = 48m².

Question 30

Answer E is correct: 112.

The area of a tile measuring 30cm² = 30 × 30 = 900cm.

The area of one larger bathroom is 4.2m × 2.4m, or 420cm × 240cm = 100,800cm. The number of tiles required is $\frac{100,800}{900} = 112$.

Question 31

Answer A is correct: (4,200 × 2,400) − (1,800 × 850).

The area that requires tiling is the area of the room (4,200mm × 2,400mm) minus the area of the shower (1,800mm × 850mm). Therefore the answer is (4,200 × 2,400) − (1,800 × 850).

Question 32

Answer C is correct: £1,122.50.

The price of 500 tiles × £2.75 = £1,375.00 − 12% discount = $\frac{1,375}{100} \times 12 = £165.00$, so £1,375.00 − £165.00 = £1,210.00.

500 tiles purchased − 430 used tiles = return of 70 tiles at £1.25 each = £87.50.

The floor layer will have paid £1,210.00 − £87.50 = £1,122.50.

Question 33

Answer B is correct: 22.

Add the number of values in the column 'number of disputes' and divide by the number of values to obtain the mean. The mean is $\frac{154}{7} = 22$.

Question 34

Answer C is correct: 25.

The mode is the number in the distribution that has the highest frequency. In this instance the number 25 appears twice and every other number only once.

Question 35

Answer E is correct: 45,840

The range of a distribution is the difference between the highest and lowest values. The highest value is 48,300 and the lowest 2,460, therefore 48,300 − 2,460 = 45,840.

Question 36

Answer A is correct: On average, redundancy had more days lost than any other reason for disputes.

Mental calculations can quickly dismiss all of the options with the exception of Answer A in relation to pay and redundancy. The average days lost per dispute for pay is $\dfrac{48,300}{52} = 928.8$. For redundancy it is $\dfrac{26,125}{24} = 1088.5$.

3. Abstract Reasoning practice subtest 1

Question number	Correct response	Question number	Correct response	Question number	Correct response
1	Set B	26	Neither Set	51	Set B
2	Neither Set	27	Set A	52	Set A
3	Set A	28	Set B	53	Set B
4	Set B	29	Neither Set	54	Set A
5	Neither Set	30	Set A	55	Set B
6	Neither Set	31	Set B	56	Set A
7	Neither Set	32	Neither Set	57	Set B
8	Set B	33	Set A	58	Set B
9	Set A	34	Neither Set	59	Neither Set
10	Set B	35	Set A	60	Set A
11	Set B	36	Set A	61	Neither Set
12	Set A	37	Set B	62	Set B
13	Neither Set	38	Neither Set	63	Set A
14	Set A	39	Neither Set	64	Neither Set
15	Neither Set	40	Set A	65	Set A
16	Set B	41	Set A	66	Set B
17	Set B	42	Neither Set	67	Set A
18	Set A	43	Set B	68	Neither Set
19	Set A	44	Set B	69	Set A
20	Neither Set	45	Set A	70	Neither Set
21	Set A	46	Set B	71	Set A
22	Set B	47	Set B	72	Neither Set
23	Neither Set	48	Set A	73	Neither Set
24	Set A	49	Neither Set	74	Set B
25	Neither Set	50	Set B	75	Set B

Questions 1–5

The shapes in Set A all contain three shapes within each other, the outer and inner shapes have solid straight lines, the middle shape has a dotted outline and is curved or part curved. The shapes in Set B also contain three shapes within each other, the outer two shapes have curved or part curved lines and the inner shape has straight lines. The use of black shading and the use of the same shape are distracters. Therefore:

Test shape 1 belongs to Set B as it contains three shapes within each other, the outer two shapes are curved and the inner shape has straight lines.

Test shape 2 belongs to Neither Set as the inner shape would need a solid outline in order to belong to Set A.

Test shape 3 belongs to Set A as it contains three shapes within each other, the outer and inner shapes have solid straight lines, the middle shape has a dotted outline and is curved.

Test shape 4 belongs to Set B as it contains three shapes within each other, the outer two shapes are curved or part curved and the inner shape has straight lines.

Test shape 5 belongs to Neither Set as it contains four shapes within each other.

Questions 6–10

The shapes in Set A all contain at least one white and one grey shaded circle. The shapes in Set B all contain at least one white star and one white square. The use of multiple white, black or grey shapes are all distracters. The answers are therefore as follows.

Test shape 6 belongs to Neither Set as one of the circles would need to be shaded grey in order to belong to Set A.

Test shape 7 belongs to Neither Set as the star would need to be white in order to belong to Set B.

Test shape 8 belongs to Set B as it contains at least one white star and one white square; the circles are incorrect for Set A as one would need to be shaded grey.

Test shape 9 belongs to Set A as it contains at least one white and one grey shaded circle.

Test shape 10 belongs to Set B as it contains at least one white star and one white square; the circles are incorrect for Set A as one would need to be shaded grey.

Questions 11–15

The shapes in Set A all contain two groups of shapes, one group containing two shapes within each other and the other group containing three shapes within each other. The shapes in Set B all contain three shapes within each other, the inner and outer shapes have straight lines and the middle shape has curved lines. The use of curved shapes and straight shapes in Set A, and the use of the same or differing shapes and black or grey shading in both sets are all distracters. The answers are therefore as follows.

Test shape 11 belongs to Set B as it contains three shapes within each other, the inner and outer shapes have straight lines and the middle shape has curved lines.

Test shape 12 belongs to Set A as it contains two groups of shapes, one group containing two shapes within each other and the other group containing three shapes within each other.

Test shape 13 belongs to Neither Set as one of the groups of shapes would need to have three shapes within each other in order to belong to Set A.

Test shape 14 belongs to Set A as it contains two groups of shapes, one group containing two shapes within each other and the other group containing three shapes within each other.

Test shape 15 belongs to Neither Set as the middle and inner shapes would need to be the other way round in order to belong to Set B.

Questions 16–20

The shapes in Set A all contain shapes with straight lines apart from one which has curved lines. The shapes in Set B all contain shapes with curved lines apart from one which has straight lines. The number and size of the shapes and black or grey shading are all distracters. The answers are therefore as follows.

Test shape 16 belongs to Set B as it contains shapes with curved lines apart from one which has straight lines.

Test shape 17 belongs to Set B as it contains shapes with curved lines apart from one which has straight lines.

Test shape 18 belongs to Set A as it contains shapes with straight lines apart from one which has curved lines.

Test shape 19 belongs to Set A as it contains shapes with straight lines apart from one which has curved lines.

Test shape 20 belongs to Neither Set as it contains an equal number of straight and curved line shapes which is not a characteristic of either set.

Questions 21–25

The shapes in Set A all comprise four sections. The shapes in Set B all comprise six sections. The number of shapes and the holes in the centre of the 'doughnut' shapes are distracters. The answers are therefore as follows.

Test shape 21 belongs to Set A as the shapes comprise four sections. Test shape 22 belongs to Set B as the shape comprises six sections.

Test shape 23 belongs to Neither Set as it contains five sections.

Test shape 24 belongs to Set A as the shape comprises four sections.

Test shape 25 belongs to Neither Set as it contains shapes that comprise four and six sections and therefore has the attributes of both sets.

Questions 26–30

The shapes in Set A are all made up of four straight lines. The shapes in Set B are all made up of five straight lines. The answers are therefore as follows.

Test shape 26 belongs to Neither Set as it is made up of eight straight lines. Test shape 27 belongs to Set A as it is made up of four straight lines.

Test shape 28 belongs to Set B as it is made up of five straight lines.

Test shape 29 belongs to Neither Set as it is made up of six straight lines. Test shape 30 belongs to Set A as it is made up of four straight lines.

Questions 31–35

The shapes in Set A all contain three shapes that overlap, creating two overlaps. The shapes in Set B all contain four shapes that overlap, creating three overlaps. The use of black and the number of shapes are distracters. The answers are therefore as follows.

Test shape 31 belongs to Set B as it contains four shapes that overlap, creating three overlaps.

Test shape 32 belongs to Neither Set as it contains five shapes that overlap, creating four overlaps.

Test shape 33 belongs to Set A as it contains three shapes that overlap, creating two overlaps. Test shape 34 belongs to Neither Set as it contains no overlapping shapes.

Test shape 35 belongs to Set A as it contains three shapes that overlap, creating two overlaps.

Questions 36–40

The shapes in Set A all contain at least one unique white shape which is not repeated in black. The shapes in Set B all contain at least one unique black shape which is not repeated in white. The use of Xs is a distracter. The answers are therefore as follows.

Test shape 36 belongs to Set A as the shape contains one unique white shape. Test shape 37 belongs to Set B as the shape contains one unique black shape.

Test shape 38 belongs to Neither Set as it does not contain any unique white or black shapes. Test shape 39 belongs to Neither Set as it contains two black shapes that are the same.

Test shape 40 belongs to Set A as the shape contains one unique white shape.

Questions 41–45

The shapes in Set A all contain at least two shapes the same on a diagonal. The shapes in Set B all contain at least two shapes the same on either the vertical or the horizontal. The use of black or white, the size of the shapes and direction changes, i.e. diagonals, are all distracters. The answers are therefore as follows.

Test shape 41 belongs to Set A as the shape contains two crosses on the diagonal.

Test shape 42 belongs to Neither Set as it contains two hearts on the diagonal and on the horizontal and vertical and therefore has the attributes of both sets.

Test shape 43 belongs to Set B as the shape contains two square shapes on the horizontal. Test shape 44 belongs to Set B as the shape contains two flag shapes on the vertical.

Test shape 45 belongs to Set A as the shape contains two octagons on the diagonal.

Questions 46–50

The shapes in Set A all contain shapes that have at least one right angle. The shapes in Set B all contain shapes with no right angles. The use of shading, the number of shapes and the use of 3D are all distracters. The answers are therefore as follows.

Test shape 46 belongs to Set B as the shape contains shapes without right angles. Test shape 47 belongs to Set B as the shape contains shapes without right angles.

Test shape 48 belongs to Set A as the shape contains shapes that all contain at least one right angle.

Test shape 49 belongs to Neither Set as it contains three shapes with at least one right angle and one shape with none, and therefore has the attributes of both sets.

Test shape 50 belongs to Set B as the shape contains shapes without right angles.

Questions 51–55

The shapes in Set A cannot be drawn without lifting the pen or pencil off the paper or retracing any line. The shapes in Set B can be drawn without lifting the pen or pencil off the paper or retracing any line. The answers are therefore as follows.

Test shape 51 belongs to Set B as it can be drawn without lifting the pen or pencil off the paper.

Test shape 52 belongs to Set A as it cannot be drawn without lifting the pen or pencil off the paper.

Test shape 53 belongs to Set B as it can be drawn without lifting the pen or pencil off the paper.

Test shape 54 belongs to Set A as it cannot be drawn without lifting the pen or pencil off the paper.

Test shape 55 belongs to Set B as it can be drawn without lifting the pen or pencil off the paper.

Questions 56–60

The shapes in Set A all contain a large shape that is reflected within by a small white shape. The shapes in Set B all contain a large shape that is reflected within by a small black shape. The number of small shapes used and the fact that some small shapes are outside the large shapes are all distracters. The answers are therefore as follows.

Test shape 56 belongs to Set A as the large white heart is reflected within by a small white heart.

Test shape 57 belongs to Set B as the large white doughnut shape is reflected within by a small black doughnut shape.

Test shape 58 belongs to Set B as the large white arrowed square is reflected within by a small black arrowed square.

Test shape 59 belongs to Neither Set as the large white circle contains both a white and black small circle and therefore has the attributes of both sets.

Test shape 60 belongs to Set A as the large white lightning flash is reflected within by a small white lightning flash.

Questions 61–65

The shapes in Set A all contain a shape with a black section, which is reflected outside the shape by a white shape. The shapes in Set B all contain a shape with a black section, which is not reflected outside by the white shape. The answers are therefore as follows.

Test shape 61 belongs to Neither Set as it does not contain a shape outside the main shape.

Test shape 62 belongs to Set B as the black section is not reflected in the white shape on the outside of the main shape.

Test shape 63 belongs to Set A as the black section is reflected in the white shape on the outside of the main shape.

Test shape 64 belongs to Neither Set as the black section is reflected as a black shape outside the main shape.

Test shape 65 belongs to Set A as the black section is reflected in the white shape on the outside of the main shape.

Questions 66–70

The shapes in Set A are all made up of curved lines. The shapes in Set B are all made up of straight lines. The use of black and white, the number of shapes used and whether shapes are within others or not, are all distracters. The answers are therefore as follows.

Test shape 66 belongs to Set B as the shapes are all made up of straight lines. Test shape 67 belongs to Set A as the shapes are all made up of curved lines.

Test shape 68 belongs to Neither Set as the shapes are made up of both curved and straight lines. Test shape 69 belongs to Set A as the shapes are made up of curved lines.

Test shape 70 belongs to Neither Set as the shapes are made up of both straight and curved lines.

Questions 71–75

The shapes in Set A all contain shapes that have three other shapes within. The shapes in Set B all contain shapes that have two other shapes within. The use of two groups of shapes is a distracter. The answers are therefore as follows.

Test shape 71 belongs to Set A as the shape contains three shapes within.

Test shape 72 belongs to Neither Set as one shape has two shapes within and the other shape has three shapes within; therefore, it has the characteristics of both sets.

Test shape 73 belongs to Neither Set as the shape only has one shape within. Test shape 74 belongs to Set B as the shape has two shapes within.

Test shape 75 belongs to Set B as the shape has two shapes within.

4. Decision Analysis practice subtest 1

Question number	Correct response
1	Option B
2	Option C
3	Option D
4	Option A
5	Options B & C
6	Option E
7	Option B
8	Option C
9	Option B
10	Option E
11	Option D
12	Option A
13	Option C
14	Options A & E
15	Options B & D
16	Option B
17	Option B
18	Option E
19	Option C
20	Option A
21	Options A & C
22	Option D
23	Option A
24	Option C
25	Option B
26	Option B
27	Option C
28	Options C & E

Question 1

🥾 K, 📄 K, 404, (11 99), ☺

The code combines the words 'sail increase','book increase','brother','happy smile','me'.

Option B,'Books on sailing please my brother' is the correct answer as it uses all the codes, with 'sail increase' being used as 'sailing', 'book increase' being used as 'books', 'happy smile' being used as 'please' and 'me' being used as 'my'.

Question 2

(404 606), 404, 606, G, FK, &K, ☺

The code combines the words 'brother cousin', 'brother', 'cousin', 'fight', 'ride increase', 'scooter increase', 'me'.

Option C,'My brother and cousin argue when riding their scooters', is the correct answer as it uses all the codes, with 'brother cousin' being used as 'their', 'fight' being used as 'argue', 'ride increase' being used as 'riding', 'scooter increase' being used as 'scooters' and 'me' being used as 'my'.

Question 3

(505 }), ☺, A, (Ⓟ 🚗)

The code combines the words 'sister skateboard', 'me', 'run', 'police car'.

Option D,'The police car ran over my sister's skateboard', is the correct answer as it uses all the codes, with 'sister skateboard' being used as 'sister's skateboard', 'me' being used as 'my' and 'run' being used as 'ran over'.

Question 4

(am pm), L, ☺ 👫, (J bb Υ 🍽)

The code combines the words 'morning afternoon', 'play', 'me them', 'negative breakfast lunch dinner'.

Option A, 'We play all day and forget to eat' is the correct answer as it uses all the codes, with 'morning afternoon' being used as 'all day', 'me them' being used as 'we' and 'negative breakfast lunch dinner' being used as 'forget to eat'.

Question 5

🚲 K, 101, &K, 101, AK

The code combines the words 'bike increase', 'us', 'scooter increase', 'us', 'run increase'.

Option B, 'Our bikes are faster than our scooters' and Option C, 'Our scooters aren't as fast as our bikes', are the correct answers as they use all the codes, with 'bike increase' being used as 'bikes', 'us' being used twice as 'our', 'scooter increase' being used as 'scooters', 'run increase' being used as 'faster' in Option B and just as 'fast' in Option C. However, the statements have the same meaning.

Question 6

⚐ K, hh, ⚓K, 11, ☺, M 505 ♂ ⚽ 404

The code combines the words 'bike increase', 'holiday', 'swim increase', 'happy', 'me', 'combine sister mother father brother'.

Option E, 'My family enjoy swimming and cycling on holiday', is the correct answer as it uses all the codes, with 'bike increase' being used as 'cycling', 'swim increase' being used as 'swimming', 'happy' being used as 'enjoy', 'me' being used as 'my' and 'combine sister mother father brother' being used as 'family'.

Question 7

707, ♂ , ⚽, 808

The code combines the words 'neighbour', 'mother', 'talk', 'doctor'.

Option B, 'Mum telephoned the doctor for the lady next door', is the correct answer as it uses all the codes, with 'neighbour' being used as 'lady next door', 'mother' being used as 'mum' and 'talk' being used as 'telephoned'.

Question 8

⚫l, 202, ♂ , 11, 101, ⛏ , M(202 ⚫ l)

The code combines the words 'enemies opposite', 'we', 'mother', 'happy', 'us', 'lunch', 'combine we enemies opposite'.

Option C, 'Our friends are happy when mum lets us have lunch together', is the correct answer as it uses all the codes, with 'enemies opposite' being used as 'friends', 'mother' being used as 'mum' and 'combine we enemies opposite' being used as 'together'.

Question 9

}, 202,⛨ , 707, 00

The code combines the words 'skateboard, 'we', 'them', 'neighbour', 'angry'.

Option B, 'Our neighbour was angry and took their skateboard', is the correct answer as it uses all the codes, with 'we' being used as 'our' and 'them' being used as 'their'.

Question 10

33 K, 77 I, 505, E, **&**, ☺

The code combines the words 'cry increase', 'tall opposite', 'sister', 'fall', 'scooter', 'me'.

Option E, 'My small sister fell off her scooter and cried', is the correct answer as it uses all the codes, with 'cry increase' being used as 'cried', 'tall opposite' being used as 'small', 'fall' being used as 'fell' and 'me' being used as 'my'.

Question 11

🚗 K, 202, J 💤, ☽

The code combines the words 'car increase', 'we', 'negative sleep', 'night'.

Option D, 'We had no sleep last night due to traffic', is the correct answer as it uses all the codes, with 'car increase' being used as 'traffic' and 'negative sleep' being used as 'no sleep'.

Question 12

🏊, 202, 101, 🪣 K, hh, ▶▶K

The code combines the words 'swim', 'we', 'us', 'bucket increase', 'holiday', 'spade increase'.

Option A, 'We swim and play with our buckets and spades on holiday', is the correct answer as it uses all the codes, with 'us' being used as 'our', and 'bucket increase' and 'spade increase' being used as 'buckets' and 'spades'.

Question 13

Ⓟ, 🚲, C K, Ⴤ , F

The code combines the words 'police', 'bike', 'jump increase', 'lunch', 'ride'.

Option C, 'The policeman jumped onto the bike and rode off for lunch', is the correct answer at it uses all the codes, with 'police' being used as 'policeman', 'jump increase' being used as 'jumped' and 'ride' becomes 'rode'.

Question 14

M(404 505), ⚔ , ☺, ☺, M(K 22 33 00), G

The code combines the words 'combine brother sister', 'mother', 'me', 'me', 'combine increase sad cry angry', 'fight'.

Option A, 'Mum gets very emotional when my siblings and I argue', and Option E, 'When I fall out with my siblings mother gets really upset', are the correct answers as they both combine all the codes. Option A uses 'mother' as 'mum' and 'combine increase sad cry angry' as 'very emotional', and 'combine brother sister' as 'siblings', and 'me' and 'me' as 'my' and 'I' respectively, and 'fight' as 'argue'. Option E uses 'fight' as 'fall out' and 'me' and 'me' as 'I' and 'my' respectively, with 'combine brother sister' being used as 'siblings', and 'combine increase sad cry angry' as 'really upset'.

Question 15

Options B and D, 'hot' and 'time', would be the two most useful additions to the codes when attempting to convey the message 'My family are flying off for a holiday in the sun later this year', the word 'hot' being used for 'sun' and the word 'time' being used for 'later'. The other words can be extrapolated from existing codes or are irrelevant.

Question 16

L, tt, 202, 🏃, 🎤, ☺, M{⚥ 🚤 🚗 🛹} ◎)

The code combines the words 'play', 'tomorrow', 'we', 'them', 'talk', 'me', 'combine bike boat car frisbee skateboard ball'.

Option B, 'I chat with my friends about which toys we will play with tomorrow', is the correct answer as it uses all the codes, with 'me' being used as both 'I' and 'my', 'them' being used as 'friends' and 'combine bike boat car frisbee skateboard ball' being used as 'toys'.

Question 17

K(99 44), 202, K 11, ☺, M(404 ⚥ 505 Υ)

Option B would be the best way to encode the message 'My family smile and laugh a lot because we are very happy'. This option has the correct codes by using K(99 44) 'increase smile laugh' as 'smile and laugh a lot', K 11 'increase happy' as 'very happy', and M(404 ⚥ 505 Υ) 'combine brother mother sister father' as family.

Question 18

⚥ , Υ , 707, 🍽, I 66, 🎤

The code combines the words 'mother', 'father', 'neighbour', 'dinner', 'opposite greedy', 'talk'.

Option E, 'The neighbour generously asked mum and dad to dinner', is the correct answer as it uses all the codes, with 'mother' and 'father' being used as 'mum' and 'dad', 'opposite greedy' being used as 'generously' and 'talk' being used as 'asked'.

Question 19

E, 88 ?, 101, 🚢, ⚓

The code combines the words 'fall', 'small skipping rope', 'us', 'opposite sail', 'boat'.

Option C, 'The rope fell off and our boat sank', is the correct answer as it uses all the codes, with 'fall' becoming 'fell', 'small skipping rope' being used as 'rope' and 'opposite sail' being used as 'sank'.

Question 20

K D, ^, L, 202, nn ww, I, M[☺ 👫]

The code combines the words 'increase fly', 'kite', 'play', 'we', 'now weekend', 'opposite', 'combine me them'.

Option A, 'This weekend we are having a kite-flying game against each other', is the correct answer as it uses all the codes, with 'now weekend' being 'this weekend', 'increase fly' becoming 'flying', 'play' being used as 'game', 'opposite' becoming 'against' and 'combine me them' being used as 'each other'.

Question 21

Options A and C, 'break' and 'drop', would be the two most useful additions to the codes when attempting to convey the message 'The police said that the paint poured on our car was criminal damage', the word 'break' being used for 'damage' and the word 'drop' being used for 'poured'. The other words can be extrapolated from existing codes or are irrelevant.

Question 22

M[bb Υ 🍽], 202, hh, M[⚣ Υ ☺ 404 505]

The code combines the words 'combine breakfast lunch dinner', 'we', 'holiday', 'combine mother father me brother sister'.

Option D, 'We have all our meals together when on holiday', is the correct answer as it uses all the codes, 'combine breakfast lunch dinner' being used as 'meals' and 'combine mother father me brother sister' being used as 'together'.

Question 23

#, E, 88 🗑, 88 707

The code combines the words 'paint', 'fall', 'small bucket', 'small neighbour'.

Option A, 'The child from next door fell over the tin of paint', is the correct answer as it uses all the codes, with 'fall' being used as 'fell over', 'small bucket' being used as 'tin' and 'small neighbour' being interpreted as 'child from next door'.

Question 24

K M(A C H B˳), 202, L, M(⸸ ϒ ☺ 404 505 606)

The code combines the words 'increase combine run jump climb walk swim', 'we', 'play', 'combine mother father me brother sister cousin'.

Option C, 'Our family have very active hobbies', is the correct answer as it uses all the codes, with 'increase combine run jump climb walk swim' being used as 'very active', 'we' being used as 'our', 'play' being used as 'hobbies' and 'combine mother father me brother sister cousin' being used as 'family'.

Question 25

G, 808, ☺, 505, I B, J ˳

Option B would be the best way to encode the message 'The doctor had to fight to stop my sister from drowning'. This option has the correct codes by using ☺ 'me' as 'my', I B 'opposite walk' as 'stop' and J ˳ 'negative swim' as 'drowning'.

Question 26

✐, ϒ, #, nn, ⛟, 55

The code combines the words 'crayon', 'father', 'paint', 'now', 'car', 'jealous'.

Option B, 'The paint colour of dad's new car is green', is the correct answer as it uses all the codes, with 'crayon' being used for 'colour', 'now' being used for 'new' and 'jealous' being used for 'green'.

Question 27

606, ☺404, ⬪K, ☺, H, nn ww, ☺404

Option C would be the best way to encode the message 'My brother and I are cycling uphill to our cousins this weekend'.

This option has the correct codes by using ☺404 'me brother' as 'my bother' and 'our', ☺ 'me' as 'I', ⬪K 'bike increase' as 'cycling', H 'climb' as 'uphill' and nn ww 'now weekend' as 'this weekend'.

Question 28

Options C and E, 'pet' and 'outside', would be the two most useful additions to the codes when attempting to convey the message 'My parents are cross with next door's cat and dog because they dig in our garden', the words 'pet increase' being used for 'dog' and 'cat' and the word 'outside' being used for 'garden'. The other words can be extrapolated from existing codes or are irrelevant.

5. Verbal Reasoning practice subtest 2

Question number	Correct response	Question number	Correct response
1	C	23	C
2	A	24	B
3	B	25	C
4	A	26	A
5	A	27	B
6	B	28	A
7	C	29	C
8	A	30	C
9	C	31	C
10	B	32	A
11	C	33	B
12	A	34	A
13	A	35	A
14	C	36	C
15	C	37	B
16	A	38	A
17	C	39	C
18	A	40	B
19	C	41	C
20	B	42	B
21	A	43	C
22	C	44	A

Passage I: question 1

C. Can't Tell

This may be the case but cannot be stated with certainty from the information contained in the passage. The passage refers to a trust hospital and it can be inferred that inspections of such hospitals are under the direction of the Healthcare Commission. However, no mention is made of National Health Service hospitals.

Passage I: question 2

A. True

Two examples are provided in the passage to support that statement: 'An audit by the hospital's own trust also found that only 6 out of 10 staff were washing their hands properly, but the trust's board was not informed' and 'The board had also been informed that attendance for mandatory infection control training by staff was acceptable, but in fact it was low'.

Passage I: question 3

B. False

The 22 cases of *C. difficile* are a statement of fact. The passage actually provides information contrary to the statement: 'The hospital has a good record on MRSA and *Clostridium difficile*' and 'These breaches of the government's hygiene code gave the Commission cause for concern, in spite of the low incidence of infections'.

Passage I: question 4

A. True

The statement is true and can be inferred from the following part of the passage: 'In the endoscopy suite it was not clear whether flexible tubes that are inserted into the body for diagnosis and treatment were ready for sterilisation or had already been decontaminated, even though this had previously been brought to the hospital's attention.' This strongly suggests an external inspection as opposed to an inspection by the trust itself. Where the trust has carried out its own inspections, these are clearly identified in the passage.

Passage II: question 5

A. True

In the last two sentences the passage talks about 'culture shock' and our reaction to another culture resulting in 'fear, which can lead to distrust and hostility'.

Passage II: question 6

B. False

This is a very general statement, and although armed conflicts might more often than not result from cultural differences, this may not always be the case. For example, a threat to survival or the actions of egomaniacs may result in conflict.

Passage II: question 7

C. Can't Tell

This might be the case, although to an extent that it would tend to contradict the essence of the passage. However, without further information, such as comparative studies with other countries, a true or false answer could not be determined.

Passage II: question 8

A. True

This is essentially the tenet of the passage as it actually states that 'Within those groups we have shared prejudices about other teams …'.

Passage III: question 9

C. Can't Tell

The passage provides two examples – the jatropha tree and algae – from which oil for use with kerosene jet fuel is being tested. It does not state that these are the only sources of alternative oil and further information would be required to clarify this.

Passage III: question 10

B. False

This answer is false as it distinctly states in the passage that this will 'not mean an end to the use of kerosene jet engines, as the amount of jatropha that would be needed to power the entire aviation section can never be produced in a sustainable way'.

Passage III: question 11

C. Can't Tell

In relation to algae, the passage states that they 'can be grown in arid regions and virtually anywhere'. However, for the jatropha tree the passage states that this is 'grown on marginal land in India, Mozambique, Malawi and Tanzania'. Although it may be the case that the jatropha tree can be grown in arid regions of the world and virtually anywhere, further information would be required before this can be stated as fact.

Passage III: question 12

A. True

This is true as the passage actually states that 'environmentalists argue that manufacturing biofuels can produce more emissions than they absorb when growing'.

Passage IV: question 13

A. True

This statement can be accepted as accurate as there is no mention in the passage of universities relaxing their entry criteria and there is no doubt that the additional 35,000 students had been accepted in defiance of the 13,000 government cap.

Passage IV: question 14

C. Can't Tell

Although it might be assumed that the university population is still mainly students under 25, this is not made explicit in the passage. The only real reference made is to the fact that 'There were an additional 60,000 applications for places in the current year, comprising a 10% increase in students overall but a 19.5% rise among students over 25 years of age.' However, this does not provide details of what numbers the increases were based on.

Passage IV: question 15

C. Can't Tell

Although redundancy and job insecurity may be a factor that has increased the number of over-25s going to university, no reasons for the increase are contained in the passage. Further information would be required before a 'true' or 'false' answer could be given.

Passage IV: question 16

A. True

This can be accepted from the statement 'the number of overseas students doubling in the past 10 years'. Next to the government, they are the biggest source of universities' funding.

Passage V: question 17

C. Can't Tell

The passage actually states that cars operate more efficiently above 30mph. However, there is no mention of lorries performing more efficiently above this speed and there is also no information about a maximum speed whereby efficiency decreases; this may be less than 70mph.

Passage V: question 18

A. True

The passage states: 'Also there is an understandable deep-rooted concern about Big Brother!' and implicit in this is the fact that speed limiters *might* lead to a greater infringement of civil liberties.

Passage V: question 19

C. Can't Tell

Although speed limiters are already fitted to the engines of some lorries, there is no information about this in the passage. Therefore, further information about this, together with comparative technical details concerning the pros and cons of existing and proposed speed limiters, would be required.

Passage V: question 20

B. False

The passage states that 'The Commission for Integrated Transport and the Motorists' Forum claim that accidents involving injuries could be cut by 12 per cent' or more where it was mandatory that speed limiters were fitted to vehicles. This statement envisages that there would be a reduction in accidents involving injury that would undoubtedly include vehicles driven by newly qualified drivers.

Passage VI: question 21

A. True

The passage actually states that '23 per cent of men and 15 per cent of women drink more than twice the government's recommended daily limit'. The passage also states that heavy drinkers are at an increased risk of permanent brain damage.

Passage VI: question 22

C. Can't Tell

The passage states that heavy drinkers are at an increased risk of engaging in unprotected sex. However, those who drink excessively only account for less than one-quarter of the population. In relation to unprotected sex, no figures are provided for either drinkers or other groups who do not drink excessively, so further information would be required before a true or false answer could be made.

Passage VI: question 23

C. Can't Tell

The passage states: 'Alcohol-related brain damage is an increasing burden on the NHS, and patients who do not die early with the condition …'. However, no comparative figures are provided with other illnesses, diseases or demographic factors that may be relevant. Further information would be required to support this statement.

Passage VI: question 24

B. False

The passage states that '23 per cent of men and 15 per cent of women drink more than twice the government's recommended daily limit'. If 15 per cent of women were heavy drinkers, for men to be twice as likely to be heavy drinkers the figure would need to be 30 per cent of men, i.e. 15 × 2, and not 23 per cent as given.

Passage VII: question 25

C. Can't Tell

In relation to 'bad parenting' the passage states: 'There are the possible positive and negative effects of … good and bad parenting.' It does not elaborate in relation to health matters of children in later life and further information would be required.

Passage VII: question 26

A. True

This is specifically stated in the passage 'more frequent occurrence of delirium with infection at the extremes of the age spectrum'.

Passage VII: question 27

B. False

The passage states: 'Early upbringing will also influence health in later life. There are the possible positive and negative effects of … parental smoking and alcohol use …'. The question states that 'Parental smoking or alcohol abuse has no adverse effect …'. This is incorrect as it may have an adverse effect.

Passage VII: question 28

A. True

The passage clearly states: 'Generally, older people see their health as functioning even in the presence of chronic disease while young people see health more as fitness.'

Passage VIII: question 29

C. Can't Tell

In relation to offenders undertaking community service the passage states that 'such sentences may result in fewer people being sent to prison'; note the word 'may'. Further information would be required to answer this question either as true or false.

Passage VIII: question 30

C. Can't Tell

Although the fact that 'the government considers that any shame felt by offenders is the shame ... of having committed an offence', clearly this doesn't mean that all offenders feel this shame; neither can we assume that none of these offenders feel ashamed. We have no way of knowing who feels ashamed and who does not, so the answer must be 'Can't Tell'.

Passage VIII: question 31

C. Can't Tell

The final sentence of the passage covers this statement, i.e. 'the Probation Service has highlighted the fact that there have been a number of attacks on offenders undertaking community service and that the use of bright orange bibs is almost certain to increase the risk'. Although the Probation Service considers an increase in attacks highly likely, as yet there is no evidence to substantiate this and further information would be required.

Passage VIII: question 32

A. True

This is actually stated within the passage 'putting offenders in stocks; that it is about shaming people'.

Passage IX: question 33

B. False

This is obviously false as the 200 pigs would still be producing 100 tons of carbon equivalent each year irrespective of the tax.

Passage IX: question 34

A. True

The last line of the passage states that cattle and pig farms going out of business would have 'a knock-on effect of widescale closures of food outlets across the country'. This indicates that there would be a shortage of pig and cattle products if the farms closed, and this shortage would mean many food outlets had nothing to sell.

Passage IX: question 35

A. True

This is true, as clearly stated in the second sentence of the passage: 'They consider this an environmental issue and say that farmers should be charged for rising levels of methane and other polluting nitrous gases emitted by farm animals.'

Passage IX: question 36

C. Can't Tell

Although farm animals' belching and flatulence do have a carbon footprint, it is not clear from the passage how 'significant' this actually is. It is difficult to assess what 100 tons of carbon equivalent is, as there are no comparative measures.

Passage X: question 37

B. False

The passage states: 'After being released from prison, 11 per cent of offenders are back in prison two years later. During the two-year period overall nearly half (46 per cent) of offenders started another prison sentence at some point.' This means that of the 46 per cent, a number started another prison sentence two years after being released.

Passage X: question 38

A. True

The final sentence states 'compared with 42 per cent for the average JSA claimant'.

Passage X: question 39

C. Can't Tell

The passage states: 'After being released from prison, 11 per cent of offenders prison are back in prison two years later.' From this it can be deduced that 89 per cent of offenders are not back in prison two years after their release. However, they may not have been apprehended for offences committed, and therefore further information would be required.

Passage X: question 40

B. False

The passage states: 'On average, offenders leaving prison spent 48 per cent of the next two years on out-of-work benefits.' The 47 per cent relates to offenders on out-of-work benefits two years after their release from prison.

Passage XI: question 41

C. Can't Tell

Although the passage states, 'As might be expected, the vast majority of people who have both low incomes and live in very energy-inefficient housing are in fuel poverty', specific measures for increasing energy efficiency such as loft insulation and double-glazing are not mentioned, and therefore further information would be required.

Passage XI: question 42

B. False

The passage states: 'It is thus a measure which compares income with what the fuel costs "should be" rather than what they actually are.'

Passage XI: question 43

C. Can't Tell

This is not specifically referred to in the passage. There is no mention in the statement in relation to people in rural areas on 'low income', and further information would be required.

Passage XI: question 44

A. True

The passage actually states that 'two of the low-income groups with high rates of fuel poverty are single-person households of working age'.

6. Quantitative Reasoning practice subtest 2

Question number	Correct response	Question number	Correct response
1	C	19	C
2	E	20	A
3	D	21	A
4	B	22	D
5	C	23	A
6	A	24	D
7	B	25	B
8	E	26	D
9	C	27	E
10	B	28	C
11	A	29	B
12	D	30	C
13	D	31	D
14	B	32	D
15	E	33	E
16	D	34	A
17	D	35	D
18	B	36	B

Question 1

Answer C is correct: £382.50.

The cost of the theatre company per session is £37.50, so 12 sessions cost £37.50 × 12 = £450.00. 85% of £450 = $\frac{450}{100} \times 85 = £382.50$.

Question 2

Answer E is correct: £35.50.

The range of a distribution is the difference between the highest and lowest values. The highest value is £37.50 and the lowest value of £2.00, therefore the range is £37.50 − £2.00 = £35.50.

Question 3

Answer D is correct: 28%.

In relation to shop training, the user cost is £32.50 and the charity cost is £23.25. The 'profit' made is £32.50 − £23.25 = £9.25. The 'profit' as a percentage of user cost is $\frac{9.25}{32.50} \times 100 = 28\%$.

Question 4

Answer B is correct: £13.80.

Add the costs for each activity: theatre company £37.50 + rural craft (×2) £15.50 + badminton £2.50 + yoga £4.00 = £59.50. Personal budget of £78.20 − £59.50 = £18.70. The amount of additional money they would need to attend shop training is the cost of the training £32.50 − £18.70 = £13.80.

Question 5

Answer C is correct: 180.10 minutes.

Find the mean running time by summing the values of the top ten women runners and dividing by the number of values. Convert the running times to minutes. First sum the value of the hours = 26, convert to minutes, 26 × 60 = 1,560 minutes. Then sum the value of the minutes = 241 minutes. Add these together, so 1,560 + 241 = 1,801 minutes. Divide by the number of values, $\frac{1,801}{10} = 180.10$ minutes. $\frac{2.42 + 2.46}{2} = 2$ hours 44 minutes.

Question 6

Answer A is correct: 14 minutes.

The mode is the number in the distribution that has the highest frequency. For the men's half marathon, the time 2 hours 48 minutes is the only one to appear more than once. For the women's half marathon the time 3 hours 2 minutes is the only one to appear more than once. Therefore, the difference between the mode running times for the men's and women's half marathon is 3 hours 2 minutes − 2 hours 48 minutes = 14 minutes.

Question 7

Answer B is correct: 2 hours 44 minutes.

To find the median of a set of values where there is an even number, add the two middle values together and divide by 2. The middle two running times are 2 hours 42 minutes and 2 hours 46 minutes, so the median is $\frac{2.42 + 2.46}{2} = 2$ hours 44 minutes.

Question 8

Answer E is correct: 55%

In the men's half marathon, 4 runners had times less than 2 hours 46 minutes. In the women's half marathon, 7 runners had times less than 3 hours 5 minutes. Therefore, 4 + 7 = 11 runners out of the 20 who reached the qualifying time. So, 11 as a percentage of 20 = $\frac{11}{20} \times 100 = 55\%$.

Question 9

Answer C is correct: 41%.

Obtain the percentage by writing the first number as a fraction of the second and multiplying by 100. There are 31 clubs with a turnover in excess of £8m (23 + 8) and 75 clubs in total, so $\frac{31}{75} \times 100 = 41.33\%$, rounded down to 41%.

Question 10

Answer B is correct: A$8,500,000.

The minimum turnover in this group is £4.1m. To convert this to Australian dollars, multiply by the conversion rate, £4.1m × A$2.10 = A$8,610,000, which to the nearest A$500,000 is A$8,500,000.

Question 11

Answer A is correct: 8.

Obtain 60% of 900, which is $\frac{900}{100} \times 60 = 540$, and this leaves 900 − 540 = 360 employees. The 360 employees are spread pro rata across 44 clubs. Therefore, each of these clubs employs $\frac{360}{44} = 8.18 \text{ staff}$, which to the nearest whole number is 8.

Question 12

Answer D is correct: 1:4.

Any two numbers can be compared by writing them alongside each other separated by a ratio (:) sign. There are 15 clubs with a turnover between £6.1m and £10m (7 + 8), and there are 60 other clubs (75 − 15). Therefore, the ratio is 15:60, which can be simplified to 1:4.

Question 13

Answer D is correct: £87.75.

To apply one coat: 7.5m × 2.75m × 2 = 41.25, rounded to 42 square metres + 3.5m × 2.75m = 9.625, rounded to 10 square metres = 52 square metres. One 5-litre tin of paint covers

12 square metres, therefore the amount of paint required is 52 square metres divided by 12 square metres = 4.3 tins of paint. Double this for two coats of paint, 4.3 × 2 = 8.6 tins of paint. Therefore, 9 tins will be required at a total cost of 9 × £9.75 = £87.75.

Question 14

Answer B is correct: 4.

The width of the wall is 3.5m (350cm) and the width of the paper is 55cm, therefore $\frac{350}{55} = 6.36,$ so 7 widths of wallpaper will be required. The height of the wall is 2.75m, so 2.75m × 7 = 19.25m is the total length of wallpaper needed. Each roll of wallpaper is 5m long, therefore $\frac{19.25}{5} = 3.85$ rolls of wallpaper are required, which rounded to the highest whole number is 4.

Question 15

Answer E is correct: 35m.

For the side wall without the door, the width of the wall is 3.5m (350cm), the width of the paper is 55cm, so $\frac{350}{55} = 6.36,$ therefore 7 widths of wallpaper will be required. The height of the wall is 2.75m, so 2.75m × 7 = 19.25m is the total length of wallpaper needed for that wall.

For the side wall with the door, initially assume that there is no door, so the length of wallpaper is the same as for the other wall at 19.25m. Calculate the depth of the door that accounts for two 55cm widths of wallpaper: 1.75 × 2 = 3.5. Deduct this from the total length: 19.25m – 3.5m = 15.75m. Add these two figures together to arrive at total length of wallpaper for both side walls: 19.25 + 15.75 = 35m.

Question 16

Answer D is correct: £520.00.

Cost of paint: £9.75 × 7 = £68.25 – 20% $\left(\frac{628.25}{100} \times 20 = 13.65 \right) = £54.60.$

Cost of wallpaper: £2.65 × 8 = £21.20 – 20% $\left(\frac{21.20}{100} \times 20 = 4.24 \right) = £16.96.$

Labour costs: £18.50 × 20 = £370.00 + VAT $\left(\frac{370}{100} \times 20 = 74 \right) = £444.00.$

The total cost of the job is £54.60 + £16.96 + £444.00 = £515.56, to the nearest £10.00 is £520.00.

Question 17

Answer D is correct: 3,100.

Detected crime resulting in a charge or court summons is 49% of 1.37m, i.e.
$\dfrac{1,370,000}{100} \times 49 = 671,300.$

Detected crime resulting in spot fines, warnings and police cautions is 207,500 + 104,000 + 362,900 = 674,400.

Therefore, 674,400 – 671,300 = 3,100 more people were dealt with by spot fines, warnings or cautions than were dealt with by a charge or court summons.

Question 18

Answer B is correct: 15.15%.

There were 207,500 spot fines. Calculate 1% of total crime of 1.37m = $\dfrac{1,370,000}{100} = 13,700.$ So the percentage of spot fines is $\dfrac{207,500}{13,700} = 15.15\%.$

Question 19

Answer C is correct: 2:7.

Any two numbers can be compared by writing them alongside each other separated by a ratio (:) sign. There were 104,000 cannabis warnings and 362,900 police cautions. The ratio is 104,000:362,900 – for an approximate ratio this can be rounded to 100,000:350,000, which can be simplified to 100:350 and then to 2:7.

Question 20

Answer A is correct: 503,797.

Number of detected crimes in 10 years will increase by $\dfrac{1,370,000}{100} \times 18 = 246,600.$ and 1,370,000 + 246,600 = 1,616,600.

Last year spot fines, warnings and cautions accounted for 51% of detected crime:
$\dfrac{1,370,000}{100} \times 51 = 698,700.$
Percentage relating to police cautions is $\dfrac{362,900}{698,700} \times 100 = 51.94\%.$

In 10 years' time, 40% of detected crime results in a charge or court summons,
$\dfrac{1,616,600}{100} \times 40 = 646,640$ people, therefore spot fines, warnings and cautions account for 1,616,600 – 646,640 = 969,960.

If police cautions still account for 51.94%, the number of people cautioned will be
$\dfrac{969,960}{100} \times 51.94 = 503,797.$

Question 21

Answer A is correct: $17\frac{3}{4}$ hours.

The flight time from the UK to New Zealand via China is $11\frac{1}{4}+16=27\frac{1}{4}$ hours. Adding a stopover of 4 days (96 hours) gives $27\frac{1}{4}+96=123\frac{1}{4}$ hours.

The flight time from the UK to Australia via Dubai is $7\frac{1}{4}+14=21\frac{1}{2}$ hours. Adding a stopover of $3\frac{1}{2}$ days (84 hours) gives $21\frac{1}{2}+84=105\frac{1}{2}$ hours.

The difference in time is $123\frac{1}{4}-105\frac{1}{2}=17\frac{3}{4}$ hours.

Question 22

Answer D is correct: £4,908.75.

A single fare: UK to China = 6,250 × £0.15 = £937.50. China to New Zealand = 9,750 × £0.20 = £1,950.00. Cost of single fare to New Zealand via China = £937.50 + £1,950 = £2,887.50.

Cost of return fare is £2,887.50 × 2 = £5,775.00, −15%. Reduction of 15% is $\frac{5,775}{100}\times15$ = £866.25. Therefore, total cost = £5,775.00 − £866.25 = £4,908.75.

Question 23

Answer A is correct: 2 minutes.

Dubai flight: $7\frac{1}{2}$ hours (flying time) + 4 hours (GMT +4) + 1 hour 12 minutes delay = 12 hours 42 minutes. Dubai time = 10.00 hours + 12 hours 42 minutes = 22.42 hours Monday.

Hawaii flight: 17 hours (flying time) − 10 hours (GMT −10) + 5 hours 20 minutes = 12 hours 20 minutes. Hawaii time = 10.00 + 12 hours 20 minutes = 22.40 hours Monday.

Question 24

Answer D is correct: $26\frac{1}{2}$ hours.

The distance to Australia with a stopover in Fiji is 12,800 + 2,300 = 15,100 miles. To calculate the time for the Boeing 787, divide the number of miles by the average speed, i.e. $\frac{15,100}{570}$ = 29.49 hours, which to the nearest half hour is 26.5 or $26\frac{1}{2}$.

Question 25

Answer B is correct: 61,782.

In 1981 the population was 56,352 and in 2001 it was 59,009.

The percentage increase between 1981 and 2001 is 59,009 − 56,352 = 2,657, then $\frac{2,657}{56,352} \times 100 = 4.7\%$.

The population in 2021 would be $59,009 + 4.7\% = \frac{59,009}{100} \times 4.7 = 2,773$; 59,009 + 2,773 = 61,782.

Question 26

Answer D is correct: In the twentieth century the percentage growth rate in Northern Ireland has exceeded that in Scotland.

The percentage growth rate in Northern Ireland: 1,675 (2001) − 1,237 (1901) = 438; $\frac{438}{1,237} \times 100 = 35.4\%$.

The growth rate in Scotland: 5,123 (2001) − 4,479 (1901) = 644; $\frac{644}{4,479} \times 100 = 14.4\%$.

The percentage growth rate in Northern Ireland far exceeded that in Scotland.

Question 27

Answer E is correct: $\frac{1}{8}$.

Population in Scotland in 1941 was 5,160 and in England and Wales was 41,748.

Expressed as a fraction, $\frac{5,160}{41,748}$, which to approximate can be rounded down to $\frac{5,000}{40,000}$, divide both by 5,000 = $\frac{1}{8}$.

Question 28

Answer C is correct: 19,178.

1951 >50 population was 25%; 1991 >50 population was 31%; an increase of 6% in four decades.

Between 1991 and 2001 (one decade) the percentage increase would be $\frac{6\%}{4} = 1.5\%$, so that 31% + 1.5% = 32.5% of the UK population would be over 50.

32.5% of the 2001 UK population is $\frac{59,009}{100} \times 32.5 = 19,177.992 = 19,178$.

Question 29

Answer B is correct: 1 hour 40 minutes.

60 minutes/30mph × 20 miles = 40 minutes.

60 minutes/60mph × 40 miles = 40 minutes.

60 minutes/30mph × 10 miles = 20 minutes.

Total time = 40 + 40 + 20 = 1 hour 40 minutes.

Question 30

Answer C is correct: 210.94 miles.

Journey time 3 hours = 180 minutes.

$\dfrac{1}{4}$ of journey is $\dfrac{180}{4}$ = 45 minutes. $\dfrac{90}{60} \times 45 = 67.5$ kilometres.

$\dfrac{3}{4}$ of journey is $\dfrac{180}{4} \times 3 = 135$ minutes. $\dfrac{120}{60} \times 135 = 270$ kilometres.

Total kilometres: 67.5 + 270 = 337.5 kilometres. Convert to miles: $\dfrac{337.5}{1.6} = 210.94$ miles.

Question 31

Answer D is correct: 718.75 kilometres.

Total fuel used = 75 + $\dfrac{2}{3}$ of 75 = 125 litres. Kilometres travelled = 125 × 5.75 = 718.75 kilometres.

Question 32

Answer D is correct: 12 laps.

Distance travelled: 80mph for 3 minutes = $\dfrac{80}{60} \times 3 = 4$ miles; 110mph for 12 minutes = $\dfrac{110}{60} \times 12 = 22$ miles; 140mph for 15 minutes = $\dfrac{140}{60} \times 15 = 35$ miles. Total distance 4 + 22 + 35 = 61 miles.

No of laps completed: $\dfrac{61}{5}$ = 12.2, therefore 12 full laps completed.

Question 33

Answer E is correct: 1,150.

If $\dfrac{1}{3}$ of women's deaths = 575, then the men's deaths account for $\dfrac{2}{3}$, which is 575 × 2 = 1,150.

Question 34

Answer A is correct: Between 1985 and 2004 the average death rate for people over 70 exceeded the average death rate for people aged 31–50 by over 44%.

Over 70: 61% + 54% + 57% + 60% = 232. $\dfrac{232}{4}$ = 58%.

31–50: 10% + 15% + 16% + 14% = 55. $\frac{55}{4} = 13.75\%$.

Difference is 58% − 13.75% = 44.25%, so deaths for people over 70 did exceed the average death rate of people aged 31–50 by over 44%.

Question 35

Answer D is correct: 4:1

Between 2000 and 2004, 60% of deaths are of those aged over 70; 14% are of those aged 31–50. The ratio is therefore 60:14, which is approximately 60:15 or 4:1.

Question 36

Answer B is correct: The largest percentage change in the death rate has occurred in people aged over 70.

The largest percentage change in the death rate in any group is the 7 percentage point fall for the over-70 group between 1985 and 1989, and 1990 and 1994.

7. Abstract Reasoning practice subtest 2

Question number	Correct response	Question number	Correct response	Question number	Correct response
1	Neither Set	26	Set A	51	Set B
2	Set A	27	Set A	52	Neither Set
3	Set A	28	Neither Set	53	Neither Set
4	Neither Set	29	Set B	54	Set A
5	Set B	30	Set B	55	Set B
6	Neither Set	31	Neither Set	56	Neither Set
7	Set A	32	Neither Set	57	Neither Set
8	Neither Set	33	Set B	58	Set B
9	Set B	34	Set A	59	Neither Set
10	Set B	35	Set A	60	Set A
11	Neither Set	36	Set B	61	Set A
12	Set B	37	Neither Set	62	Set A
13	Set B	38	Set A	63	Set B
14	Set A	39	Set B	64	Neither Set
15	Set A	40	Set A	65	Set A
16	Neither Set	41	Neither Set	66	Set B
17	Set B	42	Set A	67	Set B
18	Neither Set	43	Neither Set	68	Set A
19	Neither Set	44	Set B	69	Neither Set
20	Set A	45	Set A	70	Set B
21	Set B	46	Set B	71	Neither Set
22	Neither Set	47	Neither Set	72	Neither Set
23	Set B	48	Set A	73	Set B
24	Set A	49	Set B	74	Neither Set
25	Neither Set	50	Neither Set	75	Set A

Questions 1–5

The spots on the dominoes in Set A add up to an even number; each domino has an odd number of spots; the left-hand domino has the highest value at the top and the right-hand domino has the highest value at the bottom. The spots on the dominoes in Set B add up to an odd number; the left-hand domino adds up to an odd number; the right-hand domino adds up to an even number and the highest value is at the bottom of both dominoes. The answers are therefore as follows.

Test shape 1 belongs to Neither Set as both dominoes are an even number and this does not fit the characteristics of either set.

Test shape 2 belongs to Set A as the spots on the dominoes add up to an even number; each domino has an odd number of spots; the left-hand domino has the highest value at the top and the right-hand domino has the highest value at the bottom.

Test shape 3 belongs to Set A as the spots on the dominoes add up to an even number; each domino has an odd number of spots; the left-hand domino has the highest value at the top and the right-hand domino has the highest value at the bottom.

Test shape 4 belongs to Neither Set as the values add up to an even number as in Set A, but the highest values on the two dominoes are at the bottom left and top right, which is the reverse of the requirement for Set A.

Test shape 5 belongs to Set B as the spots on the dominoes add up to an odd number; the left-hand domino adds up to an odd number; the right-hand domino adds up to an even number and the highest value is at the bottom of both dominoes.

Questions 6–10

The shapes in Set A add up to an even number and half of the shapes are black. The shapes in Set B add up to an odd number and all but one are white. The use of different shading in Set B is a distracter as are items that contain the same shape. The answers are therefore as follows.

Test shape 6 belongs to Neither Set as the shapes add up to an odd number but more than one is black.

Test shape 7 belongs to Set A as the shapes add up to an even number and half are black.

Test shape 8 belongs to Neither Set since even though the shapes add up to an odd number, there are two shapes shaded instead of just one.

Test shape 9 belongs to Set B as the shapes add up to an odd number and all but one are white. Test shape 10 belongs to Set B as the shapes add up to an odd number and all but one are white.

Questions 11–15

The two clock shapes in Set A have clockwise angles from the large hand to the small hand that add up to either 90 or 150 degrees (15 minutes or 25 minutes). The two clock shapes in

Set B have clockwise angles from the large hand to the small hand that add up to 270 degrees (45 minutes). Therefore:

Test shape 11 belongs to Neither Set as the two clock shapes have angles that add up to 120 degrees (20 minutes).

Test shape 12 belongs to Set B as the two clock shapes have angles that add up to 270 degrees (45 minutes).

Test shape 13 belongs to Set B as the two clock shapes have angles that add up to 270 degrees (45 minutes).

Test shape 14 belongs to Set A as the two clock shapes have angles that add up to 150 degrees (25 minutes).

Test shape 15 belongs to Set A as the two clock shapes have angles that add up to 90 degrees (15 minutes).

Questions 16–20

The shapes in Set A all have four enclosed areas; if a shape with a curved side overlaps one with a straight side, then the overlap is grey. The shapes in Set B all have five enclosed areas; if shapes with straight sides overlap, then the remainder of the shape is black. The answers are therefore as follows.

Test shape 16 belongs to Neither Set as the overlap area would need to be grey for Set A and there are insufficient enclosed areas for Set B.

Test shape 17 belongs to Set B as there are five enclosed areas and no overlapping straight-sided shapes.

Test shape 18 belongs to Neither Set as the remainder of the overlapping straight sided shapes should have been black in order to belong to Set B.

Test shape 19 belongs to Neither Set as the overlap between the square and the circle should have been grey in order to belong to Set A.

Test shape 20 belongs to Set A as there are four enclosed areas and the overlap between a curved and a straight side is shaded grey.

Questions 21–25

The shapes in Set A have two shapes that create one overlap and the bottom right-hand corner is always blank. The shapes in Set B have three shapes that create two overlaps and the top left-hand corner is always blank. The number of shapes and shading are distracters. The answers are therefore as follows.

Test shape 21 belongs to Set B as the Test shape has three shapes that create two overlaps and the top left-hand corner is blank.

Test shape 22 belongs to Neither Set as the Test shape has four shapes that create three overlaps which is not a requirement for either set.

Test shape 23 belongs to Set B as the Test shape has three shapes that create two overlaps and the top left-hand corner is blank.

Test shape 24 belongs to Set A as the Test shape has two shapes that create one overlap and the bottom right-hand corner is blank.

Test shape 25 belongs to Neither Set as it does not contain any overlapping shapes and there are no blank corners.

Questions 26–30

The shapes in Set A are all made up of grids which contain 40 black squares and the remaining 24 squares have 2 grey squares vertically adjacent. The shapes in Set B are all made up of grids which contain 32 black squares and the remaining 32 squares have 3 grey squares horizontally adjacent. The answers are therefore as follows.

Test shape 26 belongs to Set A as the grid contains 40 black squares and 2 grey squares vertically adjacent.

Test shape 27 belongs to Set A as the grid contains 40 black squares and 2 grey squares vertically adjacent.

Test shape 28 belongs to Neither Set as the grid only contains 24 black squares, which is an invalid requirement.

Test shape 29 belongs to Set B as the grid contains 32 black squares and 3 grey squares horizontally adjacent.

Test shape 30 belongs to Set B as the grid contains 32 black squares and 3 grey squares horizontally adjacent.

Questions 31–35

The shapes in Set A all contain a small, medium and large shape; counting double for shaded shapes, the number of lines used to create the shapes equals 17. The shapes in Set B all contain a large grey shape and two small white shapes; counting double for the small white shapes, the number of lines used to create the shapes equals 28. The answers are therefore as follows.

Test shape 31 belongs to Neither Set as it contains shapes that would require 21 lines if the shaded shape is doubled as in Set A and it does not fit the characteristics of Set B.

Test shape 32 belongs to Neither Set as it contains three shapes that are the same size, which is not a requirement for either set.

Test shape 33 belongs to Set B as it contains a large grey shape and two small white shapes; counting double for the small white shapes, the number of lines used to create the shapes equals 28.

Test shape 34 belongs to Set A as it contains a small, medium and large shape; counting double for the shaded shape, the number of lines used to create the shapes equals 17.

Test shape 35 belongs to Set A as it contains a small, medium and large shape; counting double for the shaded shape, the number of lines used to create the shapes equals 17.

Questions 36–40

The shapes in Set A all contain the same number of hearts as there are right angles in the straight-sided shapes. The shapes in Set B all contain one more circular shape than the number of straight-sided shapes without right angles. The use of black or white hearts or circles are distracters. The answers are therefore as follows.

Test shape 36 belongs to Set B as it contains one more circular shape than the number of straight-sided shapes without right angles.

Test shape 37 belongs to Neither Set as it does not contain the correct number of hearts in relation to the number of right angles.

Test shape 38 belongs to Set A as it contains the same number of hearts as there are right angles in the straight-sided shapes.

Test shape 39 belongs to Set B as it contains one more circular shape than the number of straight-sided shapes without right angles.

Test shape 40 belongs to Set A as it contains the same number of hearts as there are right angles in the straight-sided shape.

Questions 41–45

The shapes in Set A contain eight shapes (ignoring the centre shape) which rotate clockwise in the same order in each square but the rotation does not always follow from square to square, the same shapes are always white, black, grey and striped; in addition, the centre shape is always the same as the top right-hand shape but always has the colour of the top left-hand shape. The shapes in Set B contain eight shapes (ignoring the centre shape) which rotate clockwise in the same order in each square and the rotations follow clockwise starting from left to right across each row; in addition, the centre circle is grey when two circles are on the diagonal, black when two circles are on the horizontal and white when two circles are on the vertical. The answers are therefore as follows.

Test shape 41 belongs to Neither Set as the centre shape is shaded rather than white.

Test shape 42 belongs to Set A as the shapes rotate clockwise in the same order and the centre shape is a star which is striped.

Test shape 43 belongs to Neither Set as it contains three circular shapes, which is not a characteristic of either Set A or Set B.

Test shape 44 belongs to Set B as the shapes rotate clockwise in the same order and it would be the next square in the sequence if the rotation continued; in addition, the centre circle is grey as the circles are on a diagonal.

Test shape 45 belongs to Set A as the shapes rotate clockwise in the same order and the centre shape is a cross which is white.

Questions 46–50

The shapes in Set A all join together to make the same size solid circle. The shapes in Set B all join together to make the same size solid square. The black shading is irrelevant.

Test shape 46 belongs to Set B as the shapes would form the same size solid square.

Test shape 47 belongs to Neither Set as the shapes would join together to form a solid triangle. Test shape 48 belongs to Set A as the shapes would form the same size solid circle.

Test shape 49 belongs to Set B as the shapes would form the same size solid square.

Test shape 50 belongs to Neither Set as the shapes would form either a cross or a square with a hole in the centre which would be incorrect for Set B.

Questions 51–55

The shapes in Set A all contain arrows and hearts; if at least two arrows point up, the lower heart is grey; if at least two arrows point down, the upper heart is grey; arrows can be either black or white; two hearts are always white and one is always grey. The shapes in Set B all contain arrows and hearts; if at least two arrows point left, the lower heart is white; if at least two arrows point right, the upper heart is white; arrows can be either black or white; two hearts are always grey and one is always white. The answers are therefore as follows.

Test shape 51 belongs to Set B as the two arrows point right and the white heart is uppermost.

Test shape 52 belongs to Neither Set as the arrows and hearts are the wrong shades for either set.

Test shape 53 belongs to Neither Set as the arrows and hearts are the wrong shades for either set.

Test shape 54 belongs to Set A as at least two arrows point up and the grey heart is below the two white hearts.

Test shape 55 belongs to Set B as at least two arrows point left and the white heart is below the two grey hearts.

Questions 56–60

The shapes in Set A contain a single grey diamond, but where there are two diamonds the right-hand diamond is black; there are three different white shapes; if other shapes are present, they are grey circles. The shapes in Set B contain a single white diamond, but where there are two diamonds the diamond closer to the top is grey; there are two white shapes with an additional black shape which matches one of the two; if other shapes are present, they are black circles. The answers are therefore as follows.

Test shape 56 belongs to Neither Set as the uppermost diamond would need to be grey for the shape to belong to Set B.

Test shape 57 belongs to Neither Set as the diamond to the left would need to be grey for the shape to belong to Set A.

Test shape 58 belongs to Set B as it contains a grey diamond above a white diamond and two white shapes with one repeated in black.

Test shape 59 belongs to Neither Set as the lower diamond would need to be white in order to belong to Set B.

Test shape 60 belongs to Set A as it contains a single grey diamond; three different white shapes and the additional shapes are grey circles.

Questions 61–65

The shapes in Set A contain a chevron that points to the left if two or more irregular shapes are present; otherwise the arrow points right; if a diamond is present, the arrow is black. The shapes in Set B contain a chevron which points right if two or more irregular shapes are present; otherwise the arrow points left; if a heart is present, the arrow is black.

Test shape 61 belongs to Set A as it contains four irregular shapes with a white chevron pointing left as no diamond is present.

Test shape 62 belongs to Set A as it contains no irregular shapes and a black chevron pointing right as a diamond is present.

Test shape 63 belongs to Set B as it contains three irregular shapes with a black chevron pointing right as a triangle is present.

Test shape 64 belongs to Neither Set as it contains two irregular shapes with a diamond but the chevron is pointing right instead of left.

Test shape 65 belongs to Set A as it contains no irregular shapes and a white chevron pointing right as no diamond is present.

Questions 66–70

The shapes in Set A contain an arrow which points to the right if two or three irregular shapes are present; otherwise the arrow points left; if a heart is present, the arrow is black. The shapes in Set B contain an arrow that points to the left if two or three irregular shapes are present; otherwise the arrow points right; if a diamond is present, the arrow is black. The answers are therefore as follow.

Test shape 66 belongs to Set B as the shape contains three irregular shapes with a white arrow pointing left as no diamond is present.

Test shape 67 belongs to Set B as the shape contains no irregular shapes with a black arrow pointing right as a diamond is present.

Test shape 68 belongs to Set A as the shape contains two irregular shapes with a black arrow pointing right as a heart is present.

Test shape 69 belongs to Neither Set as it contains three irregular shapes with a diamond but the arrow is pointing left instead of right.

Test shape 70 belongs to Set B as the shape contains no irregular shapes with a white arrow pointing right as no diamond is present.

Questions 71–75

The shapes in Set A contain a single grey square but where there are two, the right- hand square is black; there are 3 different white shapes; if other shapes are present they are grey triangles. The shapes in Set B contain a single white square but where there are two, the square closer to the top is grey; there are two white shapes with an additional black shape which matches one of the two; if other shapes are present they are black hearts. The answers are therefore as follows.

Test shape 71 belongs to Neither Set as the uppermost square would need to be grey in order to belong to Set B.

Test shape 72 belongs to Neither Set as the square to the left would need to be grey in order to belong to Set A.

Test shape 73 belongs to Set B as it contains a grey square above a white square and two white shapes with one repeated in black.

Test shape 74 belongs to Neither Set as the lower square would need to be white in order to belong to Set B.

Test shape 75 belongs to Set A as it contains a single grey square; three different white shapes and the additional shapes are grey triangles.

8. Decision Analysis practice subtest 2

Question number	Correct response
1	Option A
2	Option B
3	Option E
4	Option C
5	Option C
6	Option D
7	Option A
8	Option E
9	Options B & C
10	Option C
11	Option C
12	Option B
13	Option D
14	Option E
15	Option A
16	Option B
17	Option C
18	Option D
19	Option E
20	Option E
21	Option D
22	Option A
23	Options A & D
24	Option B
25	Options A & E
26	Option C
27	Option D
28	Option B

Question 1

312, 213 Z, œ, U, 123, Ω

The code combines the words 'Persia', 'Greece people', 'greater', 'budget', 'Mongolia', 'army'.

Option A, 'The Greek army budget is greater than that of Persia or Mongolia', is the correct answer as it uses all the codes, with 'Greece people' being used as 'Greek'.

Question 2

Ω, + 110, ə π, 231, Ђ

The code combines the words 'army', 'negative employment', 'opposite female', 'Mesopotamia', 'conscription'.

Option B, 'Unemployed men are forced to join the Mesopotamia army', is the correct answer as it uses all the codes, with 'negative employment' being used as 'unemployed', 'opposite female' being used as 'male' and 'conscription' being used as 'forced to join'.

Question 3

Σ, ¥ (Φ œ), 101 η, Ж, Ґ η Z

The code combines the words 'government', 'combine attack greater', 'housing less', 'insurgents', 'terrorists less people'.

Option E, 'Terrorist groups and insurgents attacked government house', is the correct answer as it uses all the codes, with 'combine attack greater' being used as 'attacked', 'housing less' being used as 'house' and 'terrorists less people' being used as 'terrorist groups'.

Question 4

η, Ω, Ґ, β, T, 999 œ

The code combines the words 'less', 'army', 'terrorists', 'unlawful', 'police', 'weak greater'.

Option C, 'Terrorists broke the law and the police were powerless without the army', is the correct answer as it uses all the codes, with 'less' being used as 'without', 'unlawful' being used as 'broke the law' and 'weak greater' being used as 'powerless'.

Question 5

231, Z, χ +, œ + Љ

The code combines the words 'Mesopotamia', 'people', 'health negative', 'greater negative rich'.

Option C, 'The population of Mesopotamia suffer from absolute poverty', is the correct answer as it uses all the codes, with 'people' being used as 'population', 'health negative' being used as 'suffer' and 'greater negative rich' being used as 'absolute poverty'.

Question 6

U, η, Σ, κ, 010 œ, 101, 110, (123 312 213 231)

The code combines the words 'budget', 'less', 'government', 'gunpowder', 'policy greater', 'housing', 'employment', 'Mongolia Persia Greece Mesopotamia'.

Option D, 'Politically explosive policies on housing and jobs will cut budgets in all countries', is the correct answer as it uses all the codes, with 'less' being used as 'cut', 'government' being used as 'politically', 'gunpowder' being used as 'explosive', 'policy greater' being used as 'policies', 'employment' being used as 'jobs' and 'Mongolia Persia Greece Mesopotamia' being used as 'all countries'.

Question 7

Ω, Ω, 333, Җ œ, δ, λλ, ψ

The code combines the words 'army', 'army', 'inside', 'insurgents greater', 'converse', 'secret', 'meeting'.

Option A, 'The army are having a meeting behind closed doors to discuss insurgency within the ranks', is the correct answer as it uses all the codes, with the second 'army' being used as 'ranks', 'inside' being used as 'within', 'insurgents greater' being used as 'insurgency', 'converse' being used as 'discuss' and 'secret' being used as 'behind closed doors'.

Question 8

¥(Я Z), ψ, ¥(ə 666), λλ, T

The code combines the words 'combine peace people', 'meeting', 'combine opposite public', 'secret', 'police'.

Option E, 'Pacifists meet in private to avoid the secret police', is the correct answer as it uses all the codes. 'Combine peace people' becomes 'pacifists', 'opposite public' becomes 'private'.

Question 9

Options B and C, 'capture' and 'concur', would be the **two** most useful additions to the codes when attempting to convey the message 'Mesopotamia signed a peace treaty with Persia agreeing to release all enemy prisoners'. The word 'concur' is used for 'agreeing' and the word 'capture' is used with the existing code 'opposite' to provide the word 'release'. The other words in the message can be extrapolated from existing codes or are irrelevant.

Question 10

Σ, η, ∪ , Z, χ, γ, Ω

The code combines the words 'government', 'less', 'budget', 'people', 'health', comparison', 'army'. Option C, 'The government spending on the army exceeds that spent on citizens' health', is the correct answer as it uses all the codes. The words in the message are paraphrased within the answer.

Question 11

Ω, Σ, 010, 123, ¥(œ Φ), ¥(γ Γ)

The code combines the words 'army', 'government', 'policy', 'Mongolia', 'combine greater attack', 'combine comparison terrorists'.

Option C, 'A military junta is in charge in Mongolia and deals brutally with acts of disaffection', is the correct answer as it uses all the codes. 'Army' becomes 'military', 'government' becomes 'junta', 'policy' becomes 'in charge', 'combine greater attack' becomes 'brutally', 'combine comparison terrorists' becomes 'disaffection'.

Question 12

Persia won the last war with Mongolia and they are now our strong allies.

Option B, '312, =, Ю, 123, ¥(γ ~), ¥(ə 999), Э', is the correct answer as it uses the codes required in the statement. The code combines the words 'Persia', 'achieve', 'war', 'Mongolia', 'combine comparison day', 'combine opposite weak', 'allies'. 'Achieve' becomes 'won', 'combine comparison day' becomes 'now', 'combine opposite weak' becomes 'strong'.

Question 13

213, ¥(γ δ), Ю, 231

The code combines the words 'Greece', 'combine comparison converse', 'war', 'Mesopotamia'.

Option D, 'Greece declares war on Mesopotamia', is the correct answer as it encompasses all the codes. 'Combine comparison converse' becomes 'declares'.

Question 14

213, 010, ¥(η β), β, 101, κ, ¥(ə E), Ω, Z

The code combines the words 'Greece', 'policy', 'combine less unlawful', 'unlawful', 'housing', 'gunpowder', 'combine opposite include', 'army', 'people'.

Option E, 'Greece passed a law forbidding the storage of explosives except by military personnel', is the correct answer as it uses all the codes. 'Policy' becomes 'passed', 'combine less unlawful' becomes 'law', 'unlawful' becomes 'forbidding', 'housing' becomes 'storage', 'gunpowder' becomes 'explosives', 'combine opposite include' becomes 'except', 'army' becomes 'military', 'people' becomes 'personnel'.

Question 15

213, δ, ¥(ə ~), ¥(β Z ψ), 333, 213

The code combines the words 'Greece', 'converse', 'combine opposite day', 'combine unlawful people meeting', 'inside', 'Greece'.

Option A, 'Greece declares a night-time curfew across the country', is the correct answer as it uses all the codes. 'Converse' becomes 'declares', 'combine opposite day' becomes 'night-time', 'combine unlawful people meeting' becomes 'curfew'.

Question 16

123, 213, 110, Γ, ¥(ə 333 123 213), œ, ¥(123 213 Ω)

The code combines the words 'Mongolia', 'Greece', 'employment', 'terrorists', 'combine opposite inside Mongolia Greece', 'greater', 'combine Mongolia Greece army'.

Option B, 'Mongolia and Greece make use of terrorists from other countries to increase the size of their armies', is the correct answer as it uses all the codes. 'Employment' becomes 'make use of', 'combine opposite inside Mongolia Greece' becomes 'other countries', 'greater' becomes 'increase the size', 'combine Mongolia Greece army' becomes 'their armies'.

Question 17

Persia is demanding that some Greek soldiers face war crime charges.

Option C, '312, ¥(ə 999 δ), 213, Ω, Z, ¥(Ю β Φ)', is the correct answer as it is the best way to encode the message 'Persia is demanding that some Greek soldiers face war crime charges'.

The encoding used in the correct answer is 312 ('Persia'), 'combine ə 999 δ' ('opposite, weak, converse') becomes 'is demanding', 213, Ω, Z ('Greece', 'army', 'people') becomes 'some Greek soldiers', ¥(Ю β Φ) ('combine war unlawful attack') becomes 'face war crime charges'.

Question 18

Z, 312, Я, ψ, ¥(ə η), Φ, γ(Φ Т)

The code combines the words 'people', 'Persia', 'peace', 'meeting', 'combine opposite less', 'attack', 'comparison attack police'.

Option D, 'People in Persia holding peaceful demonstrations are often fired on by riot police', is the correct answer as it uses all the codes. 'Meeting' becomes 'demonstrations', 'combine opposite less' becomes 'often', 'attack' becomes 'fired on', 'comparison attack police' becomes 'riot police'.

Question 19

¥(η ~), Ж, κ, 213, Σ, 101,¥ (œ Z),¥ (œ Φ)

The code combines the words 'combine less day', 'insurgents', 'gunpowder', 'Greece', 'government', 'housing', 'combine greater people', 'combine greater attack'.

Option E, 'Yesterday insurgents blew up the Greek parliament building and a large number of people were killed', is correct as it uses all the codes. 'Combine less day' becomes 'yesterday', 'gunpowder' becomes 'blew up', 'government' becomes 'parliament', 'housing' becomes 'building', 'combine greater people' becomes 'large number of people', 'combine greater attack' becomes 'killed'.

Question 20

¥(+ 123 213 231 312), Φ, ¥(123 213 231 312), +, =

The code combines the words 'combine negative Mongolia Greece Mesopotamia Persia', 'attack', 'combine Mongolia Greece Mesopotamia Persia', 'negative', 'achieve'.

Option E, 'Other countries sometimes invade the Middle East but without success', is correct as it uses all the codes. 'Combine negative Mongolia Greece Mesopotamia Persia' becomes 'other countries', 'attack' becomes 'invade', 'combine Mongolia Greece Mesopotamia Persia' becomes 'Middle East', 'negative achieve' becomes 'without success'.

Question 21

γ (E Ю), ¥(œ Z Φ), 213, Ю, 231, π, δ(œ Z)

The code combines the words 'comparison include war', 'combine greater people attack', 'Greece', 'war', 'Mesopotamia', 'female', 'converse greater people'.

Option D, 'As with all wars the main casualties when Greece fought Mesopotamia were women and children', is correct as it uses all the codes. 'Comparison include war' becomes 'as with all wars', 'combine greater people attack' becomes 'main casualties', 'war' becomes 'fought', 'female' becomes 'women', 'converse greater people' becomes 'children'.

Question 22

123, λλ, T, γ(Φ Z), ¥(+ Σ), ¥(+ =), Ω, Σ, ¥(γ Φ)

The code combines the words 'Mongolia', 'secret', 'police', 'comparison attack people', 'combine negative government', 'combine negative achieve', 'army', 'government', 'combine comparison attack'.

Option A, 'The Mongolian secret police are rounding up dissidents to prevent the military government being overthrown', is correct as it uses all the codes. 'Comparison attack people' becomes 'rounding up', 'combine negative government' becomes 'dissidents', 'combine negative achieve' becomes 'prevent', 'combine comparison attack' becomes 'overthrown'.

Question 23

Options A and D, 'help' and 'protect', would be the **two** most useful additions to the codes when attempting to convey the message 'To safeguard its borders Greece often came to Mesopotamia's assistance during its wars with Mongolia'. The word 'protect' is used for 'safeguard' and the word 'help' is used for the word 'assistance'. The other words in the message can be extrapolated from existing codes or are irrelevant.

Question 24

¥(Z 312 Σ), Э, γ(Γ Z), ¥(123 213 231)

The code combines the words 'combine people Persia government', 'allies', 'comparison terrorists people', 'combine Mongolia Greece Mesopotamia'.

Option B, 'Members of the Persian government have close ties with different terrorist groups in other countries', is correct as it uses all the codes. 'Combine people Persia government' becomes 'members of the Persian government', 'allies' becomes 'have close ties', 'comparison terrorists people' becomes 'different terrorist groups', 'combine Mongolia Greece Mesopotamia' becomes 'other countries'.

Question 25

231, Ω, œ, 123, Ω, γ, 312, Ω, +, œ, 213, Ω

The code combines the words 'Mesopotamia', 'army', 'greater', 'Mongolia', 'army', 'comparison', 'Persia', 'army', 'negative', 'greater', 'Greece', 'army'.

Options A, 'The Mesopotamian army is bigger than the Mongolian army, comparative to the Persian army, but not as big as the Greek army', and E, 'Greece's army is bigger than those of Mesopotamia, Mongolia or Persia', are both correct as they use all the codes. All of the codes for this message are self-explanatory.

Question 26

¥(γ Я), ¥(+Ю), δ, œ, 213

The code combines the words 'combine comparison peace', 'combine negative war', 'converse', 'greater', 'Greece'.

Option C, 'Make love not war was a phrase first used by the ancient Greeks', is correct as it uses all the codes. 'Combine comparison peace' becomes 'make love', 'combine negative war' becomes 'not war', 'converse' becomes 'phrase', 'greater' and 'Greece' becomes 'ancient Greeks'.

Question 27

Я, ψ, Σœ, 123, 213, 231, 312, ЮФ+

Option D would be the best way to encode the message 'The heads of Mongolia, Greece, Mesopotamia and Persia are holding a peace summit with a ceasefire'. This option has the correct codes by using 'meeting' as 'summit', 'government greater' as 'heads' and 'war attack negative' as 'ceasefire'.

Question 28

œ, γ, χ, 101, 110, Љ, Љә

The code combines the words 'greater', 'comparison', 'health', 'housing', 'employment', 'rich', 'rich opposite'.

Option B, 'The difference in well being, property and occupations between the wealthy and the poor is significant', is the correct answer as it uses all the codes, with 'greater' being used as 'significant', 'comparison' being used as 'difference', 'health' being used as 'well being', 'housing' being used as 'property', 'employment' being used as 'occupations', 'rich' being used as 'wealthy' and 'rich opposite' being used as 'poor'.

Part IV

Preparing for the BioMedical Admissions Test (BMAT)

The following chapters will help you to:

- understand the purpose and the format of the BioMedical Admissions Test (BMAT);
- understand the different sections and how to tackle them;
- prepare for the test using BMAT-style questions.

Introduction

The BioMedical Admissions Test (BMAT) was designed to help admissions officers cope with the problem of rising standards among medical school and veterinary school applicants. By examining the skills required to succeed in medicine and veterinary science, such as the application of scientific knowledge, decision-making and logical argument, they can differentiate better on paper between candidates who have the same top A1 grades.

The BMAT has always generated a lot of anxiety among students who are usually unsure of the standard and importance of the test. Now that it has been joined in the admissions process by its friend the UKCAT, its purpose may seem more unclear than before, especially as only a handful of UK medical and veterinary schools require it for entry to their courses (see Table 1). The first step to performing well in the BMAT is to understand its purpose and format, then you can progress to familiarising yourself with the format of questions used and, finally, attempt practice questions and tests to build your confidence.

Whether you're reading this part of the book in a state of panic a week before the test or as a primer to familiarise yourself with the test, if you follow the advice given here you will not only alleviate a lot of your anxiety but will also pick up those extra crucial marks that can make all the difference to the success of your university application.

Table 1 Courses requiring BMAT

Institution	UCAS	Institution code
University of Cambridge	C05	A100, A101, D100
Imperial College London	I50	A100, A109, B900, B9N2
University of Oxford	O33	A100, A101, BC98
Royal Veterinary College	R84	D100, D101, D102
University College London	U80	A100
Brighton and Sussex Medical School	B74	A100
University of Leeds	L23	A100, A200

Important note: if you are also applying to universities that require you to sit the UKCAT, you must sit this in addition to the BMAT exam. Other universities may use your score for research purposes only; if this is the case, you will be notified, but be reassured that it will not be used for selection in any way during your application process. See the BMAT website for further information.

Understanding the BMAT layout and scoring

The BMAT test has three parts and is two hours long in total.

Section 1	Aptitude and Skills	1 hour
Section 2	Scientific Knowledge and Applications	30 minutes
Section 3	Writing Task	30 minutes

These are all examined at the same time, but on separate answer sheets and with separate timings – hence, you cannot run over on one part and make it up on another. Think of them as three separate exams taken during the same sitting.

Sections 1 and 2 are multiple choice or single best answer and will be marked by a computer. Some of you may not have met this style of answer sheet before, so it is important to familiarise yourself with it before the exam (visit the BMAT website at www.admissionstestingservice.org) so that you can appreciate the importance of recording the right answer in the right space. This may sound obvious but every year students miss out a question without leaving the correct space for it blank on their answer sheets. Only later do they realise what they have done, which inevitably leads to extra stress and mistakes.

Use an HB pencil for your answers (the propelling variety is good) and try not to rub out. If you do make a mistake, rub out your answer completely before you fill in your new answer. If you do not, the computer will read any remaining traces of your first answer and will assume you have chosen two solutions, thus invalidating that answer. This style of multiple-choice assessment is becoming increasingly popular among medical and veterinary schools, so it is as well to get used to the format now.

For Section 3 ('Writing Task'), use a pen and write neatly. Watch your spelling and punctuation – there are marks for these and it would be silly to throw away marks on simple points like this.

How the BMAT is marked

For Section 1 ('Aptitude and Skills') and Section 2 ('Scientific Knowledge and Applications'), BMAT converts your marks into a score reported to the nearest decimal point on a nine-point BMAT scale.

For Section 3 ('Writing Task'), your paper will be marked for content on a scale of 0–5, and a score for written English on a scale of A, C, E. Each essay is double marked and, if the mark is the same or a single point in difference, then the average is given. If there is a larger difference in marks, then it is marked for a third time. Obviously, this is rather labour-intensive for the BMAT examiners, but they do it to ensure that the marks are objective and that you won't be marked down just because one examiner doesn't agree with your arguments. A copy of your essay is sent to the institutions you applied to, and they often use it for discussion in your interview. (They will give you a copy beforehand.)

An important point to note here is that, unlike A-levels or GCSEs, you are very unlikely to score full marks on the BMAT. Figures 1, 2 and 3 show the scores from the 2010 BMAT students. As you can see, they follow a normal distribution, with very high scores being rare and low scores being even rarer. Please remember that, however badly you think you will do on the test, it is almost impossible to 'fail' the BMAT – the test has been designed so that the average candidate for medicine, such as yourself, will score around 5.0.

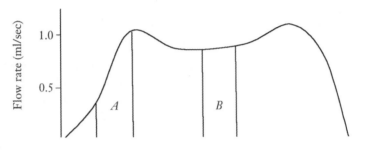

Figure 1   BMAT Section 1 scores 2010

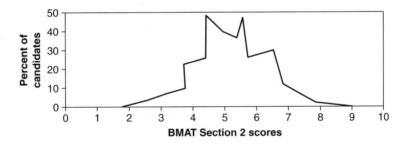

Figure 2   BMAT Section 2 scores 2010

The BMAT examiners know that only a few very exceptional applicants will score higher than 7.0, and that 6.0 represents a comparatively high score. There is, therefore, no need to panic if you find the exam difficult because it is more than likely that most other candidates will find it just as difficult. Some students do better on one section than on another, and it is for this reason that the BMAT provides a breakdown of your scores so that your assessors can get a good idea of what your strengths and weaknesses are, rather than an overall average score that does not provide them with as much information. A downside of this, however, is that you cannot spend lots of time practising one part of the test in the hope that it will boost your mark; you need to prepare for all the sections of the test to the same standard.

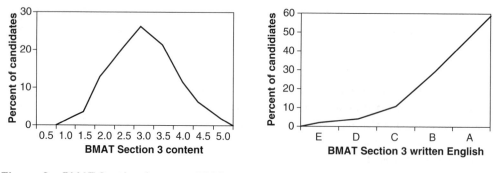

Figure 3 BMAT Section 3 scores 2010

As you can see from the above graphs, most candidates score either 'A' or 'B' for written English, although if this is something you have difficulty with, it is worth paying attention to.

The scores for context are more widely spread, with the majority of candidates scoring between 2.0 and 4.0. A small amount of preparation for Section 3 to increase your mark by 1 point will therefore increase your chances of scoring in the top percentage of your year group. More details of the criteria for awarding each score are available on the BMAT website.

How your BMAT scores will be used

How your BMAT scores will be used varies between universities. Some place a lot of weight on BMAT scores and use them as a criterion for inviting candidates for interview. Others use the BMAT as just one part of the application process, giving weight also to your personal statement, AS scores and UCAS form when deciding whether or not to invite you to interview and offer you a place. So the BMAT is important, but don't prepare excessively for it at the expense of working on your A-levels. If you get your UCAS form completed by the end of September, you will have a whole month to prepare for the BMAT.

If you are unclear about how important your BMAT score will be for your application, check out the details in the prospectus or email the applications officer at your prospective university. If you do this before you sit the test you can, first, make sure you prepare appropriately and, second, will save yourself a great deal of angst and worry if you think you have done badly on the day. The timescale for applying to sit the BMAT exam is detailed on their website. You must apply before the beginning of October, and you sit the test in early November. Results are usually available online two weeks later. Check with your school or college if you are at all unsure about the arrangements.

In the following chapters the three sections of the BMAT test are examined in detail, with advice, worked answers and practice papers to test yourself. Don't try to work through the whole test in one sitting: work on each section of the test independently, in conjunction with the sample and past papers available on the BMAT website, until you are confident that you know how to tackle the type of questions you will meet in the real test. Familiarising yourself with the type and format of the questions and practising how to solve them is absolutely the best preparation you can do.

Chapter 9
Section 1: Aptitude and Skills

35 marks/60 minutes

Multiple choice or single best answer

No calculators allowed

During your time at university you will rely heavily on problem-solving skills, reasoning and analytical thinking in order to progress with your studies and to deal with the new ideas and concepts that you will meet. This is what Section 1 is for: it attempts to find out if you have the necessary skills to cope with an undergraduate course in medicine, dentistry or veterinary science. So, although a lot of the questions may seem unrelated to what you have been studying in your AS and A-level courses, the underlying skills needed to answer them correctly are very important.

You may be panicking because you think you don't have the necessary skills, or you may have heard that you can't practise for the test because you've either 'got it' or you haven't. The BMAT itself says that 'An approach to developing these thinking skills can be taught, and the skills will improve with familiarity and practice. We encourage this because we think these skills are really worthwhile; they are useful skills in many walks of life, and very important for success in higher education.' So if you really want that university place and to do well once you get there, now is the time to invest some time in preparation.

The BMAT goes on to say: 'What you cannot do is to be taught to answer as if you were a performing seal. There are no simple shortcuts – you really do have to think the answers through.' While this is true to some extent, you can compare preparing for the BMAT with preparing for your GCSEs or A-levels. Normally, after you have finished studying the curriculum content, in order to pass the exam you work through practice and past papers. Doing the past papers won't teach you the knowledge or skills that you need to pass the exam, but familiarising yourself with the type of questions that are asked and figuring out how to apply your knowledge are vital parts of the preparation process.

This type of preparation is just what you should do for the BMAT. It is reassuring that the examiners themselves note that there is no special 'trick' to answering questions: all the knowledge you require has been taught to you already at GCSE level. What you can do is get yourself up to speed by practising lots of BMAT-style questions so that, when you get into the exam, you can question-spot and recognise how questions should be solved.

Important note: on the BMAT website there is a list of recommended reading on how to improve your thinking skills. You may find such reading beneficial, but bear in mind that these books are very wordy and not that useful for practising for the BMAT, especially if you have limited time on your hands.

Section I is worth 35 marks and tests:

- problem solving (approx. 30 mins);
- understanding argument (approx. 15 mins);
- data analysis and inference (approx. 15 mins).

This means that you have 60 minutes to get 35 marks (i.e. less than 2 minutes for each question). The marks tend to be split equally between the three question types, which are spread throughout the paper. However, the problem-solving questions take longer to read, so allow yourself a little extra time for these – but you will have to be speedy on the other types of questions.

There is no negative marking on the BMAT, so if you run short of time a guess is always better than no answer at all. For most of the multiple-choice questions you have at least a 20 per cent chance of getting it right. If you don't know an answer, fill in one answer as a guess and place a '?' by the side to come back to it later if you have the time. Never leave an answer blank because you may run out of time at the end and thus never get the chance to make a guess at it.

However short of time you are, you must always read the question carefully. While the examiners do not set questions to catch you out deliberately, the questions often require you to perform a calculation and then give the remainder as the answer, or the questions may use different units from the answer choices. If you are rushing, you may not spot these nuances and all your calculations will go to waste. Also, beware of feeling relieved that the answer you have obtained is offered as a choice – the examiners also include the most commonly worked-out incorrect answers as possible solutions in the answer sets.

On the BMAT website you will find a number of practice papers you should do in exam conditions to get a feel for what is required of you. You can also visit www.ucl.ac.uk/lapt/bmat. htm. Here you will find lots of excellent logic and problem-solving questions that test the same skills used in the BMAT – they even talk you through the solutions. Attempt the answer yourself first and then either pat yourself on the back or see where you went wrong. Rather than sit down and do them all in one mammoth session, do a few a day – that way you'll be consolidating your learning. Note that some of the questions are the same as those on the BMAT website.

Below you will find worked examples of BMAT-style questions, with a step-by-step guide on how to approach them. After these you will find a BMAT-style test with answers and explanations of how to work them out. By working through these examples you should feel much more confident in your ability to tackle the BMAT.

Example: data analysis

1. The graph opposite shows how the flow rate of liquid out of a cylinder varies with time. The area marked B is twice as large as A. Which **two** of the following are false?

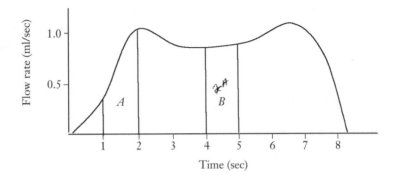

A   The rate of fluid flow after 4 seconds is twice what it is after 1 second.

B   The average rate of fluid flow is twice as great between 4 and 5 seconds, compared with 1 and 2 seconds.

C   The flow rate increases twice as rapidly between 4 and 5 seconds as it does between 3 and 4 seconds.

D   The amount of fluid flowing between 1 and 2 seconds is half as much as the amount flowing between 4 and 5 seconds.

How to solve it

First, work out what the graph is showing you – they even tell you: flow rate on the y axis, time on the x axis. Then, note that B = 2 × A (given) and realise that two of the possibilities are correct and that they want you to mark down the false answers. Don't be caught out! It is easiest to work out which ones are correct and then write down the other two.

A   The rate of fluid flow after 4 seconds is twice what it is after 1 second. We're dealing with rate of fluid flow, so read from the y axis. The flow rate at 4 seconds is around 0.9 ml/s; the flow rate after 1 second is around 0.3 ml/s. Because 0.9 is not (2 × 0.3), this is false.

B   The average rate of fluid flow is twice as great between 4 and 5 seconds, compared with 1 and 2 seconds. They have told you that the volume (area under the graph) of B is 2A. The three variables described by the graph are time, flow rate and volume. The volume has doubled, whereas the time period (1 second) is constant. Therefore the flow rate increase must be double.

C   The flow rate increases twice as rapidly between 4 and 5 seconds as it does between 3 and 4 seconds. The rate of flow is the graph line. It is flat between 3 and 4 seconds, and it's still flat between 4 and 5 seconds – i.e. the flow rate is remaining constant. Therefore this choice is false.

D   The amount of fluid flowing between 1 and 2 seconds is half as much as the amount flowing between 4 and 5 seconds. The y axis is rate of flow, the x is time. Remember that 'Rate of flow = Volume/Time'. Thus the area under the graph is volume. This is why they told you that B was twice A. So D is correct.

B and D are correct. Therefore, you have to mark down A and C on your form.

The lesson here is that, although the questions in themselves are not difficult, there are lots of easy mistakes you could make in the heat of the moment, especially when you are under time pressure. Force yourself always to read the questions carefully before you jump in and solve them: you will save yourself a lot of time and will avoid making mistakes.

Example: problem-solving

2. Mr Jones has to renew the white lines on a 1km stretch of road. Each edge of the road is marked with a solid line and there is a 'dashed' line in the centre. Drivers are warned of approaching bends by two curved arrows. Mr Jones will have to paint four curved arrows. The manufacturers have printed the following guidance on each 5-litre drum of paint:

    Solid lines – 5 metres per litre.
    Dashed lines – 20 metres per litre.
    Curved arrows – 3 litres each.

    How many drums of paint will Mr Jones require?

    A   53

    B   92

    C   93

    D   103

    E   462

How to solve it

The solid lines require 200 litres for each side of the road (1,000/5).

The dashed line requires 50 litres (1,000/20).

The arrows require 12 litres (3 × 4).

Total paint required is 462 litres (200 + 200 + 50 + 12).

Beware! Most candidates at this point will go for choice E. The question asks how many **drums** of paint you require – you have worked out the litres required.

Total drums required is 92.4 (462/5).

You will have to round up to the nearest drum. Therefore C is correct.

All the choices given here will seem correct, if you calculate the answer incorrectly. As you become more efficient at answering the questions, you will find time to double-check your answers. If a question at first seems too easy, look for the hidden twist. For example, forgetting to round up the drums may lead you incorrectly to select B, or only having a solid line on one side of the road will lead you incorrectly to select A.

Example: understanding argument

3. Vegetarian food can be healthier than a traditional diet. Research has shown that vegetarians are less likely to suffer from heart disease and obesity than meat eaters. Concern has been expressed that vegetarians do not get enough protein in their diet, but it has been demonstrated that, by selecting foods carefully, vegetarians are able amply to meet their needs in this respect.

    Which of the following best expresses the main conclusion of the above argument?

    A   A vegetarian diet can be better for health than a traditional diet.

    B   Adequate protein is available from a vegetarian diet.

    C   A traditional diet is very high in protein.

    D   A balanced diet is more important for health than any particular food.

    E   Vegetarians are unlikely to suffer from heart disease and obesity.

How to solve it

These questions are tough, mainly because it takes quite some time to read the passage and the answers. The best way to approach this is to read the passage and then to pick holes in all the choices offered. Note that all the choices could be argued to be a conclusion – the question asks for the best choice (which is often the only one you can't pick a hole in). The conclusion is sometimes a statement in the text, although it needn't necessarily be at the end.

A   A vegetarian diet can be better for health than a traditional diet. This is the first line of the passage – think of news reports, which always have their conclusions at the start. Hold this one in reserve for now.

B   Adequate protein is available from a vegetarian diet. This is mentioned in the passage, but only by selecting foods carefully. It is doubtful if this is the main conclusion.

C   A traditional diet is very high in protein. It may well be, but this is an inference from the passage – vegetarians don't get enough protein so meat eaters must do(?) This is not the main conclusion here.

D   A balanced diet is more important for health than any particular food. It doesn't say so anywhere in the passage. Don't let what you know cloud your judgement about what the passage says. This is not the main conclusion.

E   Vegetarians are unlikely to suffer from heart disease and obesity. Be careful! Vegetarians are *less* likely, not *unlikely*! There could be a 98 per cent chance, which is still less likely than 99 per cent, but still very high. Not the conclusion.

So, there is a choice between A and B. If in doubt, always go for the statement that has been mentioned explicitly in the passage. This may seem rather simple and make you second-guess, but remember there is nothing subtle about the BMAT. The best answer is A.

Now, try the practice test for Section 1. Check your answers after you have completed the entire test. There are fewer questions in this test than in the actual BMAT exam. This is so you can take your time with each question and focus on how you are working out the answers rather than using an element of guesswork. Make sure you are definitely happy with each question before moving on. Also included are explanations of how the correct answers were reached so that you can gain an understanding of how to tackle the questions and also learn from your mistakes.

Section 1 practice test

1   Happy Pharma sells two types of cough medicine, which can be bulk-bought in mixed boxes.

   24 Muco-eaze and 20 Tickle-gone costs £134.

   20 Muco-eaze and 24 Tickle-gone costs £130.

   What is the price of a single unit of Muco-eaze?

2   A dentist has appointments with 1,800 patients in a year. About 20% of his patients are female, and 50% of his male patients are over 60. He finds that, as a rule, 1 in 20 patients needs further dental work after they come for a routine check-up.

   Assuming that all his patients attend for a routine check-up in a year, what is the number of male patients under the age of 60 who will need further dental work? Give your answer to the nearest whole number.

   A   20

   B   36

   C   18

   D   72

   E   9

3   In the waiting-room of the clinic, Tom places some toy-bricks in a pile. The red brick is above the blue brick, which is above the yellow brick. The green brick is below the blue brick and above the white brick.

   The yellow brick must be:

   A   Below the white, but above the red.

   B   Above the blue, but not above the green.

   C   Below the blue, but not necessarily below the red.

   D   Below the blue, but not necessarily below the green.

4 Bob the plumber charges a flat call-out rate, plus a fixed fee per half-hour of work, charged to each complete half-hour.

Andy pays Bob £210 for $2\frac{1}{2}$ hours' work.

Brian pays Bob £150 for $1\frac{1}{2}$ hours' work.

How much will Clive pay for 1 hour of work?

5 At school sports day, Anthony finished the 5,000m race ahead of Ben, but after Charlie. Damian beat Charlie, but not Edward.

In what position did Damian finish?

A First

B Second

C Third

D Fourth

E Fifth

Questions 6 to 8 refer to the following information.

A blood transfusion laboratory audits 5,000 transfusion reactions and notes their causes, shown in the pie chart below.

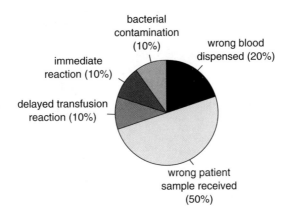

6 How many reactions were due to the wrong type of blood being dispensed?

7 After an awareness drive, the number of wrong patient samples received fell by 250. If all other categories remained constant, what percentage of the reactions is now caused by wrong patient samples? Give your answer to the nearest whole number.

8 If the number of transfusions given increases by 15%, what would be the predicted number of immediate transfusion reactions (based on original data)?

9 If you drink too much alcohol and have a hangover, you may have a headache or tremors. Some, but not all, hung-over people with a headache also have tremors. Some, but not all, hung-over people with tremors also have a headache.

Which one of the options, A to F, correctly lists the following statements in order of their probability, listing the least likely first?

1 Someone suffering from a hangover will have a headache.

2 Someone suffering from a hangover will have a headache and tremors.

3 Someone suffering from a hangover will have a headache or tremors.

A 1, 2, 3

B 1, 3, 2

C 2, 1, 3

D 2, 3, 1

E 3, 1, 2

F 3, 2, 1

10 Two nurses, Amelia and Boris, each collect blood samples from my patients on the ward and do their rounds hourly. They are both as hard working as each other and blood samples are ready to be collected all the time. Unfortunately, I can never remember at what times they visit the ward, so I just give the blood samples to the first nurse who comes along. Strangely, I discover over the year that Amelia collects more blood from me than Boris.

Amelia visits the ward at *a* minutes past the hour, and Boris visits the ward at *b* minutes past the hour. If Amelia visits the ward in the first half of the hour, which **one** of the following would explain the higher probability of Amelia coming to the ward first?

A $b > 30$

B $0 < (b - a) < 30$

C $0 < (b - a) < 60$

D $a > ba/b < 1$

E $a/b < 1$

11 The spread of HIV-AIDS is a subject which should greatly concern the human race. The march of this disease through our populations should be checked before it is too late. Our future as a species depends on the continued research and investigation into finding a cure, and we should not take comfort from

the limited success of antiretroviral drugs. We should all give generously to charities which support research into this deadly disease in order to protect the future of our children.

Which of the following is closest to the underlying assumption in the passage above?

A   HIV-AIDS is incurable.

B   Antiretroviral drugs are ineffective.

C   Donating to charity can help to cure HIV-AIDS.

D   Charities provide most of the funding for HIV-AIDS research.

12   On Paige Ward there are 20 nurses. They must all complete at least one training module in a year, but no more than four.

Each of the four modules has to be completed before moving onto the next one, in a sequential process (e.g. 1 → 2 → 3 → 4). Thirty-six modules are taken in total.

1 nurse takes module 4.

5 nurses take module 3.

How many nurses complete module 2?

A   4

B   5

C   9

D   10

E   15

13   There are 40 students in year 12 and all take biology.

75% of students study biology only.

50% study chemistry and 75% study maths.

5% of students study all three subjects and 20% study either maths or chemistry.

If 5 students study biology and maths only, how many study biology and chemistry, but not maths?

A   2

B   3

C   4

D   5

Questions 14 to 17 refer to the following article.

Is bleach to blame for childhood asthma?

In a paper published this month, a group from Bristol University demonstrate a link between childhood exposure to domestic cleaning products and the development of persistent wheeze in children, a condition which often progresses to asthma. The study followed a cohort of more than 7,000 children until the age of 3.5 as part of the Avon Longitudinal Study of Parents and Children (ALSPAC). Analysis of questionnaires delivered both during and after pregnancy formed the basis of the study, with mothers being asked a number of questions regarding health and lifestyle choices. The participants were asked how often they used common household chemicals such as bleach, disinfectant, air-freshener and cleaning products, with their responses quantified to create a quotient of total chemical burden (TCB). The analysis suggested that no single product was solely implicated in the association with infant wheezing, and the authors were not able to determine whether the observed effect was due to in utero or postnatal exposure. However, given the strong correlation between prenatal and postnatal TCB scores found, and their association with persistent wheezing, it is likely that this represents postnatal exposure with a direct inflammatory insult to the airways (rather than a prenatal priming of airway inflammation in response to postnatal exposures such as airborne allergens). The headlines therefore centre on the statistically significant link between postnatal exposure to domestic chemical products and persistent wheezing illness in young children up to the age of 3.5 years, supporting an effect on the development of airway inflammation and asthma rather than a fundamental effect on airway development in utero.

With the incidence of asthma continuing to rise (the number of sufferers has tripled between 1970 and 2000), there has been much interest in the role environmental factors may play in causing asthma. Much speculation has centred on a possible link between house-hold chemicals and asthma, especially given that the market for household cleaners has grown in line with the increased prevalence of the disease, and the observation that people, especially mothers with young children, spend most of the day indoors. However, the Avon analysis is at odds with a similar study, published in 2003, which found no association between direct exposure to domestic volatile organic compounds and wheezing illness in children aged 9–11. In defence, the authors of the Avon study speculate that in this age category 'the majority of wheezing illness is likely to be established asthma and this may have a different aetiology to wheezing illnesses that develop in early childhood'. Another consideration is that, whereas previous observational studies have consistently identified a link between chemical exposure and asthma, few interventional studies have been able to document such an association. This may be due to participant numbers, duration of exposure or, most significantly, the observed association in observational studies could be confounded by a factor which is a determinant of asthma and is also associated with exposure to volatile organic compounds.

Such a confounding factor may be cleanliness itself. A popular explanation for the increasing incidence of autoimmune diseases in childhood cites the underexposure of children to environmental antigens whilst their immune systems are developing, so that they later develop diseases of atopy. Proponents of this theory cite observations that the increased incidence of asthma has followed the spread of urbanisation from the north southwards, and no doubt could interpret the results of the Avon study to confirm that a hyper-clean environment causes asthma. While these considerations could be integrated into the relationship between chemicals and childhood wheeze, critics point to countries such as Hong Kong, Sweden and Thailand, which have comparable levels of domestic cleaner usage and yet have the lowest rates of severe childhood wheeze. In a statement Professor Andrew Peacock, of the British Thoracic Society, said: 'More long-term studies are needed before we advise pregnant women to throw out all their air fresheners.'

Answer the following questions, assuming the information in the article is accurate.

14 Which one of the following statements can we safely conclude to be accurate?

   A Being too clean causes asthma.

   B There are more asthma sufferers today than there were 30 years ago.

   C It is likely that just one product will be found to cause childhood wheezing.

   D Exposure to cleaning products in utero is more damaging than postnatal exposure.

15 The main message of the article is that:

   A Asthma is a dangerous disease in childhood.

   B There is a strong link between cleaning product use and the development of wheezing.

   C It is not possible to identify a cause-and-effect relationship between any factor and asthma.

   D Pregnant women should take care to avoid exposure to cleaning products.

16 If 10,000 people suffered from asthma in 1970, and the rate of increase mentioned in the article stays constant, how many sufferers will there be in 2030?

   A 30,000

   B 60,000

   C 90,000

   D 120,000

   E 150,000

17 Which one of the following is not expressly mentioned by the article?

   A Hong Kong, Sweden and Thailand have the lowest rates of severe childhood wheeze.

   B There is much interest in the role that environmental factors play in causing asthma.

   C The market for household cleaners has grown in line with the increased prevalence of asthma.

   D Children in the age group 9–11 suffer only from established asthma.

   E Previous observational studies have identified a link between chemical exposure and asthma.

18 Damian test drives a variety of cars and measures their speed at 50 seconds from a standing start. Their profiles are shown below.

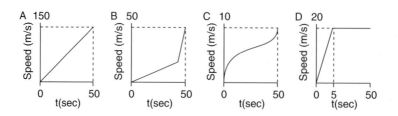

Put the cars in order of speed of acceleration:

A a b c d

B b c d a

C c a b d

D d a b c

E a d b c

19 £400 in a will is divided among five charities. The will states that no two charities are to get the same amount of money, and each is to have at least £20. The donations are to be given out according to the charity's size: the largest gets the most, the smallest the least. If these rules are adhered to, what is the largest donation that the third biggest charity can receive?

A 22

B 120

C 119

D 118

E 121

Questions 20 to 22 refer to the following information.

A medical school has student dormitories on both sides of its campus. The girls' dormitories are on the south side and the boys' dormitories are on the north side. Because of student protests, the Dean decides to integrate the dormitories and to move the first student on the alphabetical list, Miss Adams, from the south side to the north side.

The registry list of room, rent and test scores (before the move) is shown below.

South side (girls)			North side (boys)		
Student surname	Rent paid (£)	Test score	Student surname	Rent paid (£)	Test score
Adams	80	140	Hill	65	130
Brown	100	120	Ibrahim	70	145
Cowen	55	130	Jones	110	125
Docker	60	125	Kent	95	140
Evans	35	130	Long	75	120
Fetts	40	120	McNamara	70	125
Gower	50	145	Norman	85	130
Total	420	910		570	915

20 What is the average rent paid (to the nearest whole number) on the south side of the campus after Miss Adams's move?

A 56

B 57

C 58

D 59

21 By how much will the average test score on the north side of the campus rise after Miss Adams moves? Give your answer to the nearest whole number.

A 0

B 1

C 2

D 3

22 If all the rents rise by 7.5% next year, what will the total rent bill be?

A £990

B £1,039.50

C £1064.25

D £1,089

23 A wine stopper is made of aluminium with a density of 2.0g/cm³. Its dimensions
    are shown below.

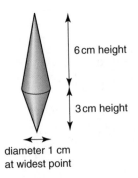

6 cm height

3 cm height

diameter 1 cm
at widest point

What is the mass of the wine stopper if the volume of a cone is described by $\frac{1}{3}\pi r^2$?
Give your answer as a value of π.

END OF TEST

Section 1 practice test: answers

Question number	Correct response	Comments	Marks
1	£3.50		1
2	B		1
3	D		1
4	£120		1
5	B		1
6	1,000		1
7	47%		1
8	575		1
9	C		1
10	B		1
11	C		1
12	D		1
13	B		1
14	B	If plus any other answer, no mark	1
15	C		1
16	C		1
17	D		1
18	D		1
19	D		1
20	B		1
21	B		1
22	C		1
23	1.5π		1

Section 1 practice test: explanation of answers

1 Happy Pharma: £3.50

Muco-eaze = x, Tickle-gone = y

A $24x + 20y = 134$

B $20x + 24y = 130$

A − B = $4x − 4y = 4$

∴ $x = 1 + y$

a. $24(1 + y) + 20y = 134$ b. $20x + (24 × 2.5) = 130$
$24 + 24y + 20y = 134$ $20x = 70$
$44y = 110$ $x = 3.5$
$y = 2.5$

Check in a: $84 + 50 = 134$

∴ Muco-eaze = £3.50.

2 Dentist and his patients: B

1,800 patients, 20% female (thus 80% male); 50% male patients are over 60 (thus 50% of 80% of 1,800 patients are under 60); 1/20 consult; $1,440 × 0.5 × 1/20 = 36$.

3 Tom and his bricks: D

The only way to do this one is by a diagram. Once you have done this, it is clear that the only possible answer is D.

Possible combinations:

```
R   R   R
B   B   B
Y   G   G
G   Y   W
W   W   Y
```

4 Bob the plumber: £120.

A Andy $x + 5y = 210$
B Brian $x + 3y = 150$

A − B: $2y = 60$ ∴ each half hour = £30

Clive pays $60 + (2 × 30) = £120$.

5 School sports day: B

A diagram helps:

(E)   Damian did not beat Edward.

(D)   Damian beat Charlie.

(C)   Anthony finished after Charlie.

(A)   Anthony finished ahead of Ben.

(B)

Blood bank (6–8)

6 1,000

20% of 5,000

7 47%

Wrong patient = 2,500 − 250 = 2,250

2,250/4,750 = 47.4 = 47%.

8 575

New number of transfusions = 5,750

10% = 575.

9 Hangovers and headaches: C (2, 1, 3)

'Or' is more probable than specific illness, which in turn is more probable than 'and'. Watch that you list them in the correct order (i.e. and<specific<or).

10 Amelia and Boris: B

There is a lot of wording in this question, but many of the statements allow you to eliminate the given answer choices. Note that a and b are probabilities relating to Amelia and Boris.

A   This choice does not explain why Amelia should come first as it is stated that blood samples become available at all times (i.e. not just in the first half of the hour).

B   This choice is correct. Imagine Amelia comes at 29 minutes past (so within the first half of the hour, as stated). In order for B to be fulfilled, Boris must visit the ward between 30 and 58 minutes past (note the < symbol is used, not ≤) i.e. Amelia will always come first.

C   Although this choice also describes the time condition as in B, it will not explain why Amelia comes first. If we use the example time for Amelia as in B ($a = 29$), the value of b could be anything between 30 and 88. Any value >60 would mean Boris visited the ward before Amelia, because the difference in minutes would mean he visits in the next hour, before Amelia.

D   A lot of people will choose this one because it seems to describe that Amelia comes before Boris. However, the probability of Amelia and Boris visiting the ward is stated to be the same; what we are trying to find out is a description of why Amelia comes first (i.e. a condition of time).

E The same explanation as above holds for this answer; the probability of visiting the ward is actually $a = b$.

11 HIV-AIDS: C

The clue is in the last sentence when it says 'we should all give generously to charities ... to protect the future of our children'. Thus, it is assuming that this money will help cure HIV-AIDS. The others aren't that convincing either. With this type of question, if you cannot decide between two answers, always go with your original 'hunch': experience shows that it is generally correct.

12 Nurses and training: D

			Modules
1		10	10
1 + 2	c	5	10
1 + 2 + 3	b	4	12
1 + 2 + 3 + 4	a	1	4
			36

It is easiest to draw a table.

1 nurse takes module 4, so must have taken 1, 2 and 3 as well (modules left = 32). (a)

5 nurses take module 3 (including the one who also did module 4) so 4 nurses took 12 modules. (b)

This means that 15 nurses must have taken the remaining 20 modules: the only way this is possible is if 10 took only 1, and 5 took 2. (c)

∴ the number of nurses taking module 2 is 5 + 4 + 1 = 10.

13 Biology class: B

This is very wordy, but is much simpler if you use a venn diagram (see numbered steps below).

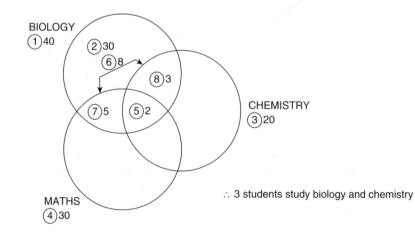

Bleach and asthma (14–17)

This is a long article, so look at the questions first, then you will know what you are looking for when you read it.

14 B

B is the only factual statement from the article, and thus we can assume it to be accurate (that's why the question introduction says 'assuming the information in the article is accurate').

15 C

The article doesn't come to any conclusions regarding the link between cleaning products and asthma. Thus the other three statements are incorrect.

16 C

Easy: 10,000 × 3 × 3 = 90,000

17 D

Be careful: in this age group, the majority of wheezing illness is *likely* to be established asthma. It is not a fact expressly mentioned by the article that children aged 9–11 suffer only from established asthma.

18 Damian and acceleration: D

This is easy.

$$a = \frac{(\Delta s)}{t}$$

$$A = \frac{150}{50} = 3$$

$$B = \frac{50}{50} = 1$$

$$C = \frac{10}{50} = 0.5$$

$$D = \frac{20}{5} = 4$$

Just be careful for D that you don't do 20 (the speed reaches 20m/s at 5 seconds).

19 Charity donations: D

Pay careful attention to the instructions here. Note that it says 'the *largest* donation that the third biggest charity can receive'. This means you have to give 4 and 5 the minimum (£21 and £20, respectively). This then leaves you with £359: £121, £120 and £118. Note that it can't be £119 as you would then have to give two amounts of £120, which is forbidden.

Boys and girls (20–22)

This looks horrible, but most of the adding up has been done for you.

20 B

$(420 - 80)/6 = 56.666\ (57)$

21 B

Before move: $915/7 = 130.7$

After move: $(915 + 140)/8 = 131.6$. Difference $= 0.9\ (1)$

22 C

Total rent $= 420 + 570 = 990$

$7.5\% = 5\% + 2.5\% = 49.50 + 24.75$

Total $= £1,064.25$

23 Wine stopper: 1.5π

Luckily, the equation is given to you.

Work the volume out first.

$$6\text{ cm cone} = \frac{1}{3}\pi r^2 h \qquad 3\text{ cm cone} = \frac{1}{3}\pi r^2 h$$

$$= \frac{1}{3}\pi(0.25 \times 6) \qquad = \frac{1}{3}\pi(0.25 \times 3)$$

$$= \frac{1}{3}\pi \times 1.5 \qquad = \frac{1}{3}\pi \times 0.75$$

$$\text{Total} = \frac{1.5\pi + 0.75\pi}{3} = \frac{2.25\pi}{3}$$

$$\text{Mass} = \frac{2.25\pi}{3} \times 2 = \frac{4.5\pi}{3} = 1.5\pi$$

Chapter 10
Section 2: Scientific Knowledge and Applications

27 marks/30 minutes

Multiple choice or single best answer

No calculators allowed

On first glance, Section 2 of the BMAT looks to be the most difficult, due to its reliance on testing factual scientific and mathematical knowledge. Remember that the standard is only GCSE level, and the examiners are looking for this level of ability in your tackling scientific problems rather than, for example, a detailed knowledge of the periodic table. Don't worry if you have not studied the subject further than GCSE level and feel a little rusty; as each of the subject areas is similarly weighted, you are likely to make up in one area what you lose in another and, with practice, you will be surprised at how much of your past studies you remember.

A number of subject areas will not be tested (as stated by the BMAT). These are green plants as organisms (i.e. no photosynthesis); products from organic sources; products from metal ores and rocks; products from air; changes to the Earth and atmosphere; the Earth and beyond; and seismic waves. Looking at what is left in the GCSE syllabuses, combined with what aptitudes the BMAT aims to test, enables us to make an educated guess as to those subject areas that will be tested in the exam, including the following.

- Human biology
- Cells and cellular processes
- Basic maths – equations, fractions, multiplication, algebra (remember, no calculators)
- Basic physics equations
- Balancing chemical equations

Probably, these are all topics that you're studying or skills that you are using at the moment, but if you know you are weak in certain areas, such as your ability to do maths without a calculator or balancing equations, then get your old books out. Otherwise, what you really need to practise is time management – the challenge to obtain 27 marks in 30 minutes means you have to be speedy, accurate and decisive.

Again, note that there is no negative marking, so always give an answer. Work on the basis of 1 minute per question and, if you get stuck, move on after making a guess – you can return to it later if you have time. Remember that all the other candidates will be in the same boat as you time-wise, and an educated guess after reading a question will be better than going back through the paper in the last 30 seconds and filling in the questions you missed with wild guesses. There will also be lots of questions to which you know the answers immediately, so this will give you a little more time for the questions you find more difficult.

It's usually best not to work out answers in your head as, under the pressure of the exam, mistakes are easily made, and it also makes it difficult for you to check your answers if you have time on your hands later. The question paper can be used for all your working, but be aware that this is purely for your own benefit – you will only receive credit for answers correctly transferred and validly marked on the answer sheet.

Have a look at the past papers on the BMAT website to get an idea of what format the questions will take and what standard of knowledge you have to achieve. Below, you will find some specimen questions to familiarise yourself with, together with their answers and solutions. These are just a flavour of the types of questions that could come up.

Some of the questions on the BMAT will be harder, some a little easier. Always look for the underlying rule or equation you have been taught that will allow you to solve the problem. Once you realise which equation or rule to apply, things will be a lot simpler. When you are familiar with the type of questions in Section 2, try the practice test at the end of this chapter and the ones on the BMAT website.

Example: maths

1. Simplify the following expression.

$$\frac{8a^3b \times 4a^2b^4}{2ab^2}$$

Answer

$$\frac{32a^5b^5}{2ab^2}$$
$$= 16a^4b^3$$

Remember, with powers you subtract when they are divided, and add when they are multiplied.

2. Give the value of A in the figure below.

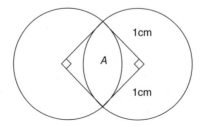

A $1 - \pi/4$

B $\pi - 1/2$

C $1 - \pi/2$

D $\pi/2 - 1$

Answer

A bit tricky, but not if you realise that the area of a quarter of this circle is $\pi/4$ (πr^2 is the area of a circle – always look at the answers to give you a clue). The area of the square is 1 ($1 \times 1 = 1$). Within the square there are effectively two quarter circles – total area $\pi/2$ ($2 \times \pi/4$) – which overlap giving the area A:

$\pi/2 - A = 1$

$A = -1 + \pi/2$

$\therefore A = \pi/2 - 1$ (answer D)

Beware answer C, which results from incorrectly rearranging the equation. As always, look for the trick to the question, and then solve it quickly and accurately.

Example: chemistry

3.   Calculate the relative formula mass, M_r, of ammonium sulphate, $(NH_4)_2SO_4$. (N=14, H=1, S=32, O=16).

Answer

N=28, H=8, S=32, O=64

$M_r = 132$.

Example: physics

4.   A brick rests on a ledge and has a potential energy of 75J. When it falls, it hits the ground with a speed of $\sqrt{50}$ m/s.

What is the mass of the brick? (Discount air resistance.)

A   3g

B   30g

C   300g

D   3000g

Answer

Potential energy (PE) = kinetic energy (KE)

$$KE = \frac{1}{2} MV^2$$

$$75 = 0.5 \times m \times (\sqrt{50})^2$$

$$75 = 25m \therefore m = 3$$

As standard units are used, mass is in kilograms, therefore m = 3000g = D.

Example: biology

The diagram shows the inside of a human heart.

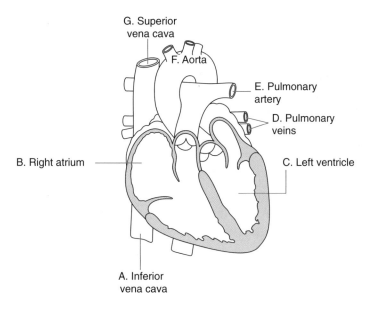

G. Superior
vena cava

F. Aorta

E. Pulmonary
artery

D. Pulmonary
veins

B. Right atrium

C. Left ventricle

A. Inferior
vena cava

5. Which vessel has the highest pressure during systole (contraction) of the heart?

6. Blood enters the inferior vena cava (A). Which of the following options best describes its subsequent route through the heart?

Ⓐ	A	G	B	E	D	C
Ⓑ	A	B	E	D	C	F
Ⓒ	A	B	E	C	D	F

Answers

5. This requires some knowledge of the human heart. Note that it says which *vessel*, not structure, has the highest pressure during systole.

    The vessels to choose from are A, G, D, E and F. You should know that veins have lower pressures than arteries (with the exception of the pulmonary vein and artery). The left ventricle generates most of the blood pressure during systole, therefore the aorta (F) is the correct answer.

6. Blood flows from the right side of the heart to the left, via the lungs, then to the body via the aorta. Therefore, B is the only correct option.

Section 2 practice test

Time allowed: 30 minutes

1 A tuning fork is being tested for accuracy.

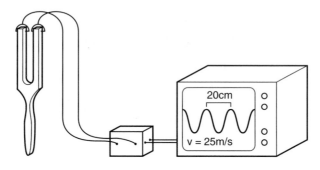

Tim records the velocity and wavelength as shown on the screen. Give the frequency of the tuning fork's oscillation in hertz (Hz).

2 $5 \times 10^3 \div 2 \times 10^{-2}$.

Solve the equation above, giving your answer to the nearest whole number.

3 A solid block weighs 200 N and has the dimensions shown below.

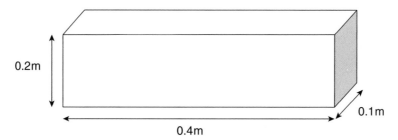

If the block can stand on any of its faces, what is the smallest pressure that the weight of the block will exert on the ground?

4 Below is a diagram depicting the knee-jerk reflex.

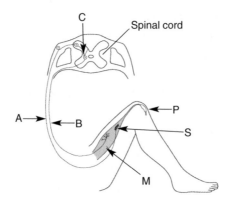

Place the letters in the correct order to describe the pathway of the stimulus and nerve impulse.

A S, M, B, C, A

B S, A, C, B, P

C P, S, A, C, B

D P, S, B, C, A

E P, B, C, A, S

5 Study the voltage–current graphs below.

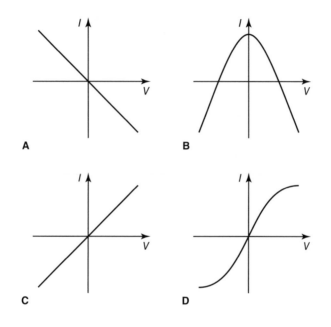

A

B

C

D

Which graph describes the resistance in:

i. a resistor;

ii. a filament lamp?

6 A medical student takes a history from patient A and constructs a family pedigree.

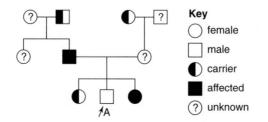

Key

○ female

□ male

◑ carrier

■ affected

? unknown

What is the percentage probability that patient A is affected by the disease?

A 100%

B 75%

C 66%

D 50%

E 33%

F 25%

7 Which **two** of the following elements form compounds that are coloured?

A Copper

B Sodium

C Calcium

D Magnesium

E Iron

8 Which of the following is not found in the urine of a normal healthy adult? (Circle your answer.)

A uric acid

B ammonia

C urea

D glucose

E sodium chloride

9 Nitrogen (N_2) and hydrogen (H_2) react to make ammonia (NH_3).

A factory uses 28 tonnes of nitrogen in 2 hours. How much ammonia will be produced at maximal efficiency? ($N=14$, $H=1$)

10 In a particle accelerator a particle of mass 0.01 g travels at 400 m/s. If the particle comes to rest on a sensor in 1×10^{-4} seconds, what force is exerted on the sensor? Give your answer to the nearest whole number.

11

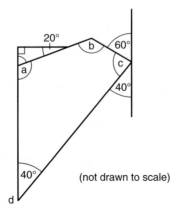

(not drawn to scale)

What is the value of angle b?

A   110°

B   130°

C   150°

D   160°

12   Rearrange the formula to make x the subject.

$$y - 2 = \sqrt{\dfrac{2}{x} + 1}$$

13   The diagram below shows a pregnant uterus.

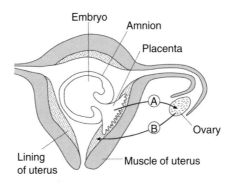

Circle the name of hormone A and draw a line under the name of hormone B.

    Oestrogen   FSH   Adrenaline

            Human chorionic gonadotrophin (HCG)

    LH   Progesterone   Oestradiol

Questions 14–17 are based on the information below.

Ranil tests two substances, A and B, to find out what they contain. He knows that A is a sodium salt and that B is a chloride. His tests and results are shown below.

Test	Result
Add dilute hydrochloric acid to solid A	A gas X is given off which turns limewater cloudy
Add sodium hydroxide solution to solid B and warm	A gas Y is given off which turns litmus paper blue

14 Select the name of gas X.

    A Chlorine

    B Carbon dioxide

    C Chloride

    D Hydrogen

15 Select the name of solid A.

    A Sodium carbonate

    B Sodium chloride

    C Sodium hydroxide

    D Sodium peroxide

16 Select the name of gas Y.

    A Nitrous oxide

    B Nitrogen

    C Hydrogen

    D Ammonia

17 Select the name of solid B.

    A Nitrogen chloride

    B Nitrogen hydroxide

    C Nitrous oxide

    D Ammonium chloride

18 Which of the following factor pairs describe the equation $c^2 - 3c - 10$?

    A $(c + 2)(c + 5)$

    B $(c - 2)(c + 5)$

    C $(c - 2)(c - 5)$

    D $(c + 2)(c - 5)$

19 The line below has an intersection with the line $y = 2x + 4$.

    Where do the graphs intersect? (Give your answer as co-ordinates.)

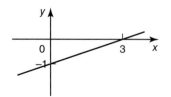

Questions 20–22 are based on the following diagram and labels.

Label the diagram of the thorax using the labels provided. They may be used once, more than once, or not at all.

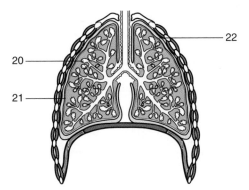

A Bronchiole

B Visceral pleura

C Liver

D Trachea

E Rib

F Lobe

G Blood

H Bone

I Alveolus

J Parietal pleura

K Intercostal muscle

L Diaphragm

23 Look at the table of hormones involved in glucose homeostasis. Which combinations of hormones would be seen in a healthy individual?

	Blood sugar	Insulin	Glucagon
A	↓	↑	↑
B	↑	↓	↑
C	↓	↓	↑
D	↑	↑	↓
E	↓	↓	↓

24 Which of the following formulae for ethanol is correct?

A C_2H_6

B CH_2OH

C C_2H_5OH

D $C_2H_5OH_2$

Section 2 practice test: answers

Question number	Correct response	Comments	Marks
1	125 Hz		1
2	250,000		1
3	2,500 Pa		1
4	C		1
5	(i) C (ii) D	Both for 1 mark	1
6	D		1
7	A and E	Both correct for 1 mark	1
8	Glucose		1
9	34 tonnes		1
10	40 N	1 mark for units	2
11	B		1
12	$x = \dfrac{2}{(y-3)(y-1)}$		1
13	A = HCG; B = progesterone	Both correct for 1 mark	1
14	B		1
15	A		1
16	D		1
17	D		1
18	D		1
19	(−3, −2)		1
20	I		1
21	B		1
22	J		1
23	C and D		2
24	C		1

Section 2 practice test: explanation of answers

1 Tuning fork: 125 Hz

velocity (V) = frequency(f) × wavelength(l)

V = f × λ (where velocity is in m/s, frequency is in Hz and wavelength is in m)

25 = f × 0.2 (note 20 cm = 0.2 m)

$$f = \frac{25}{0.2} = 125Hz$$

2 Exponents: 250,000

$$\frac{5 \times 10^3}{2 \times 10^{-2}} = 2.5 \times 10^5$$ (remember to add the powers, and negative denominators become positive)

2.5 × 10^5 = 250,000

3 Solid block: 2,500 Pa

They would probably give you a choice of answers for this one, but it may be more fun to work it out yourself. The smallest pressure will result from the block resting on its largest area:

0.4 × 0.2 = 0.08

Pressure = Force/Area

Pressure = 200/0.08 = 2,500 Pa – always remember your units.

4 Knee jerk: C

Patella tap (P) is sensed by the sensory nerves in the muscle (S) which is then relayed via the afferent nerves (A) to the spinal cord (C) and then down the efferent nerves (B) to the muscle (M), which contracts to move the leg.

5 Resistance graphs: C, D

  i.   Resistors have a steady resistance producing a straight-line positive graph ($R = V/I$)

  ii. Filament lamps are non-ohmic – their resistance increases as they heat up, also in a positive manner.

6 Family tree: D

This is a recessive trait, like cystic fibrosis, or sickle cell disease.

The mother of A must be a carrier to produce an affected sister.

No children will be unaffected; they have a 50% chance of being a carrier and a 50% chance of being affected.

7 Coloured compounds: A and E

A knowledge one here. Think back to your practical sessions or, if stumped, then think sensibly – copper and iron are both coloured metals.

8 Kidney: glucose

The kidney acts as an ultrafiltration and dialysis system – glucose is too large to cross the normal renal capsule.

9 Ammonia factory: 34 tonnes

First, write down the equation.

N_2 $+ 3H_2$ $= 2NH_3$

I mole   : 3 moles   : 2 moles

$2 \times 14 = 28$ g $: 3 \times 2 = 6$ g   : 34 g

28 tonnes   : 6 tonnes   : 34 tonnes.

Take care with these sorts of equations. There weren't any charges to worry about, but there could easily be in a different question.

10 Particle accelerator: 40 N

$f = ma$: $a = \Delta s/t = 400/1 \times 10^{-4}$

$f = 1 \times 10^{-5} \times 400/1 \times 10^{-4}$ (remember mass is in kg)

$= 40$ N (don't forget the units)

11 Angles: B.

Remember angles in a triangle and along a line add up to 180°, and angles in a quadrilateral add up to 360°.

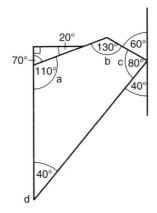

12 Rearrangement: $x = \dfrac{2}{(y-3)(y-1)} + 1$

$y - 2 = \sqrt{\dfrac{2}{x} + 1}$

$(y-2)^2 = \dfrac{2}{x} + 1$

$$y^2 - 4y + 4 = \frac{2}{x} + 1$$

$$y^2 - 4y + 3 = \frac{2}{x}$$

$$x = \frac{2}{y^2 - 4y + 3}$$

$$\therefore x = \frac{2}{(y-3)(y-1)}$$

13 Pregnant uterus: A = HCG, B = progesterone

HCG is secreted from the implanted blastocyst to inhibit further ovulation, while progesterone is secreted by the ovary to maintain the lining of the womb and to support the process of implantation. Unfortunately this is another knowledge-based question, although you could probably have a good guess from the answers supplied. If you have no idea of the answer, then the best thing is to guess and move on rapidly: spend the time on some of the questions that require you to work out the answer.

14–17 Chemical reactions: B, A, D, D

Carbon dioxide turns limewater cloudy.

Only a carbonate produces CO_2 when it reacts with acid.

Ammonia gas turns damp litmus paper blue (it is alkaline).

Ammonia gas is produced from ammonium chloride when mixed with sodium hydroxide.

18 Factorising quadratics: D

This is a very quick and easy question. Just make sure you don't get yourself confused between B and D.

19 Equations of lines: (–3, –2)

The equation of the line is

$$y = mx + c$$

$$y = \frac{1}{3}x - 1$$

Intersection: $\frac{1}{3}x - 1 = 2x + 4$

$$-\frac{5}{3}x = 5$$

$$-5x = 15 \therefore x = -3$$

$$2x + 4 = y$$

$$-6 + 4 = y \therefore y = -2$$

20–22 Apparatus of breathing: I, B, J

The only mistake you might make is confusing the visceral and parietal pleura. Remember 'visceral' is a word for organs, so the visceral pleura abuts the lungs.

23   Insulin and glucagon: C and D

Remember that the job of insulin is to decrease blood sugar by taking it into cells, whereas glucagon releases stored insulin into the blood.

24   Ethanol: C

The formula is C_2H_5OH.

Chapter 11
Section 3: Writing Task

Choose one of four questions

30 minutes inclusive of planning and writing

Only one-page response allowed

Most BMAT candidates neglect to prepare for the final section of the test, either sacrificing the time for more preparation on the first two sections or believing that it isn't the type of task you can prepare for. If you have already looked at the questions in the specimen papers, you will have realised that they are very different from the type of factual essay you are used to writing in biology exams. Indeed, they seem more at home in a philosophy admissions exam than the BMAT.

However, the very fact that Section 3 is different from your normal A-level essays means that you should invest time in preparing for it – this section of the BMAT has been included specifically to test the skills that will be vital for your biomedical degree. An excellent answer on this section of the BMAT will demonstrate that you can:

- recognise and resolve conflict;
- formulate and provide valid support for logical arguments;
- consider alternative explanations for difficult ideas.

Looked at in this way, Section 3 suddenly seems a lot more relevant to your application than you probably thought it was. After you are happy with the question format and answer strategy of the first two sections of the BMAT, you should turn your attention to some proper preparation for the Writing Task. Time spent in preparation will reap bigger rewards than practising the same old multiple-choice questions again and again until you can do them in your sleep.

In order to prepare for the Writing Task, it is best to try to get your hands on the broadsheet newspapers and to keep up to date with the topical medical and ethico-legal debates. For example, there are always debates about whether the NHS should fund the purchase of unproven drug treatment regimens (think about the benefit for one versus the cost to many) or about court cases regarding ventilating terminally ill patients (which have to balance the right to life against the right to have a peaceful and private death). This isn't really the type of research that you can do on the night before the BMAT exam; not only will effective preparation allow you to incorporate convincing examples into your essays, but it will also help you to think critically and to challenge information that is presented to you.

The best way you can prepare for this section of the BMAT is to invest in a notebook, divide each page in two and write down 'for' and 'against' arguments for each biological/medical/

ethical/legal debate that you come across. Not only will this help you to clarify your ideas, but it will also provide you with a fantastic revision prompt for the night before the BMAT. Although the issues you choose may not be asked about explicitly, you will build up a large library of examples, allowing you to answer the BMAT question that most appeals to you, as opposed to the only one that you could write two lines about.

As an added incentive, any time spent in researching for the BMAT won't be wasted. These sorts of ethical and biomedical debates make ideal interview topics, and interviewers will give credit to a candidate who can back up his or her arguments with elegant and relevant examples, compared with one who justifies his or her response with 'I just think it's wrong'.

However, in order to turn the brilliant examples you will collect into sparkling essays, you need to practise essay planning. Below you will find a breakdown of a BMAT-style Section 3 question that describes how you should order and arrange your essay and how to incorporate scientific examples effectively. Also included in this chapter is a Section 3 practice test, complete with suggested answers in the form of spider diagrams. You will appreciate that every answer is different, and it is how you incorporate your ideas into your essays that counts in the end (and in your score). If you work through these examples and practise arranging your answers as described, you can feel confident that you are effectively prepared for the final section. It cannot be emphasised enough that you will receive a score directly proportional to the time and effort you invest in preparation, so make sure you prioritise wisely.

It is also worth having a look at the BMAT marking criteria for Section 3, which is available on the BMAT website. From this, you will see that there are separate marking criteria for quality of content and quality of English. Before you get stuck in, consider that the final section is as much a test of how well you can follow instructions as of what you can actually write. The following points may seem obvious, but the low average scores for the BMAT Section 3 suggest that perhaps they aren't.

Read the questions carefully

Take the time to read all the question choices and to decide which one of the choice of four questions you could answer the best. You would be surprised at the number of candidates who simply choose the first question on the paper (often in sheer relief that they can actually answer it). The question that seems impossible at first may offer a wealth of possibility on the second reading.

Plan your essay

You must always write an essay plan. Half an hour is plenty of time for you to write a single page of A4, so I would advise spending ten minutes of the time choosing your question carefully, and planning and thinking of examples. There is nothing worse than getting half-way through your answer and realising that you have completely run out of points to make, leading to repeating yourself or leaving half of the answer space empty. More frequently, candidates run out of time or space on the sheet and have to miss out the conclusion, which is as vital a part of your answer as the examples that you give.

Planning an essay allows you to write an effective introduction and conclusion: there is no need to use the age-old trick of leaving a space at the start of your essay to write the introduction at the end if you have planned your entire answer in advance.

Answer the question

Always answer the question(s) asked. You have probably heard this a hundred times before but, unfortunately, too many candidates run off at a tangent and neglect to answer the question in hand (which scores them few or no marks). If the examiners don't ask about it, they don't want to hear about it. That's not to say that you can't cleverly draw pre-prepared examples into your answer, but be aware that, unless you explicitly answer the question, and answer all parts, your answer will be marked little higher than an incomplete or absent answer. Try ticking the questions off as you answer them in your plan to ensure you incorporate all of them into your answer.

Avoid bias

Consider both sides of the question and/or argument. The examiners deliberately set questions that do not have a definite or right answer, which means that you have to present both sides of the argument. If you read some of the sample answers on the website you will notice that, often, they aren't very balanced and, as a result, they seem rather shallow and uninformed.

Include a couple of points in support of the argument and a couple against, and follow them up with your own opinions on the matter. Even if the question seems to ask just for your opinion, you must always present evidence as to why you think this in the form of examples, and always demonstrate that you have considered alternative answers to the problem. It is very important to show the examiner that you do not harbour any unfair prejudices – you do want them to let you into medical, dental or vet school, after all.

Answer within the space provided

Use all the space provided but no more. Following instructions is important, and they have provided you with just one sheet of ruled A4 so that you write no more and no less. However, each year failure to plan the essay adequately causes many students to run out of space and to torture the examiner with teeny-tiny mouse-size script snaking its way up the margins, over the page and on to the desk. Unlike in AS exams, the examiners aren't impressed by the expanse of your knowledge and will definitely mark you down for your failure to follow instructions and demonstration of poor planning. An excellent answer can be produced easily within the confines of one page, so when the lines stop, so do you.

First of all, let's consider how we would go about tackling some BMAT-type questions.

In the scientific world, advancements can only be made if mistakes are allowed to happen.

Explain what you think is meant by this statement: Can scientific advancements be made without mistakes being made first? What do you think determines whether a scientific outcome is a mistake or advancement?

Note that there are lots of 'mini-questions' in the main question, aimed at helping you to consider all aspects of your answer. The best way to cover these is to use them as the basis of your introduction, main body and conclusion. Also, make sure you take note of the trigger words in each question, which you may find helpful to underline.

Explain what <u>you</u> think is meant by this statement.

This is the perfect opportunity to grab the examiner's attention and acts as the introduction to your essay. Don't be afraid to state the obvious – they don't use trick questions. Below is one possible answer.

Scientific advancements arise as the result of many years of study and research and, in order to find the correct answer to a problem, you often have to make many mistakes first.

Although this is a good start, the answer fails to incorporate a personal touch (they are asking what you think, after all) and also does not explain why mistakes have to be made (as opposed to the fact that they are just a part of research). A better answer would be something like the following.

I believe that this statement is describing the fact that, in science, there is no proof: a hypothesis can only be demonstrated to be wrong. In order to move forward, we have to demonstrate that all other theories are wrong. One way that this happens is through the process of making mistakes, and hence making mistakes becomes a vital part of scientific discovery.

This forms a concise and elegant introduction to your essay and will also lead nicely into some examples. It gives a flavour of what is to come and should tie in well with a conclusion. It also shows that you have planned your answer: it is often only when you start to plan examples for and against an argument that you realise what the original statement means.

Can scientific advancements be made without mistakes being made first?

This question should form the basis of the main body of your essay. It is just asking to be answered with lots of examples for and against (after you have done a few of this type of question, you will realise that they are all the same and the mini-questions will practically walk you through your answer).

It is probably easier to think of examples where mistakes had to be made for scientific advancement to be possible, and then to consider examples when they didn't. It may be that you find one half of the argument much harder than the other, and this will probably point you in the direction of what your conclusion should be.

This question is asking for scientific examples, but even if the question doesn't explicitly ask, try to choose examples that have some relevance to medicine or biomedical science – this is the BMAT, after all. The best examples you could choose are the ones that could be argued both ways.

Scientific advancements with mistakes.

- *Drug testing*: at all stages of drug trials scientists are looking for side-effects and problems with the drugs. If there are, this means the drug is not fit for its designed purpose, which means there has been a 'mistake'. New drugs can only be developed by learning from these mistakes and refining the drug formula. Specific example: drug trial for thalidomide led to the recognition that isomeric forms of drugs can be dangerous.

- *Transplants*: in the past, organ transplantation often led to rejection – the ultimate failure or 'mistake'. This prompted scientists to research why rejection was happening, leading to the scientific advancement of tissue-matching donor organs with recipients.

Scientific advancements without mistakes.

- *Fleming's discovery of penicillin*: Fleming discovered penicillin growing in his laboratory; the drug is still used today.

- *Early Renaissance scientists dissecting human cadavers pushed forward the knowledge of anatomy*: by actually observing the structures they could make no mistakes in describing them, although they did not understand all the functions of the organs or the changes that occurred at death.

What do you think determines whether a scientific outcome is a mistake or an advancement?

This question is asking you to write a conclusion, incorporating the points you have already made. An average BMAT candidate will either neglect to answer this question properly or give an inarticulate answer. You should concentrate on two or three points you can use to draw everything together.

- Expected or not expected.
- Future work.
- Limits of current knowledge.

Here you have three examples of what determines whether a scientific outcome is a mistake or advancement. State them categorically and use your existing examples to back them up – this adds to the feeling that you have planned an integrated essay.

There are a number of factors that determine whether a scientific outcome is a mistake or advancement. First, it depends whether the outcome is expected or not expected. If, during a drug trial, it is expected that a reaction will occur, then if this reaction happens the outcome will add to scientific knowledge and become an advancement. If a reaction is not expected it could be classed as a mistake, but often investigation into why this mistake happened results in scientific advancement.

Secondly, it is often only future discoveries that confirm the status of a scientific outcome: there are always examples of fortuitous discoveries in science, such as Fleming discovering penicillin growing in his laboratory. However, it was only through future work, involving mistakes, that this discovery became a practical scientific advancement.

Lastly, the limits of current knowledge determine our perception of whether it is a mistake or advancement. It is only when the correct solution is reached that we realise where we had been going wrong, such as in the knowledge of organ rejection. It is only in retrospect and with the knowledge acquired from such experiments that we can classify them as mistakes. Therefore scientific progress relies on outcomes that are both mistakes and advances.

Notice how the questions are summarised in the last line of the answer. This is a trick you will all be familiar with from GCSE English, and it works here too in leading the examiner to believe you have answered the question more directly and concisely than you may have actually done. Just be careful that you don't rely on it solely as a conclusion: the examiners are familiar with this trick and will award you nothing for your efforts.

Have a look at the answer written by previous BMAT students on the website. Try to count the number of points raised and the examples given. Often even the answers that receive the best marks only contain a few examples, so you can see how much they will do for your score. If you doubt that you could produce such a coherent argument, incorporating ready-prepared ideas will be much more effective than trying to think up examples on the spot. Also remember that exam conditions have the effect of making you write faster, so you don't need to worry about incorporating all your examples in the time allowed.

Now that you have seen how to break down a question into its component parts, you should practise answering sample questions yourself, ensuring that all the questions are answered and that your essay hangs together well. After you have done a few questions you will realise that they all follow the same basic outline, with the multiple subquestions acting as prompts for your introduction, main arguments and conclusion.

Once you are familiar with the approach to essay writing, rather than spending your preparation time in writing out page-long answers, I suggest you prepare spider diagrams to generate essay plans. This also has the benefit of being quick and easy to do in the BMAT exam itself, allowing you to draw links and contrasts between your arguments and to stay focused on the question. You can also tick off the points and examples as you progress through your essay, which helps significantly with time management.

Have a look at the example spider diagrams for the sample questions below to gain an understanding of how they can be used effectively. If you feel a bit unsure about essay writing, then you could use the example spider diagrams as a basis for your practice essays so that you can get a feel for how much of the contents you can incorporate into your essay in the 20–25 minutes of writing time you have during the exam. When you are confident in turning essay plans into great essays, then your remaining preparation can focus on generating spider diagrams and collecting examples.

At the end of this chapter we have included three more specimen tests for you to use either for spider diagram or essay practice, and you can also use the BMAT past papers as a basis for your spider diagrams. If you do use the BMAT past papers, remember that, while the style of the questions changes very little, the actual question topics will change, so it isn't wise to spend too much time preparing answers and examples for the specific questions in the past papers.

Example essay questions

1. **'Stop moaning! The pain is there to help you!'**

What does the above statement imply? Give examples that illustrate how pain can be beneficial and others that illustrate the opposite. How can you explain the differences in the function of pain?

2. **In the modern age of science, the laws of natural selection no longer apply to humans.**

What do you understand by the statement above? Can you suggest examples where natural selection still applies and examples where it does not? What factors affect whether natural selection applies to a species?

3. **Health and disease are points along a continuum, rather than separate states.**

Explain what the meaning of this statement is. Do you agree with this statement? Advance arguments in support of and in opposition to this statement. What determines the balance between health and disease?

4. **The Animal Welfare Act (2006) makes owners and keepers responsible for ensuring that the welfare needs of their animals are met.**

What welfare needs do animals have? Are there any possible conflicts between upholding the welfare needs of animals and the rights of owners/keepers? Should animals have the same rights as humans?

Example essay questions: suggested answers

1 'Stop moaning! The pain is there to help you!'

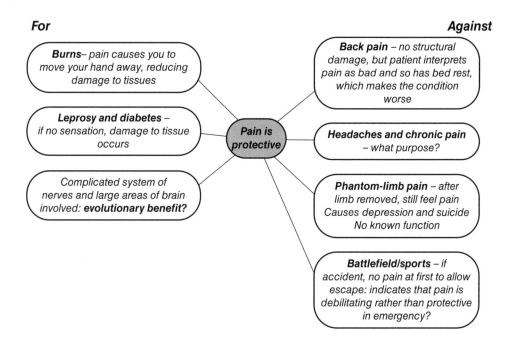

For   *Against*

Burns– *pain causes you to move your hand away, reducing damage to tissues*

Back pain – *no structural damage, but patient interprets pain as bad and so has bed rest, which makes the condition worse*

Leprosy and diabetes – *if no sensation, damage to tissue occurs*

Pain is protective

Headaches and chronic pain *– what purpose?*

Complicated system of nerves and large areas of brain involved: **evolutionary benefit?**

Phantom-limb pain – *after limb removed, still feel pain Causes depression and suicide No known function*

Battlefield/sports – *if accident, no pain at first to allow escape: indicates that pain is debilitating rather than protective in emergency?*

Statement implies

Pain is largely assumed by lay people to be a negative and harmful process, but the fact that complex pain pathways and mechanisms exist in humans may indicate it is protective and therefore of evolutionary benefit. The statement is also indicating that it is of a day-to-day benefit.

How can you explain the differences?

- Lack of knowledge (e.g. headache may serve some protective function).

- Pain may be so vital that mechanisms are 'hard-wired' into brain and independent of limbs, etc. (e.g. phantom limb pain).

- Psychological aspect of pain: different people in different circumstances feel the same pain differently (e.g. a broken leg on the sports field may hurt less than if someone attacks you).

- Different situations: pain sensation in the feet is wanted – lost in diabetes – but chronic pain that appears to serve no purpose is unwanted.

2 **In the modern age of science, the laws of natural selection no longer apply to humans.**

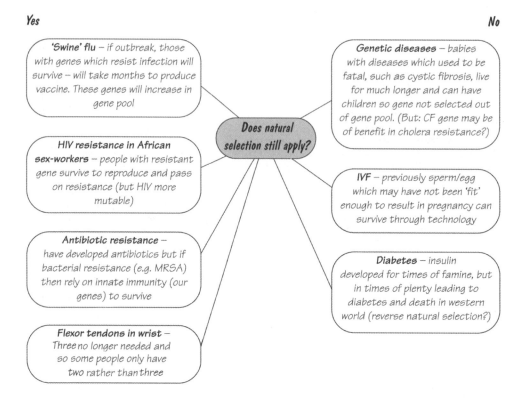

Yes   *No*

'Swine' flu – *if outbreak, those with genes which resist infection will survive – will take months to produce vaccine. These genes will increase in gene pool*

HIV resistance in African sex-workers – *people with resistant gene survive to reproduce and pass on resistance (but HIV more mutable)*

Antibiotic resistance – *have developed antibiotics but if bacterial resistance (e.g. MRSA) then rely on innate immunity (our genes) to survive*

Flexor tendons in wrist – *Three no longer needed and so some people only have two rather than three*

Does natural selection still apply?

Genetic diseases – *babies with diseases which used to be fatal, such as cystic fibrosis, live for much longer and can have children so gene not selected out of gene pool. (But: CF gene may be of benefit in cholera resistance?)*

IVF – *previously sperm/egg which may have not been 'fit' enough to result in pregnancy can survive through technology*

Diabetes – *insulin developed for times of famine, but in times of plenty leading to diabetes and death in western world (reverse natural selection?)*

Statement means

Natural selection = Darwin's theory of 'survival of the fittest' – i.e. those best adapted to their environment survive and pass on their genes. In the modern age these rules may not apply due to medical and scientific support which effectively adapts the environment for us.

What factors affect whether natural selection applies?

- Environment – the difference with humans is that we can change our environment to a large extent. But when the environment changes, it takes time for us to adapt.

- Reproduction – now assisted (e.g. IVF: can increase disease genes).

- Mixing of gene pool.

- Mutation rate – much slower in humans – we have evolved mechanisms to prevent DNA mutation.

- Time – generation time is much longer in humans; see changes slowly.

3 Health and disease are points along a continuum, rather than separate states.

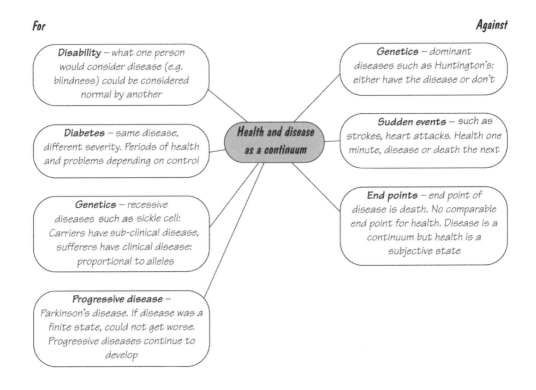

For

Disability – what one person would consider disease (e.g. blindness) could be considered normal by another

Diabetes – same disease, different severity. Periods of health and problems depending on control

Genetics – recessive diseases such as sickle cell: Carriers have sub-clinical disease, sufferers have clinical disease: proportional to alleles

Progressive disease – Parkinson's disease. If disease was a finite state, could not get worse. Progressive diseases continue to develop

Health and disease as a continuum

Against

Genetics – dominant diseases such as Huntington's: either have the disease or don't

Sudden events – such as strokes, heart attacks. Health one minute, disease or death the next

End points – end point of disease is death. No comparable end point for health. Disease is a continuum but health is a subjective state

Statement means

Health is often considered as the absence of disease. Hence, one cannot exist without the other. It is the loss of full health that, for most people, constitutes disease, and the impact of this loss of health can vary greatly between individuals.

What determines the balance between health and disease?

- Individual perception
- Perception of society
- Medical advances 'normalise' some diseases so they seem less severe (e.g. diabetes)
- Nature and nurture

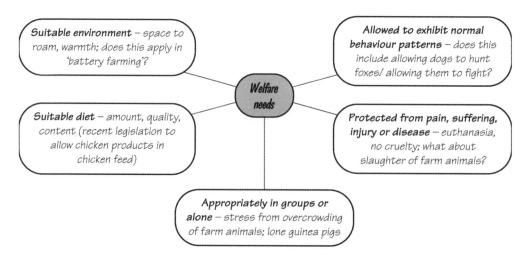

Spider diagram nodes:

Suitable environment – space to roam, warmth; does this apply in 'battery farming'?

Allowed to exhibit normal behaviour patterns – does this include allowing dogs to hunt foxes/ allowing them to fight?

Welfare needs

Suitable diet – amount, quality, content (recent legislation to allow chicken products in chicken feed)

Protected from pain, suffering, injury or disease – euthanasia, no cruelty; what about slaughter of farm animals?

Appropriately in groups or alone – stress from overcrowding of farm animals; lone guinea pigs

4 The Animal Welfare Act (2006): Owners' and keepers' responsibility

Remember to think about both pets and livestock!

Should animals have the same rights as humans?

Should the right to life without cruelty be universal?

Should animals have the right to be protected from suffering? Does this include slaughtering animals, and the issue of euthanasia which is not possible in humans?

Now you have some idea of how to break down the questions and understand how to use a spider diagram, have a go at creating spider diagrams and writing essays using the practice tests at the end of this chapter. There are no correct answers, but enlist your family, friends and teachers to help look over your essay plans and essays – after all, you want to try to achieve the broadest perspective on your outlook, and they will be able to suggest ideas and examples that you may never have thought of.

Although it is tempting to concentrate on the questions to which you already know you could give a good answer, attempt some of the ones that look less attractive. In the exam it will seem like all the questions are horrible and impossible to answer so, if you practise answering some that you find more difficult at this stage, you will be well prepared by the time you come to take the BMAT.

Section 3 practice test

Time allowed: 30 minutes

Practice test A

YOU MUST ANSWER <u>ONLY</u> ONE OF THE FOLLOWING QUESTIONS

1. **'Extreme remedies are very appropriate for extreme diseases' – Hippocrates, 'Aphorisms'**

   'There are some remedies worse than the disease' – Publilius Syrus

Which of these statements do you agree with? Give some examples in support of these arguments. How can we reconcile these differing aspects of remedies?

2. **'A cost to an individual can be justified by a benefit to the group.'**

Do you agree with this hypothesis? Outline arguments in support of and in opposition to this statement. What factors influence the rights of an individual over that of the group?

3. **'You can only believe in what you know to be true.'**

What relevance does this statement have to scientific thought? Advance an argument against this idea. What other factors influence scientific belief?

4. **'As medicine advances, so too does the bill.'**

What do you think is meant by this statement? Can you give examples of where this statement is correct/incorrect? What factors affect the costs of medical science?

END OF TEST

Practice test B

YOU MUST ANSWER ONLY <u>ONE</u> OF THE FOLLOWING QUESTIONS

1. **'The right to life carries with it the right to death.'**

Discuss the implications of this statement. In what circumstances would you agree with this idea, and in what circumstances would you disagree? What factors would influence the possession of such rights?

2. **'If a man will begin with certainties, he shall end in doubts, but if he will be content to begin with doubts, he shall end in certainties' – Francis Bacon**

What do you interpret this statement to mean? Can you think of any examples where he is right? Can you ever know something for certain?

3. **'Medicine is an art form rather than a scientific discipline.'**

Do you agree with this statement? In what ways could medicine be considered an art form, and in what ways could it be considered a scientific discipline?

4. **'A scientific man ought to have no wishes, no affections, – a mere heart of stone'– Charles Darwin**

What does Darwin mean by this statement? Do you think he is right? Give examples in science, human or animal medicine to support your answer.

END OF TEST

Practice test C

YOU MUST ANSWER ONLY <u>ONE</u> OF THE FOLLOWING QUESTIONS

1. **'The ability to laugh is what makes us human.'**

What different meanings could this statement have? Advance arguments for the genetic versus the environmental effect on our personality development.

2. **'All perceived benefits carry with them a known risk.'**

Discuss, with examples, whether this statement is true. How could we resolve the conflict between benefit and harm?

3. **'Genes control our lives.'**

Explain what the statement above means. Advance an argument in support of and in opposition to the statement. How can we identify the role that genes play in our lives?

4. **'That knowledge which is popular is not scientific.'**

What do you think the author means by this statement? Give examples of scientific advancements which have been popular and/or unpopular. How can we achieve public understanding of scientific principles?

END OF TEST

Chapter 12
After the BMAT

Depending on the university you applied to and the style of interview, you may be asked about your essay when you go for interview, as the BMAT sends each of the universities a copy of your Section 3 script along with your marks for Sections 1 and 2. The interviewers won't ask you about spelling and grammar, but they may ask you about your essay, especially if they thought it was well written or had some good ideas (which should be the case after all your hard work). They will always give you a copy of your answer, but it's always useful to have had a refresher read beforehand. Therefore it is advisable to spend 10 minutes after you come out of the exam jotting down the spider diagram you used for your essay, along with the major examples. Not only will this keep your mind off which questions your friends got right and you didn't, but it will also serve as an aide-memoire when you are preparing for your interview, because it is almost guaranteed that you won't remember anything about your BMAT test by the time your interview comes around a month or two later. It may well be that you never hear anything further about your BMAT exam, but ten minutes spent now will at least stop you worrying about the possibility of having to talk about your essay later on.

Good luck for the big day. If you have prepared to the best of your ability, then you can be satisfied that you will fulfil your potential, however tough the exam. This effort and the skills that you learn will stand you in good stead for your future career.